Pharmacogenetics

Pharmacogenetics

EDITED BY

Ian P. Hall

University Hospital of Nottingham
Nottingham, U.K.

Munir Pirmohamed

University of Liverpool
Liverpool, U.K.

Taylor & Francis
Taylor & Francis Group
New York London

Taylor & Francis is an imprint of the
Taylor & Francis Group, an informa business

Published in 2006 by
Taylor & Francis Group
270 Madison Avenue
New York, NY 10016

Printed in the United States of America on acid-free paper
10 9 8 7 6 5 4 3 2 1

International Standard Book Number-10: 0-8247-2884-X (Hardcover)
International Standard Book Number-13: 978-0-8247-2884-7 (Hardcover)
Library of Congress Card Number 2005046644

Library of Congress Cataloging-in-Publication Data

Pharmacogenetics / edited by Ian P. Hall, Munir Pirmohamed.
p. cm.
Includes bibliographical references and index.
ISBN-13: 978-0-8247-2884-7 (alk. paper)
ISBN-10: (invalid) 082472884x (alk. paper)
1. Pharmacogenetics. I. Hall, Ian P. II. Pirmohamed, Munir.

QP909.P53 2006
615'.19--dc22 2005046644

informa
Taylor & Francis Group
is the Academic Division of Informa plc.

Visit the Taylor & Francis Web site at
http://www.taylorandfrancis.com

Foreword

Pharmacogenetics seeks to determine how a person's genetic makeup affects their response to medicines. Rapid advances in genetic technologies have opened up the possibility of genetic testing on a large scale at an affordable cost, thus facilitating the exploitation of pharmacogenetics not only in assessing risks, benefits, and indications of medicines, but also as a valuable tool in drug discovery.

Since the beginning of modern drug therapy, it has been realized that dose is a poor predictor of therapeutic response and that there is substantial variability in both therapeutic efficacy and the occurrence of adverse effects of most medicines. One of the main aims of clinical pharmacology is to understand the basis of this variability. Whether it is due to differences in drug disposition caused by variations in absorption, distribution, transport, metabolism, or elimination, or by differences in end-organ responsiveness, many studies have shown that genetic variability is a most important determinant of each of these.

In the field of drug discovery, the application of genetics was originally focused on the discovery of novel disease genes that could become the targets for new drug discovery programs. But the rapid expansion of understanding of the variability of human DNA sequences has given rise to an appreciation that this approach may be more challenging than originally thought. Currently, more use is made of population-based genetic association studies to identify disease intervention targets.

As the recent report of the Royal Society "Personalised Medicines: Hopes and Realities" makes abundantly clear, it is easy to exaggerate the importance of pharmacogenetics on clinical practice. While there are a few medicines on the market where there is evidence for the benefits of genetic testing for patient selection, mainly in the field of cancer, there are as yet no marketed products that are the result of genetic-based discovery. It seems likely that this situation will radically change, but the time scale is not yet clear. It seems more likely that, for the foreseeable future, the impact of pharmacogenetics will be most profound in the development of diagnostic tests that will allow for the better use of medicines, both in terms of efficacy and safety.

This book is a timely account of the state of the science and clinical application of pharmacogenetics. Its format should make it attractive and easy to use for the clinician in search of detailed information about specific disease areas, and also for those wishing to be updated in the field of pharmacogenetics in general.

Alasdair Breckenridge
Medicines and Healthcare Products Regulatory Agency
London, U.K.

Preface

This book aims to provide a comprehensive account of pharmacogenetics with particular reference to its potential role in specific disease areas. While there have been previous books on pharmacogenetics, these have concentrated on the broader principles (often almost exclusively dealing with pharmacokinetic issues). We felt that a book that provides an account of the generic issues and then provides a disease-area-by-disease-area account would be of value.

This approach has an obvious advantage in that a reader specifically interested in the possible role of pharmacogenetics in dealing with patients with cardiovascular disease, for example, will be able to find all the relevant information in a single chapter, as opposed to having to read about specific enzymes or receptor systems and pick out those bits of information relevant to the disease area. It has, however, caused some difficulty in editing the text because obviously some issues (e.g., the role of cytochrome P450 polymorphism) are generic to many disease areas. In general, we left essential information in each chapter to ensure that the reader can gain all the relevant details without constantly having to cross-refer to other chapters. This means that there is a small amount of repetition in some of the chapters, but wherever possible we have reduced this to the minimum required to maintain the flow of the text.

The other obvious difficulty in this fast-moving subject area is ensuring that the account is up to date. While many of the broad issues have not changed over recent years, many new studies are underway. We tried to ensure that the book is as comprehensive as possible.

Looking through the contents readers will note that there is no specific chapter dealing with neurological disease; however, the relevant issues are dealt with either in the chapter on adverse drug reactions (anticonvulsants) or psychiatric disease. Similarly, the relatively small amount of information on renal disease pharmacogenetics is covered in the sections on metabolic and cardiovascular disease.

We hope that this book provides a useful starting point for both clinicians and non-clinicians with an interest in pharmacogenetics. This is an exciting time to be involved in the study of pharmacogenetics. Although the concept of personalized prescribing has been around for about 50 years, the next 10 years will prove whether or not this approach to improving the effectiveness of prescribing by achieving high efficacy while reducing the risk of severe adverse drug reactions is a viable generic approach to patient management.

Ian P. Hall
Munir Pirmohamed

Contents

Contributors

Guruprasad Padur Aithal Queen's Medical Centre University Hospital, Nottingham, U.K.

Ana Alfirevic Department of Pharmacology and Therapeutics, University of Liverpool, Liverpool, U.K.

Maria J. Arranz Section of Clinical Neuropharmacology, Institute of Psychiatry—King's College, London, U.K.

Ian N. Bruce arc Epidemiology Unit, University of Manchester, Manchester, U.K.

John R. Cockcroft Wales Heart Research Institute, Cardiff University, Cardiff, U.K.

Simon Constable Department of Pharmacology and Therapeutics, University of Liverpool, Liverpool, U.K.

David N. Cooper Institute of Medical Genetics, Cardiff University, Cardiff, U.K.

Romano Danesi Division of Pharmacology and Chemotherapy, Department of Oncology, University of Pisa, Pisa, Italy

Filippo De Braud Clinical Pharmacology and New Drug Development Unit, European Institute of Oncology, Milano, Italy

Laurent A. Decosterd Division of Clinical Pharmacology, University of Lausanne, Lausanne, Switzerland

Mario Del Tacca Division of Pharmacology and Chemotherapy, Department of Oncology, University of Pisa, Pisa, Italy

Antonello Di Paolo Division of Pharmacology and Chemotherapy, Department of Oncology, University of Pisa, Pisa, Italy

Robert Dingwall Institute for the Study of Genetics, Biorisks and Society, University of Nottingham, Nottingham, U.K.

Charles Eby Department of Medicine, Washington University School of Medicine, Saint Louis, Missouri, U.S.A.

Brian Gage Department of Medicine, Washington University School of Medicine, Saint Louis, Missouri, U.S.A.

Hakon Hakonarson Division of Inflammation and Pharmacogenomics, deCODE Genetics, Inc., Reykjavik, Iceland

Eva Halapi Division of Inflammation and Pharmacogenomics, deCODE Genetics, Inc., Reykjavik, Iceland

Ian P. Hall Division of Therapeutics and Molecular Medicine, University Hospital of Nottingham, Nottingham, U.K.

Samantha L. Hider arc Epidemiology Unit, University of Manchester, Manchester, U.K.

Reinhold Kerb Experimental Medicine, Astra Zeneca, Mölndal, Sweden

Robert W. Kerwin Section of Clinical Neuropharmacology, Institute of Psychiatry—King's College, London, U.K.

Belle L. Lee University of California, San Francisco, California, U.S.A., and Division of Infectious Diseases, Department of Clinical Research, University Hospital, Berne, Switzerland

Stephen B. Liggett Departments of Medicine and Physiology, University of Maryland School of Medicine, Baltimore, Maryland, U.S.A.

Dalu Mancama Section of Clinical Neuropharmacology, Institute of Psychiatry—King's College, London, U.K.

Paul Martin Institute for the Study of Genetics, Biorisks and Society, University of Nottingham, Nottingham, U.K.

Howard L. McLeod Department of Medicine, Washington University School of Medicine, Saint Louis, Missouri, U.S.A.

Catharine Morgan arc Epidemiology Unit, University of Manchester, Manchester, U.K.

B. Kevin Park Department of Pharmacology and Therapeutics, University of Liverpool, Liverpool, U.K.

Munir Pirmohamed Department of Pharmacology and Therapeutics, University of Liverpool, Liverpool, U.K.

Andrew Smart Institute for the Study of Genetics, Biorisks and Society, University of Nottingham, Nottingham, U.K.

Alaisdair C. Stamps UCB-Celltech, Slough, U.K.

Amalio Telenti Institute of Microbiology, University Hospital, University of Lausanne, Lausanne, Switzerland

Jonathan A. Terrett Medarex, Inc., Milpitas, California, U.S.A.

Wendy Thomson arc Epidemiology Unit, University of Manchester, Manchester, U.K.

Monika Werner GSK Glaxo Smith Kline Beecham, Munich, Germany

Matthias Wjst Gruppe Molekulare Epidemiologie, GSF—Forschungszentrum für Umwelt und Gesundheit, Neuherberg/Munich, Germany

Yasmin Clinical Pharmacology Unit, University of Cambridge, Cambridge, U.K.

1

Identification of Treatment Response Genes

Eva Halapi and Hakon Hakonarson
Division of Inflammation and Pharmacogenomics, deCODE Genetics, Inc., Reykjavik, Iceland

INTRODUCTION

Genetic diversity contributes to both disease susceptibility and variability in response to drug therapy. Pharmacogenomics is a discipline focused on examining the genetic basis for individual variations in response to therapeutics (1–4). Although the task of developing individualized medicines tailored to patient's genotypes poses a major scientific challenge, pharmacogenomics is already starting to influence how physicians/scientists design clinical trials and its impact on the practice of medicine is forthcoming (5,6). Recent evidence suggests that most prescribed medications are effective in no more than 60% of the individuals in whom they are used, and a significant number of patients also develop major adverse effects. Better understanding of the genetic factors that regulate patient's responsiveness to drugs is therefore needed to elucidate the molecular mechanisms involved and allow for development of new therapeutic strategies that match each patient and the most suitable drug (7–9).

While drug treatment constitutes the mainstay of medicine, for most drugs, there is considerable variability in patient's therapeutic response (2,3). In other cases, unforeseen serious side effects may occur (10,11). For the patient this represents a dangerous and potentially life-threatening situation, and, at the societal level, adverse drug reactions are the most common cause of hospital admissions in the elderly and represent a leading cause of disease and death (12). In some cases, genetic variations have been shown to influence both efficacy and safety profiles, as in the case of dicumarol, warfarin, or isoniazid, wherein patient variation in response to these drugs can largely be attributed to polymorphisms in the CYP450 gene family that confer rapid versus slow acetylation of these drugs (10). Since genetic variations can lead to differences in the regulatory functions of genes, variability in their mRNA and/or protein expressions may follow. Pharmacogenomics is charged with measuring these differences in mRNA and protein messages in response to drugs, and although relatively few examples of success exist, this approach holds the promise that we may be able to profile these variations in individuals' genetic makeup and accurately predict response to drugs addressing both efficacy and safety issues (3,4,6,9,10).

In recent years, microarray technology has revolutionized almost all fields of biomedical research by enabling high-throughput gene expression profiling in a single experiment, thereby allowing thousands of genes in different species to be examined in the context of organ differentiation and development in search for disease susceptibility genes and new targets in drug discovery. With the use of expression microarray, the future holds the promise that we may soon gain more global understanding of gene expression changes with respect to disease susceptibility and progression and that biomarkers will become increasingly used as diagnostic and prognostic indicators of treatment response and also provide new insights into the process of new target discovery.

A brief overview of some of the key examples of pharmacogenetic effects follows. This is designed to give the reader an initial idea of the potential for pharmacogenetic effects to contribute to disease management. Fuller accounts of the range of pharmacogenetic effects relevant to each major disease group can be found in the chapters that follow.

PHARMACOGENETICS OF METABOLIZING ENZYMES: CYP450 AND DRUG TRANSPORTER GENES

The cytochrome P450 (CYP450) enzyme system is involved in various metabolic and biosynthetic processes and constitutes a superfamily of heme enzymes found in most organisms (i.e., bacteria to humans). These enzymes are estimated to account for the biotransformation of approximately 60% of the most commonly prescribed drugs in the United States. A few representative examples are discussed in the following, and additional details on some of these examples (and others) are contained in later chapters.

CYP2D6

Three main phenotypes have been identified that relate to the oxidative metabolisms of drug substrates by CYP2D6. The slow metabolizers (with defective CYP2D6 alleles), the normal metabolizers (wild type), and the ultra-rapid metabolizers all have variable number of genes for the functional CYP2D6 enzyme (13–15). Within the Caucasian population, approximately 7% of the CYP2D6 alleles are defective, resulting in potentially increased concentration of various drug metabolites at conventional therapeutic doses. Some of the most commonly used drugs, such as the beta-adrenoceptor blockers and tricyclic antidepressants, are substrates for CYP2D6 (13–15). The latter are known to cause adverse reactions that are attributed to increased levels of tricyclic antidepressants. These include, but are not limited to, such events as life-threatening arrhythmias and other cardiotoxic effects that result from decreased activity of CYP2D6 metabolism. Diagnostic tests are now available to identify beforehand those who are at risk.

CYP2C9

Three defective alleles have been reported in the CYP2C9 enzyme, two of which confer decreased activity. Their frequency ranges from 1% to13% in different populations (13–15). Substrates of CYP2C9 include nonsteroidal anti-inflammatory drugs and hypoglycemic agents (13–15). The clinical relevance of CYP2C9 is particularly noticed in the metabolism of drugs that are used to treat Type II diabetes, wherein decreased clearance of these drugs may result in severe hypoglycemia. Another relevant example is *S*-warfarin, where major bleeding may occur (10).

CYP2C19

CYP2C19 is a highly polymorphic enzyme system, with approximately 3% of the Caucasians having allele variation that renders them as slow metabolizers. In contrast, almost 20% of the Asian population carries the slow allele. Allele 9 confers total abolishment of enzymatic activity (13–15). For most pharmacological compounds that are substrates for CYP2C19, this poses a limited problem because the majority of the drugs are metabolized by several CYP450 enzymes. An important exemption is the drug omeprazole, which is only partially metabolized by CYP3A4 and shows up to 12-fold larger area under the concentration–time curve (AUC) in slow versus fast metabolizers (13–15).

Drug Transporters

Blood and tissue concentrations of most drugs are influenced by interindividual variation in the structure and function of the metabolizing enzyme and transporter genes. Transporters are genes that control drug uptake, distribution, and elimination. The multidrug resistance gene (*MDR1*) encodes for a P-glycoprotein (PgP), which belongs to the large adenosine triphosphate (ATP)-binding cassette (ABC) protein. The *MDR1* gene was originally discovered as the protein causing cross-resistance of tumors to many different cytotoxic agents (16). Multiple substrates are transported by PgP, including the chemotherapeutics tamoxifen and mitoxantrone, the antibiotics cefotetan and cefazolin, the immunosuppressant cyclosporin A, the antiarrytmic drug quindine, the cardiac stimulants digoxin, and such opioid drugs as morphine, to name a few (17). Many cancers are known to overexpress the PgP protein, and this has been correlated with poor prognosis, particularly in patients with leukemia (18). Several SNPs have been reported in the MDR1 gene, some of which have been correlated with PgP protein expression, notably including the C/T polymorphism in exon 26 (19). In a recent study (20), antiviral response to nelfinavir and efavirenez was shown to correlate with the allelic variant, 3435C/T, of the *MDR1* gene. Patients who were homozygotes, carrying two copies of the 3435 T allele, demonstrated lower serum concentration, faster recovery in CD4 T cell count, and more rapid decrease in viral load, suggesting that the MDR1 3435C/T variant may be predictive of immune recovery after antiviral treatment in HIV patients (20). Approximately 50% of Caucasians are heterozygote (C/T) at the 3435 MDR1 polymorphic site, while a homozygote state (C/C) or (T/T), is seen in 25% of individuals, respectively. In contrast, the frequency of the CC genotype in African Americans is 67% to 83%, whereas the frequency of the TT allele is very low. Increased expression of PgP has also been correlated with variation in clinical response to glucocorticoids in patients with inflammatory bowel disease (21) and systemic lupus erythematosus (22). Collectively, these studies suggest that there are important variations in the *MDR1* gene that regulate tumor resistance, immune function, and metabolism of multiple drugs.

PHARMACOGENETIC TARGETS IN CANCER

For most cancers, conventional histopathologic evaluation, encompassing tumor grade and stage, is inadequate to accurately predict the biological behavior of the tumor (23–25). Considerable effort is underway to identify and characterize the biological potential of various cancers at the molecular level. The need to predict response to therapy and determine which tumors are most likely to progress or recur or which invasive tumors will metastasize has prompted intensive efforts in search for prognostic biomarkers and markers that correlate with patients' responses to anticancer therapy.

Estrogen and Progesterone Receptors

In the United States and other western societies, approximately one in 10 women develops breast cancer. Given the unacceptably high mortality rate of approximately 40%, it is critically important that the most effective therapy at any given time is administered to each patient. Although both adjuvant chemo- and hormonal therapies reduce the risk of metastasis by approximately one-third, the best indicators for clinical progression available today, including lymph node status, tumor size and histological grade, are unable to accurately predict the outcome.

SERM

The presence of estrogen and/or progesterone receptors on tumors is considered favorable because these patients are eligible for hormonal treatment. Tamoxifen, is a selective estrogen-receptor modulator (SERM), which acts as an estrogen antagonist in normal breast tissue and breast cancer cells but as an antagonist in liver and bone cells. Apart from lowering serum cholesterol and preventing postmenopausal osteoporosis (26), tamoxifen is the most effective and extensively used hormonal treatment for all stages of breast cancer. More recently, the drug was approved for prevention of breast cancer in high-risk individuals. In a recent meta-analysis, which included information on 37,000 women in 55 clinical trials of adjuvant tamoxifen therapy for five years (27), reduction in recurrence and mortality rates were 47% and 26%, respectively, over a 10-year period. Fifty percent decrease was also observed in the incidence of contralateral breast cancer in patients receiving tamoxifen, regardless of the ER status of the primary tumor (27). Several SERMs are currently in clinical trials. Toremifene is a relatively new SERM drug with properties similar to that of tamoxifen. However, unlike tamoxifen, toremifene does not seem to increase the risk of endometrial cancer. Based on information available to date, the Food and Drug Administration (FDA) has restricted the use of toremifene to postmenopausal women with metastatic breast cancer. Raloxifene is another antiestrogen SERM that has received approval for the treatment of osteoporosis in women beyond menopause.

Aromatase Inhibitors

Aromatase, a cytochrome P-450 enzyme that catalyzes the conversion of androgens to estrogens, is the major source of estrogen synthesis in postmenopausal women. Inhibition of aromatase, the terminal step in estrogen biosynthesis, provides a mechanism to intervene in hormone-dependent breast cancer in postmenopausal women. Compared to tamoxifen, both nonsteroidal (such as anastrozole and letrozole) and steroidal (such as exemestane) aromatase inhibitors (AIs) provide superior efficacy and better toxicity profile as first- and second-line therapy of metastatic disease. Early results from the ATAC study (anastrozole, tamoxifen, alone or in combination trial), encompassing 9300 women with early-stage disease at 381 research and medical centers in 21 countries, suggest that anastrozole is superior to tamoxifen as measured by disease-free survival in receptor-positive patients and in reducing the incidence of contralateral breast cancer (28).

ER Antagonists

Fulvestrant (faslodex) is a potent antiestrogen drug that mediates its effects by estrogen receptor (ER) downregulation. It acts as a pure antiestrogen and exhibits none of the negative side effects associated with the partial agonist activity of tamoxifen and related drugs. It has been shown to have comparable efficacy to that of the oral AI, anastrozole, in postmenopausal women with advanced breast cancer who have failed to respond to tamoxifen or related drugs (29). It therefore provides the clinician with an alternative therapeutic strategy following the development of tamoxifen resistance. Fulvestrant might also be beneficial as a follow-on therapy after tamoxifen in an adjuvant setting to palliate some of the concerns surrounding a long-term therapy with tamoxifen (five years).

Antiestrogens are among the most potent therapies in preventing cancer and reducing the risk of recurrence in high-risk patients and in treating metastatic disease. Thus, ER expression has become a valuable marker in predicting treatment response in breast cancer.

Epidermal Growth Factor Receptor Family

Epidermal Growth Factor Receptor

The epidermal growth factor (EGF) pathway has been identified as a key regulator of cell growth and replication (30,31). Cumulative evidence shows that the epidermal growth factor receptor (EGFR) pathway is actively involved in a wide variety of solid tumurs, including non–small cell lung cancer (NSCLC), prostate cancer, breast cancer, stomach cancer, colon cancer, ovarian cancer, and tumors of the head and neck (30–32). Overexpression of the EGFR in cancer cells has been associated with more advanced disease, development of metastatic phenotypes, and poor prognosisents (32). Iressa™, a new tyrosine kinase inhibitor, directly blocks the signals for cell growth and division and is currently licensed for the treatment of inoperable or recurrent NSCLC in Asia and is being tested in clinical trials for other solid tumors (33). Other drugs targeting the EGFR are Tarceva™ and Erbitux™, which are currently in clinical trials.

HER2/neu

HER2/neu has been shown to be overexpressed in 20% to 30% of breast cancer patients (34,35). Recent evidence supports a clear association between HER2 overexpression and reduced overall and disease-free survival, especially in patients with node-positive disease (34–38). Tumors displaying HER2 amplification show a correlation with poor prognosis (39,40). Thus, the greatest value of HER2 as a predictive marker lies in the prediction of response to therapies that target HER2, notably herceptin. Indeed, patients with strongly HER2-positive breast cancer get significant clinical benefits from herceptin therapy, and HER2 testing has become an integral part of the optimal management of breast cancer patients. It is important to determine HER2 status of all primary breast cancers at the time of diagnosis and recurrence because HER2 overexpression and amplification can be used to identify patients for herceptin therapy (41). Thus, HER2 has approached a clinically validated status as a prognostic factor and also as a predictive factor for response to therapy, and it is already part of the routine assessment for breast cancer patients. A prior knowledge of HER2 status is therefore an absolute requirement for herceptin therapy.

Thiopurine *S*-Methyltransferase

The thiopurine *S*-methyltransferase (*TPMT*) gene metabolizes thiopurine medications, such as mercaptopurine, azathioprine, and thioguanine. *TPMT* activity is polymorphic with 10% of the subjects being heterozygous and about 1/300 with low or deficient activity (42,43). Patients with low or deficient *TPMT* activity are at high risk for severe hematological toxicity from standard doses of thiopurine medications. Thus, it is important to be able to identify those patients who are at risk for such complications. The molecular basis for altered *TPMT* activity is well characterized with three distinct alleles accounting for up to 95% of both heterozygous and homozygous mutant patients (43). However, significant ethnic differences have been identified in both the frequency of low *TPMT* activity and in the mutations that account for them (43). Although extended clinical studies are needed to better understand and quantitate the dosing of these drugs, TPMT genotype-specific dosing guidelines have been proposed for the use of mercaptopurine in leukemia patients (44). Given the severity of thiopurine medication-related toxicity in *TPMT*-deficient patients, screening of the entire patient populations for *TPMT* polymorphism prior to prescribing these drugs has been shown to be cost-effective. By determining thiopurine transferase activity in patients before they receive thiopurines, enzyme efficacy can be determined beforehand and life-threatening complications, which are strongly related to the genetically determined activity of this enzyme, can be avoided. Accordingly, screening for genetic variations in the *TPMT* gene presents an ideal model for the translation of genomic information to guide patient therapeutics.

N-Acetyltransferase (NAT)

NAT was first identified as the enzyme responsible for inactivation of the antitubercular drug isoniazid (45). NAT also plays an important role in carcinogen metabolism. The *N*-acetylation metabolizing pathway is a major route for the conjugative metabolism of many drugs and chemicals (46). Functional polymorphisms in the *NAT* gene were initially associated with differences in the susceptibility to occupational and smoking-related bladder cancer (47). Based on the substrate, individuals can be phenotyped as either "fast" or "slow" acetylators. Individuals with the slow phenotype are homozygotes for the slow allele, whereas subjects with the fast phenotype are either heterozygotes or homozygotes for the fast allele. The frequency of slow acetylator varies worldwide, ranging from 5% to 10% in Asia and reaching 90% frequency in certain European populations (13). Two functionally relevant human *NAT* genes, *NAT1* and *NAT2*, have been identified that are highly polymorphic and are encoded at multi-allelic loci. The relationship between these polymorphisms and the resulting phenotypes is well established (48).

PHARMACOGENETIC TARGETS IN CENTRAL NERVOUS SYSTEM DISORDERS

Although pharmacotherapy in patients with affective disorders has improved the outcome of millions of patients worldwide, medical treatment of mental depression is efficacious in no more than two-thirds of the cases, and there are no biological markers of treatment response. Apart from identification of genomic markers of treatment response, which would constitute an enormous clinical advantage of public health value, the application of pharmacogenmoics may also uncover new targets for the development of novel and hopefully more efficacious drugs with favorable side-effect profile.

Serotonin Transporter

Selective serotonin reuptake inhibitors (SSRIs) are widely used for the treatment of depression because of their efficacy and relatively favorable side-effect profile compared with those of the tricyclic antidepressants. SSRIs act by interfering with the activity of the serotonin transporter (SERT) (49). A number of polymorphisms have been reported in the *SERT* gene (50–52), and genetic variations in the SERT promoter have been linked to altered functions, such as the association between the short (S) allele (44 bp deletion) of the SERT-PR site and poor response to fluvoxamine and paroxetine in patients treated for major depression (53,54).

Dopamine Transporter

Attention deficit/hyperactivity disorder (ADHD) affects between 3% and 5% of school-age children. Treatment of major symptoms, such as inattention, hyperactivity, and impulsive behavior, has been effectively achieved using psychostimulants, of which methylphenidate (Ritalin®) is the most commonly prescribed in the United States. These drugs are beneficial in many cases; however, inter-individual variation in clinical response and adverse events is well documented (55–57). Methylphenidate binds to and directly inhibits the dopamine transporter (DAT1). Accordingly, variations in genes involved in dopamine action and metabolism (such as *DAT1, D2*, and the *D4* receptor genes) have been examined in search for explanation of the variability in clinical response to methylphenidate and other psychostimulants in ADHD patients. A recent study (58) demonstrated significant association between the 10/10 genotype in DAT1 and lack of response to methylphenidate but failed to demonstrate any association with polymorphism in the dopamine receptors (58). These results have recently been confirmed in a larger patient cohort (59).

Dopamine and Serotonin Receptors

Clozapine is a potent drug in the treatment of schizophrenia; however, not all patients benefit from treatment, and some patients react adversely to therapy while others fail to respond adequately. Several studies have reported an association between clozapine response and polymorphisms in the dopamine receptor 3 (*D3*) gene (60–62), dopamine receptor 4 (*D4*) gene (63,64), and in the serotonin receptor 2A (65,66) and 5A genes (67). In a recent study, Arranz et al. (68) screened for the combination of upto 19 polymorphisms that predicted clinical response to clozapine in schizophrenic patients with high accuracy. These 19 single-nucleotide polymorphisms (SNPs) were located in eight receptor genes and one transporter gene, including the α2A-adrenoceptor, dopamine D3 receptor, 5-HT2A, 5-HT2C, 5-HT3A, 5-HT5A, histamine H1 receptor, histamine H2 receptor, and the serotonin transporter gene. A combination of six polymorphisms, including the 5-HT2A 102T/C, His452Tyr, 5-HT2C-330GT/-244CT, Cys23Ser, 5-HTTLPR, H2-1018G/A, predicted clinical response with 76.86% accuracy ($\chi^2 = 35.8$; $P = 0.0001$) with sensitivity of 95.89 ($\pm$0.04), suggesting that these polymorphisms could be used to identify patients who are most likely to show a satisfactory improvement with treatment.

Apolipoprotein E

Apart from its role in cardiovascular disease, the apoliprotein E (ApoE) protein has also been associated with late onset and sporadic Alzheimer's disease (AD) (69,70). In the central nervous system (CNS), ApoE plays a key role in mobilization and redistribution of cholesterol and phospholipids during membrane remodeling (70). In a study assessing the influence of the ApoE genotype on therapeutic response to tacrine (acetylcholinesterase inhibitor) in a responder/nonresponder cohort, more than 80% of ApoE4 negative carriers demonstrated marked clinical response to tacrine, as measured by the AD assessment scale (ADAS), whereas ApoE4 positive carriers presented ADAS scores that were worse compared with the baseline levels (69). The ApoE genotype has also been implicated in modulating response to drugs targeting vasopressinergic activity (71). Thus, ApoE is emerging as a potentially useful marker in predicting clinical response to tacrine.

PHARMACOGENETIC TARGETS IN RESPIRATORY DISORDERS

There are four major classes of asthma pharmacotherapy currently in widespread use (72): (*i*) β_2-agonists (β-agonist) used by inhalation for the relief of airway obstruction (e.g., albuterol, salmeterol, fenoterol); (*ii*) glucocorticoids for both inhaled and systemic use (e.g., fluticazone, beclomethasone, triamcinolone, prednisone); (*iii*) theophylline and its derivatives; and (*iv*) inhibitors and receptor antagonists of the cysteinyl-leukotriene pathway (e.g., montelukast, pranlukast, zafirlukast, zileuton). The following section summarizes pharmacogenetic work reported on β-agonists and inhibitors of the cysteinyl-leukotriene pathway in asthma; comprehensive accounts of these effects are contained in the chapter on respiratory disease.

β_2 Adrenergic Receptor

Four polymorphisms of the coding block of β_2 adrenergic receptor (β_2AR) have been found, three of which result in receptors that have different properties compared with the wild-type (73). These polymorphisms include Arg16 $\rightarrow$ Gly, Gln27 $\rightarrow$ Glu, Val34 $\rightarrow$ Met, and Thr164 $\rightarrow$ Ile, of which the first two are the most common. Most studies have found no differences in the frequencies of these polymorphisms between asthma patients and healthy nonasthmatic controls (74,75). Thus, the genetic variability of the β_2AR does not appear to play a major causative role in asthma. However, these polymorphisms, although not causative, could modify the disease. Other studies have assessed the relationship between β_2AR polymorphisms at positions 16 and 27 and atopy, including IgE levels (76). A significant association between the Glu27 form of the β_2 receptor and log serum IgE was reported, suggesting that β_2AR polymorphisms may act to modify the asthmatic phenotype (77).

Several studies have assessed the modulatory role of β_2AR polymorphisms on the treatment response to β-agonists (2,78) in relation to bronchial hyperreactivity (79) and control of asthma (80). These studies demonstrate that certain β_2AR polymorphisms affect the clinical response to β-agonist therapy, which may impact the asthmatic phenotype, rendering these variants candidates that may ultimately provide for individualized therapy in asthma.

Leukotriene Pathway Pharmacogenetics

The leukotrienes are eicosatetraenoic acid compounds that are derived from arachidonic acid and exhibit a wide range of pharmacological and physiological actions (81). Three enzymes are exclusively involved in the formation of the leukotrienes, including the 5-lipoxygenase (ALOX5), the leukotriene C4 synthase (LTC4), and LTA4 epoxide hydrolase. ALOX5 is the central enzyme required for the production of both the cysteinyl-leukotrienes (LTC4, LTD4, and LTE4) and the potent neutrophil chemo-attractant, LTB4. Drugs that inhibit ALOX5 activity or antagonize the action of the cysteinyl-leukotrienes at their receptor site have been shown to attenuate broncho-constriction in asthma patients (82).

Mutations in the *ALOX5* gene were found to have significant functional consequences in the context of promoter–reporter constructs and patients with variable number of tandem repeats (VNTRs) other than the wild-type (i.e., five repeats of the sequence −GGGCGG− in the core promoter) have been shown to have diminished transcription of the *ALOX5* gene and produce lower levels of leukotrienes (83,84).

The leukotriene LTC4 synthase is another enzyme with a known SNP in its promoter region (A −444C) with a C allele frequency that is reportedly higher in patients with severe asthma (71,72), wherein the −444C variant is associated with enhanced cysteinyl-leukotriene production, suggesting that patients with the A/A genotype may have leukotriene-driven asthma. These findings provide possible evidence that, apart from the ALOX5, there may be another pharmacogenetic locus that can modulate the leukotriene pathway. Whether DNA sequence variants that are associated with decrease in cysteinyl-leukotriene synthesis will also be associated with a decreased response to therapy remains to be determined.

PHARMACOGENETIC TARGETS IN CARDIOVASCULAR DISEASE

Atherosclerosis is, at least in part, attributed to an underlying immune-mediated process with onset early in life, ultimately leading to severe clinical manifestations, such as myocardial infarction, unstable angina, and cerebral stroke. The increased incidence of cardiovascular events in the western societies is attributed to the underlying immune process, which is amplified by additional cardiovascular risk factors, such as hypercholesterolemia, hypertension, smoking, diabetes, and obesity, which by themselves have their own genetic background. This section provides a summary of some of the key issues; for a full discussion, see the chapter on cardiovascular disease.

Apolipoprotein E

Statins act primarily by inhibiting hydroxy-methylglutaryl coenzyme A (HGM-CoA) reductase activity (85–87). Although statins are among the most effective cholesterol-lowering agents available, hyperlipidemic individuals display marked variability in lipid-lowering response which may, at least in part, be due to genetic differences (88). Among the multiple candidate genes that have been shown to be involved in lipid metabolism, most attention has been focused on the ApoE locus. ApoE is essential for the normal catabolism of triglyceride-rich lipoprotein constituents. Three major ApoE isoforms are encoded by three common alleles at the ApoE locus (89). Genetic variations in the *ApoE* gene at the ApoE locus have been associated with plasma lipoprotein concentrations in both fasting and in the postprandial states (89,90). In this regard, the E2 allele is associated with lower and the E4 allele with higher total plasma cholesterol and low-density lipoprotein (LDL) cholesterol levels compared with the E3 allele, whereas ApoE E2 carriers have been reported to be more responsive to lipid-lowering statin therapy (91). The ApoE E4 allele has been shown in some studies to be associated with increased response to dietary intervention.

Angiotensin-Converting Enzyme

Angiotensin-converting enzyme (ACE) plays a critical role in blood pressure regulation. Restenosis after coronary artery stent is a major health problem that is primarily attributed to intimal hyperplasia, which can be attenuated by ACE inhibitors. Identification of patients who are at higher risk of developing restenosis is therefore desirable. In this regard, an insertion/deletion (I/D) polymorphism in intron 16 of the *ACE* gene has attracted significant attention due to its correlation with serum ACE activity (92). An association was recently reported between carriers of the D allele and reduced risk of restenosis following coronary stenting (93,94).

MICROARRAY AND DISEASE RESPONSE GENES

Studies using commercially available whole genome or targeted arrays as well as "in-house" spotted arrays have generated a wealth of information that importantly contributes to our understanding of human biology in health and disease. These studies are particularly important in addressing molecular pathways involved in organ differentiation and development. More recently, their value in screening for disease susceptibility genes and new drug targets has become evident (95–99). Indeed, the DNA microarray technique has proven to play a fundamental role in high-throughput screening of the genome. Microarrays are commonly used for global assessment of mRNA expression levels in various tissues and cell culture systems (100–107) and also for polymorphism scoring (108–111). The two major technology platforms for microarray analysis consists of: (i) spotted microarrays in which pre-synthesized single- or double-stranded DNA are bound onto glass slides and; (ii) high density oligonucleotide arrays where sets of oligomers are synthesized directly on wafers using photolabile nucleotide chemistry (95–98,112). More novel application for this technology, includes the array-based comparative genomic hybridization (CGH) (113,114) and high-density protein microarrays (115,116), which allow for assessment of protein–protein, protein–DNA, protein–RNA, and protein–ligand interactions.

As the last decade has witnessed an explosion in various applications of microarray, an attempt to cover this area thoroughly is not feasible, so the following section highlights only a few studies aiming at identifying genes that may serve as biomarkers of treatment response and also as possible new drug targets.

Predicting Treatment Response/Clinical Outcome

Apart from their important contribution to cancer classification (103,107), DNA microarrays have been utilized to define distinct gene expression profiles that are associated with treatment response to various anticancer drugs in diseases, such as diffuse large B-cell lymphomas (107,117) and primary breast cancer (104–106).

Approximately 35% to 40% of diffuse large B-cell lymphomas respond to anthracyclins. By analyzing molecular signatures using cDNA arrays, Alizadeh et al. (107) demonstrated that diffuse large B-cell lymphoma consisted of two major groups: a germinal center B-cell-like type and an activated B-cell-like type. Patients with germinal centre B-cell-like diffuse large B-cell lymphoma demonstrated significantly better 5-year overall survival of 76%, compared with 16% of those with the activated form.

More recently, Rosenwald et al. (117), distinguished three different subtypes of gene expression profiles—germinal center B-cell-like, activated B-cell-like, and a type-3 profile—in biopsies from 240 diffuse large B-cell lymphomas. Clinical and gene expression data were then used to identify genes that predicted the outcome. A molecular predictor consisting of 17 genes was constructed using gene expression data from 160 patients, and the predictor was validated on an independent set of 80 patients. Accordingly, the gene expression profiling approach generates valuable biomarkers that allow physicians to target patients who are most likely to benefit from conventional therapy and focus on alternative therapy in those who do not.

In a study by van't Veer et al. (105), the expression patterns of 98 primary tumors from young patients with lymph node-negative breast cancer were examined, and a set of 70 genes, "classifier," whose expression profile correlated most accurately with the shortest interval to appearance of distant metastases (i.e., poor prognosis signature), was identified and then analyzed in a larger cohort of patients. The latter study included 295 primary breast cancer patients (106), who were either lymph node-negative or -positive. Of those, 180 tumors were assigned the poor prognosis profile, and 115 were classified as having a good prognosis profile. The mean overall 10-year survival rate was 54.6% and 94.5% in the poor and favorable tumor expression profile cohorts, respectively. Interestingly, lymph node involvement did not correlate with the expression profile, whereas patient's age, ER status, and histological grade were associated with specific expression profile patterns, with younger age and higher histological grade being more prevalent in the poor prognosis group, whereas positive ER status was indicative of a favorable prognosis profile.

In a study by Sotiriou et al. (118), fine-needle aspirates from breast tumors were used to investigate whether sufficient RNA for microarray analysis could be obtained and whether specific gene expression profiles could be used to distinguish between patients with differential response to chemotherapy. Although a small set of patients were analyzed, the authors identified a set of 37 genes that distinguished response status from lack of response in pretreatment samples. As drug resistance to chemotherapy poses a major problem, establishment of predictive markers for drug response are of great value. The use of neoadjuvant treatment of advanced breast cancer prior to operation is growing, and biomarkers of response would facilitate the selection of patients who are eligible for such treatment. Many breast cancer patients receive unnecessary treatment for possible tumor spread after the removal of the primary tumor. Molecular profiling would offer more accurate predictions of who may need such treatment.

Discovery of Novel Drug Targetable Genes

Several studies have made an attempt to associate glucocorticoid (GC) resistance to known polymorphic variations in genes that constitute the GC response pathway (119–123). Although both structural and functional alterations in the glucocorticoid receptor units or their response elements are important determinants of glucocorticoid responsiveness, no relevant clinical prediction has emerged from these studies. In a recent study using microarray to examine gene expression profiles in peripheral blood cells (PBM) cells obtained from asthmatic patients who were either glucocorticoid therapy responders or nonresponders, glucocorticoid responders could be separated from nonresponders with more than 85% accuracy using only a few genes (124). The glucocorticoid-resistant patients were also clustered into families and examined for linkage (125).

A set of genes unique for psoriatic skin disease was recently reported in a study using DNA microarray. By comparing lesional and uninvolved skin from patients with psoriasis, a set of 159 genes that showed twofold or greater difference in their expression level was defined. Of these, several were mapped to disease-associated loci (126). The gene set predicted expression patterns unique to normal versus lesional skin with 100% accuracy, and a subset of these genes was also useful for monitoring treatment response (126).

Microarray has also been applied in combination with genetic linkage studies to dissect out disease susceptibility genes in experimental models. A recent study using quantitative trait loci (QTL) analysis in a mouse model of experimental allergic asthma revealed two distinct loci on chromosome 2 that controlled allergen-induced airway hyperresponsiveness (AHR), *abhr1* and *abhr2* (127). In a study comparing expression profiles in

RNA from lung obtained from susceptible (A/J), resistant (C3H/HeJ), and backcross mice with various phenotypes, Karp et al. (128) identified 21 differently expressed genes, including complement factor 5 (*C5*) that mapped to either locus. Expression levels of *C5* were significantly higher in AHR-resistant mice than in AHR-susceptible mice. Sequence analysis of the *C5* gene in the parental strain revealed a 2 bp deletion in the 5′ untranlated region of A/J mice, resulting in reduced *C5* mRNA level and lack of functional C5 protein (128). In a backcross progeny, more extreme AHR was seen in mice that were homozygotes for the susceptible A/J-derived C5 allele, compared with the low responders that were heterozygotes. The authors concluded that C5 deficiency might interfere with monocyte/macrophage production of interleukin-12, thereby altering immunoregulatory mechanisms that determine susceptibility to asthma (128).

Linkage analysis in combination with microarray expression analysis has also been applied to identify candidate genes in cardiovascular disease. In this regard, a QTL regulating high-density lipoprotein cholesterol (HDL-C) phenotype, was localized in baboons at chromosome 18 (129). An array consisting of genes from the chromosomal region was created by assembling a contig of bacterial artificial chromosome (BAC) clones for the region of interest. This chromosomal region is highly conserved between species allowing human BACs to be used to assemble the contig (129). Liver cDNA from sibling baboons of contrasting HDL_1-C phenotypes that were exposed to different diets was used to screen for differently expressed genes. The authors identified 53 differentially expressed genes of keen interest (129).

In a recent study, Lock et al. (130) selected genes that were expressed differently in acute and chronic lesions obtained from autopsy samples of patients with multiple sclerosis (MS). The genes were used as targets for therapy in experimental autoimmune encephalitis (EAE), an experimental model for MS. Of note, the granulocyte colony-stimulating factor (GM-CSF) was overexpressed in acute plaques but not in chronic plaques, whereas the Fcγ receptor was upregulated in chronic plaques and not increased in acute plaques. Administration of GM-CSF prior to induction of EAE halted the onset and lowered the disease score compared with the control. EAE was also ameliorated in FcγR knockout mice compared with the wild-type mice (130).

CONCLUSION

The powerful combination of genetic linkage and microarray expression profiling presents an integrated approach that is likely to facilitate discovery of genes involved in common complex disease processes and the regulation of therapeutic response to drugs, thereby facilitating the development of new drugs, DNA-based disease diagnostic products, and pharmacogenomic tests to the market. Such tests will play an important role in delivering more personalized medicine, contributing to the development of more effective means of diagnosing and treating disease by matching each patient and the most suitable drug. Accordingly, the new scope of genetics is charged with the promises to transform the practice of medicine by enabling physicians to assess the risks of disease, permit early detection of disease, determine likely responses to medication, choose the best courses of therapy, and have at their disposal new therapies that target the disease process itself. This chapter has provided a general introduction to the subject and given some key examples of what is currently known about the potential value of pharmacogenetic information and the potential use of such information in the near future. The following chapters in this book consider both general issues and disease-specific pharmacogenetics in detail.

REFERENCES

1. Roden D. Principles in pharmacogenetics. Epilepsia 2001; 42(suppl 5):44–48.
2. Tan S, Hall I, Dewar J, Dow E, Lipworth B. Association between beta 2-adrenoceptor polymorphism and susceptibility to bronchodilator desensitisation in moderately severe stable asthmatics. Lancet 1997; 350:995–999.
3. Roses A. Pharmacogenetics and the practice of medicine. Nature 2000; 405:857–865.
4. McLeod H, Evans W. Pharmacogenomics: unlocking the human genome for better drug therapy. Annu Rev Pharmacol Toxicol 2001; 41:101–121.
5. Roberts R, Begg E, Joyce P, Kennedy M. How the pharmacogenetics of cytochrome P450 enzymes may affect prescribing. N Z Med J 2002; 22:137–140.
6. Grant S. Pharmacogenetics and pharmacogenomics: tailored drug therapy for the 21st century. Trends Pharmacol Sci 2001; 22:3–4.
7. Marton M, DeRisi J, Bennett H, Iyer V, Meyer M, Roberts C, Stoughton R, Burchard J, Slade D, Dai H, Bassett DJ, Hartwell L, Brown P, Friend S. Drug target validation and identification of secondary drug target effects using DNA microarrays. Nature Med 1998; 4:1293–1301.
8. Curran M. Potassium ion channels and human disease: phenotypes and drug targets? Curr Opin Biotechol 1998; 9:565–572.
9. Roses A. Pharmacogenetics and future drug development and delivery. Lancet 2000; 355:1358–1361.
10. Aithal G, Day C, Kesteven P, Daly A. Association of polymorphisms in the cytochrome 450 CYP2C9 with warfarin dose requirement and risk of bleeding complications. Lancet 1999; 353:717–721.
11. Rodondi N, Darioli R, Ramelet A, Hohl D, Lenain V, Perdrix J, Wietlisbach V, Riesen W, Walther T, Medinger L, Nicod P, Desvergne B, Mooser V. High risk for hyperlipidemia and the metabolic syndrome after an episode of hypertriglyceridemia during 13-cis retinoic acid therapy for acne: a pharmacogenetic study. Ann Intern Med 2002; 136:582–589.
12. Vogel C, Peiter A, Feuring M, Wehling M. Drug therapy in the old age. Drug effects in the elderly. MMW Fortschr Med 2001; 143:33–35.
13. Puga A, Nebert D, McKinnon R, Menon A. Genetic polymorphisms in human drug-metabolizing enzymes: potential uses of reverse genetics to identify genes of toxicological relevance. Crit Rev Toxicol 1997; 27:199–222.
14. Venkatakrishnan K, Von Moltke L, Greenblatt D. Human drug metabolism and the cytochromes P450: application and relevance of in vitro models. J Clin Pharmacol 2001; 41:1149–1179.
15. Hasler J, Estabrook R, Murray M, Pikuleva I, Waterman M, Capdevila J, Holla V, Helvig C, Falck J, Farrell G, Kaminsky L, Spivack S, Boitier E, Beaune P. Human cytochromes P450. Mol Aspect Med 1999; 20:1–137.
16. Chen C, Chin J, Ueda K, Clark D, Pastan I, Gottesman M, Roninson I. Internal duplication and homology with bacterial transport proteins in the mdr1 (P-glycoprotein) gene from multi-drug-resistant human cells. Cell 1986; 47:381–389.
17. Brinkmann U, Roots I, Eichelbaum M. Pharmacogenetics of the human drug-transporter gene MDR1: impact of polymorphisms on pharmacotherapy. Drug Discov Today 2001; 15:835–839.
18. Dhooge C, De Moerloose B, Laureys G, Kint J, Ferster A, De Bacquer D, Philippe J, Benoit Y. P-glycoprotein is an independent prognostic factor predicting relapse in childhood acute lymphoblastic leukaemia: results of a 6-year prospective study. Br J Haematol 1999; 105:676–683.
19. Hoffmeyer S, Burk O, von Richter O, Arnold H, Brockmoller J, Johne A, Cascorbi I, Gerloff T, Roots I, Eichelbaum M, Brinkmann U. Functional polymorphisms of the human multidrug-resistance gene: multiple sequence variations and correlation of one allele with P-glycoprotein expression and activity in vivo. Proc Natl Acad Sci USA 2000; 97:3473–3478.

20. Fellay J, Marzolini C, Meaden E, Back DJ, Buclin T, Chave J, Decosterd L, Furrer H, Opravil M, Pantaleo G, Retelska D, Ruiz L, Schinkel AH, Vernazza P, Eap CB, Telenti A for The Swiss HIV Cohort Study. Response to antiretroviral treatment in HIV-1-infected individuals with allelic variants of the multidrug resistance transporter 1: a pharmacogenetics study. Lancet 2002; 359:30–36.
21. Diaz-Borjon A, Richaud-Patin Y, Alvarado de la Barrera C, Jakez-Ocampo J, Ruiz-Arguelles A, Llorente L. Multidrug resistance-1 (MDR-1) in rheumatic autoimmune disorders. Part II: increased P-glycoprotein activity in lymphocytes from systemic lupus erythematosus patients might affect steroid requirements for disease control. Joint Bone Spine 2000; 67:40–48.
22. Farrell R, Murphy A, Long A, Donnelly S, Cherikuri A, O'Toole D, Mahmud N, Keeling P, Weir D, Kelleher D. High multidrug resistance (P-glycoprotein 170) expression in inflammatory bowel disease patients who fail medical therapy. Gastroenterology 2000; 118:279–288.
23. Smith B. Approaches to breast-cancer staging. N Engl J Med 2000; 342:580–581.
24. Braun S, Pantel K, Muller P, Janni W, Hepp F, Kentenich C, Gastroph S, Wischnik A, Dimpfl T, Kindermann G, Riethmulle G, Schlimok G. Cytokeratin-positive cells in the bone marrow and survival of patients with stage I, II, or III breast cancer. N Engl J Med 2000; 342:525–533.
25. Donckier J, Roelants V, Pochet J. Staging of non-small-cell lung cancer with positron-emission tomography. N Engl J Med 2000; 343:1572–1573.
26. O'Regan M, Jordan V. The evolution of tamoxifen therapy in breast cancer: selective oestrogen-receptor modulators and down regulators. Lancet Oncol 2002; 3:207–214.
27. EBCTC Group. Tamoxifen for early breast cancer: an overview of the randomised trials. Lancet 1998; 351:1451–1467.
28. Buzdar A. Anastrozole (Arimidex) in clinical practice versus the old 'gold standard', tamoxifen. Expert Rev Anticancer Ther 2002; 2:623–629.
29. Bross P, Cohen M, Williams G, Pazdur R. FDA drug approval summaries: fulvestrant. Oncologist 2002; 7:477–480.
30. Goustin A, Leof E, Shipley G, Moses H. Growth factors and cancer. Cancer Res 1986; 46:1015–1029.
31. Aaronson S. Growth factors and cancer. Science 1991; 254:1146–1153.
32. Salomon D, Brandt R, Ciardiello F, Normanno N. Epidermal growth factor-related peptides and their receptors in human malignancies. Crit Rev Oncol Hematol 1995; 19:183–232.
33. Ranson M. ZD1839 (IressaTM): for more than just non-small cell lung cancer. Oncologist 2002; 7(suppl 4):16–24.
34. Slamon D, Clark G, Wong S, Levin W, Ullrich A, McGuire W. Human breast cancer: correlation of relapse and survival with amplification of the HER-2/neu oncogene. Science 1987; 235:177–182.
35. Slamon D, Godolphin W, Jones L, Holt J, Wong S, Keith D, Levin W, Stuart S, Udove J, Ullrich A. Studies of the HER-2/neu proto-oncogene in human breast and ovarian cancer. Science 1989; 244:707–712.
36. Hynes N. Amplification and overexpression of the erbB-2 gene in human tumors: its involvement in tumor development, significance as a prognostic factor, and potential as a target for cancer therapy. Semin Cancer Biol 1993; 4:19–26.
37. Hynes N, Stern D. The biology of erbB-2/neu/HER-2 and its role in cancer. Biochem Biophys Acta Rev Cancer 1994; 1198:165–184.
38. Ross J, Fletcher J. The HER-2/neu oncogene in breast cancer: prognostic factor, predictive factor, and target for therapy. Stem Cells 1998; 16:413–428.
39. Borg A, Tandon A, Sigurdsson H, Clark G, Fernö M, Fuqua S, Killander D, McGuire W. HER2/neu amplification predicts poor survival in node positive patients. Cancer Res 1990; 50:6701–6707.
40. Farabegoli F, Ceccarelli C, Santini D, Baldini N, Tafurelli M, Marrano D, Trere D, Derenzini M. c-erbB-2 overexpression in amplified and non-amplified breast carcinoma samples. Int J Cancer 1999; 84:273–277.

41. Bast R Jr, Ravdin P, Hayes D, Bates S, Fritsche HJ, Jessup J, Kemeny N, Locker G, Mennel R, Somerfield M for the American Society of Clinical Oncology Tumor Markers Expert Panel: 2000 Update of recommendations for the use of tumor markers in breast and colorectal cancer: clinical Practice Guidelines of the American Society of Clinical Oncology. J Clin Oncol 2001; 19:1865–1878.
42. Krynetski E, Tai H, Yates C, Fessing M, Loennechen T, Schuetz J, Relling M, Evans W. Genetic polymorphism of thiopurine S-methyltransferase: clinical importance and molecular mechanisms. Pharmacogenetics 1996; 6:279–290.
43. McLeod H, Siva C. The thiopurine S-methyltransferase gene locus—implications for clinical pharmacogenomics. Pharmacogenomics 2002; 3:89–98.
44. McLeod H, Krynetski E, Relling M, Evans W. Genetic polymorphism of thiopurine methyltransferase and its clinical relevance for childhood acute lymphoblastic leukemia. Leukemia 2000; 14:567–572.
45. Evans D. Genetic variations in the acetylation of isoniazid and other drugs. Ann NY Acad Sci 1968; 151:723–733.
46. Weber W, Hein H. Arylamine N-acetyltransferases. Pharmacol Rev 1985; 37:25–70.
47. Cartwright R, Glashan R, Rogers H, Ahmad R, Barham-Hall D, Higgins E, Kahn M. Role of N-acetyltransferase phenotypes in bladder carcinogenesis: a pharmacogenetic epidemiological approach to bladder cancer. Lancet 1982; 8303:842–845.
48. Upton A, Johnon N, Sandy J, Sim E. Arylamine N-acetyltransferases of mice, men and microorganisms. Trends Pharmacol Sci 2001; 22:140–146.
49. Hiemke C, Hartter S. Pharmacokinetics of selective serotonin reuptake inhibitors. Pharmacol Ther 2000; 85:11–28.
50. Serretti A. Pharmacogenetics in affective disorders. Eur J Pharmacol 2002; 438:117–128.
51. Heils A, Teufel A, Petri S, Stöber G, Riederer P, Bengel D, Lesch P. Allelic variation of human serotonin transporter gene expression. J Neurochem 1996; 66:2621–2624.
52. Heils A, Mossner R, Lesch K. The human serotonin transporter gene polymorphism-basic research and clinical implications. J Neural Transm 1997; 104:1005–1014.
53. Smeraldi E, Zanardi R, Benedetti F, Di Bella D, Perez J, Catalano M. Polymorphism within the promoter of the serotonin transporter gene and antidepressant efficacy of fluvoxamine. Mol Psychiatry 1998; 6:508–511.
54. Yu YW, Chen TJ, Lin CH, Hong CJ. Association study of the serotonin transporter promoter polymorphism and symptomatology and antidepressant response in major depressive disorders. Mol Psychiatry 2002; 88:1115–1119.
55. Masellis M, Basile VS, Mugalia P, Özdemir V, Macciardi FM, Kennedy JL. Phychiatric pharmacogenetics: personalizing physchostimulant therapy in attention-deficit/hyperactivity disorder. Behav Brain Res 2002; 130:85–90.
56. Kelly KL, Rapport MD, DuPaul GJ. Attention deficit disorder and methylphenidate: a multistep analysis of dose-response effects on children's cardiovascular functioning. Int Clin Psychopharmacol 1988; 3:167–181.
57. Barkley RA, McMurray MB, Edelbrock CS, Robbins K. Side effects of methylphenidate in children with attention deficit hyperactivity disorder: a systemic, placebo-controlled evaluation. Pediatrics 1990; 86:184–192.
58. Winsberg BG, Comings DE. Association of the dopamine transporter gene (DAT1) with poor methylphenidate response. J Am Acad Child Adolesc Psychiatry 1999; 38:1474–1477.
59. Roman T, Szobot C, Martins S, Biederman J, Rohde LA, Hutz MH. Dopamine transporter gene and response to methylphenidate in attention-deficit/hyperactivity disorder. Pharmacogenetics 2002; 12:497–499.
60. Scharfetter J, Chaudhry H, Hornik K, Fuchs K, Sieghart W, Kasper S, Aschauer H. Dopamine D3 receptor gene polymorphism and response to clozapine in schizophrenic Pakastani patients. Eur Neuropsychopharmacol 1999; 10:17–20.
61. Shaikh S, Collier D, Sham P, Ball D, Aitchison K, Vallada H, Smith I, Gill M, Kerwin R. Allelic association between a Ser-9-Gly polymorphism in the dopamine D3 receptor gene and schizophrenia. Hum Genet 1999; 97:714–719.

62. Malhotra A, Goldman D, Buchanan R, Rooney W, Clifton A, Kosmidis M, Breier A, Pickar D. The dopamine D3 receptor (DRD3) Ser9Gly polymorphism and schizophrenia: a haplotype relative risk study and association with clozapine response. Mol Psychiatry 1998; 3:72–75.
63. Cohen B, Ennulat D, Centorrino F, Matthysse S, Konieczna H, Chu H, Cherkerzian S. Polymorphisms of the dopamine D4 receptor and response to antipsychotic drugs. Psychopharmacology 1999; 141:6–10.
64. Hwu H, Hong C, Lee Y, Lee P, Lee S. Dopamine D4 receptor gene polymorphisms and neuroleptic response in schizophrenia. Biol Psychiatry 1998; 44:483–487.
65. Arranz M, Collier D, Sodhi M, Ball D, Roberts G, Price J, Sham P, Kerwin R. Association between clozapine response and allelic variation in 5-HT2A receptor gene. Lancet 1995; 346:281–282.
66. Arranz M, Munro J, Owen M, Spurlock G, Sham P, Zhao J, Kirov G, Collier D, Kerwin R. Evidence for association between polymorphisms in the promoter and coding regions of the 5-HT2A receptor gene and response to clozapine. Mol Psychiatry 1998; 3:61–66.
67. Birkett J, Arranz M, Munro J, Osbourn S, Kerwin R, Collier D. Association analysis of the 5-HT5A gene in depression, psychosis and antipsychotic response. Neuroreport 2000; 11:2017–2020.
68. Arranz M, Munro J, Birkett J, Bolonna A, Mancama D, Sodhi M, Lesch K, Meyer J, Sham P, Collier D, Murray R, Kerwin R. Pharmacogenetic prediction of clozapine response. Lancet 2000; 355:1615–1616.
69. Poirier J, Delisle M, Quirion R, Aubert I, Farlow M, Lahiri D, Hui S, Bertrand P, Nalbantoglu J, Gilfix B, Gauthier S. Apolipoprotein E4 allele as a predictor of cholinergic deficits and treatment outcome in Alzheimer disease. Proc Natl Acad Sci USA 1995; 92:12260–12264.
70. Poirier J. Apolipoprotein E: a pharmacogenetic target for the treatment of Alzheimer's disease. Mol Diagn 1999; 4:335–341.
71. Richard F, Helbecque N, Neuman E, Guez D, Levy R, Amouyel P. APOE genotyping and response to drug treatment in Alzheimer's disease. Lancet 1999; 349:539.
72. Palmer L, Silverman E, Weiss S, Drazen J. Pharmacogenetics of asthma. Am J Respir Crit Care Med 2002; 165:861–865.
73. Liggett S. The pharmacogenetics of beta2-adrenergic receptors: relevance to asthma. J Allergy Clin Immunol 2000; 105:S487–S492.
74. Reihsaus E, Innis M, MacIntyre N, Liggett S. Mutations in the gene encoding for the beta 2-adrenergic receptor in normal and asthmatic subjects. Am J Respir Cell Mol Biol 1999; 8:334–449.
75. Dewar J, Wheatley A, Venn A, Morrison J, Britton J, Hall I. Beta2-adrenoceptor polymorphisms are in linkage disequilibrium, but are not associated with asthma in an adult population. Clin Exp Allergy 1998; 28:442–448.
76. Dewar J, Wilkinson J, Wheatley A, Thomas N, Doull I, Morton N, Lio P, Harvey J, Liggett S, Holgate S, Hall I. The glutamine 27 b2 adrenoceptor polymorphism is associated with elevated immunoglobulin E levels in asthmatic families. J Allergy Clin Immunol 1997; 100:261–265.
77. Coqueret O, Dugas B, Mencia-Huerta J, Braquet P. Regulation of IgE production from human mononuclear cells by 2-adrenoreceptor agonists. Clin Exp Allergy 1995; 25:304–311.
78. Martinez F, Graves P, Baldini M, Solomon S, Erickson R. Association between genetic polymorphisms of the beta2-adrenoceptor and response to albuterol in children with and without a history of wheezing. J Clin Invest 1997; 100:3184–3188.
79. D'amato M, Vitiani L, Petrelli G, Ferrigno L, di Pietro A, Trezza R, Matricardi P. Association of persistent bronchial hyperresponsiveness with 2-adrenoceptor (ADRB2) haplotypes. Am J Respir Crit Care Med 1998; 158:1968–1973.
80. Hancox R, Sears M, Taylor D. Polymorphism of the 2-adrenoceptor and the response to long-term 2-agonist therapy in asthma. Eur Respir J 1998; 11:589–593.
81. Samuelsson B, Dahlen S, Lindgren J, Rouzer C, Serhan C. Leukotrienes and lipoxins: structures, biosynthesis, and biological effects. Science 1987; 237:1171–1176.
82. Drazen J, Israel E, O'Byrne P. Treatment of asthma with drugs modifying the leukotriene pathway. N Engl J Med 1999; 340:197–206.

83. In K, Asano K, Beier D, Grobholz J, Finn P, Silverman E, Silverman E, Collins T, Fischer A, Keith T, Serino K, Kim S, De Sanctis G, Yandava C, Pillari A, Rubin P, Kemp J, Israel E, Busse W, Ledford D, Murray J, Sega A, Tinkleman D, Drazen J. Naturally occurring mutations in the human 5-lipoxygenase gene promoter that modify transcription factor binding and reporter gene transcription. J Clin Invest 1997; 99:1130–1137.
84. Silverman E, Du J, De Sanctis G, Radmark O, Samuelsson B, Drazen J, Collins T. Egr-1 and Sp1 interact functionally with the 5-lipoxygenase promoter and its naturally occurring mutants. Am J Respir Cell Mol Bio 1998; 19:316–323.
85. (LIPID) Study Group. Prevention of cardiovascular events and death with pravastatine in patients with coronary heart disease and a broad range of initial cholesterol levels. N Engl J Med 1998; 339:1349–1357.
86. Sacks F, Pfeffer M, Moye L, Rouleau J, Rutherford J, Cole T, Brown L, Warnica J, Arnold J, Wun C-C, Davies B, Braunwald E for the Cholesterol and Recurrent Events Trial investigators. The effect of pravastatine on coronary events after myocardial infarction in patients with average cholesterol levels. N Engl J Med 1996; 335:1001–1009.
87. Downs J, Clearfield M, Weis S, Whitney E, Shapiro D, Beere P, Langendorfer A, Stein E, Kruyer W, Gotto AJ. Primary prevention of acute coronary events with lovastatine in men and women with average cholesterol levels. JAMA 1998; 279:1615–1622.
88. Ordovas J, Schaefer E. Genes, variation of cholesterol and fat intake and serum lipids. Curr Opin Lipidol 1999; 1:15–22.
89. Davignon J, Gregg R, Sing C. Apolipoprotein E polymorphism and atherosclerosis. Arteriosclerosis 1988; 8:1–21.
90. Zannis V, Just P, Breslow J. Human apolipoprotein E isoprotein subclasses are genetically determined. Am J Hum Genet 1981; 8:11–24.
91. Ordovas J, Lopez-Miranda J, Perez-Jimenez F, Rodriguez C, Park J, Cole T, Schaefer E. Effect of apolipoprotein E and A-IV phenotypes on the low density lipoprotein response to HMG CoA reductase inhibitor therapy. Atherosclerosis 1995; 113:157–166.
92. Rigat B, Hubert C, Alhenc-Gelas F, Cambien F, Corvol P, Soubrier F. An insertion/deletion polymorphism in the angiotensin I-converting enzyme gene accounting for half the variance of serum enzyme levels. J Clin Invest 1990; 186:1343–1346.
93. Okumura K, Sone T, Kondo J, Tsuboi H, Mukawa H, Tsuzuki M, Imai H, Kamiya H, Mabuchi Y, Matsui H, Hayakawa T. Quinapril prevents restenosis after coronary stenting in patients with angiotensin-converting enzyme D allele. Circ J 2002; 66:311–316.
94. Amant C, Bauters C, Bodart J, Lablanche J, Grollier G, Danchin N, Hamon M, Richard F, Helbecque N, McFadden E, Amouyel P, Bertrand M. D allele of the angiotensin I-converting enzyme is a major risk factor for restenosis after coronary stenting. Circulation 1997; 96:56–60.
95. Debouck C, Goodfellow P. DNA microarrays in drug discovery and development. Nat Genet 1999; 21(suppl 1):48–50.
96. Cheung V, Morley M, Aguilar F, Massimi A, Kucherlapati R, Childs G. Making and reading microarrays. Nat Genet 1999; 21(suppl 1):15–19.
97. Clarke P, te Poele R, Wooster R, Workman P. Gene expression microarray analysis in cancer biology, pharmacology, and drug development: progress and potential. Biochem Pharmacol 2001; 62:1311–1336.
98. Holloway A, van Laar R, Tothill R, Bowtell D. Options available—from start to finish—for obtaining data from DNA microarrays II. Nat Genet 2002; 32(suppl 1):481–489.
99. Gerhold DL, Jensen RV, Gullans SR. Better therapeutics through microarrays. Nat Genet 2002; 32(suppl 1):547–551.
100. Schena M, Shalon D, Davis RW, Brown PO. Quantitative monitoring of gene expression patterns with a complementary DNA microarray. Science 1995; 270.
101. Schena M, Shalon D, Heller R, Chai A, Brown PO, Davis RW. Parallel human genome analysis: microarray-based expression monitoring of 1000 genes. Proc Natl Acad Sci USA 1996; 93:10614–10619.

102. Lockhart DJ, Dong H, Byrne MC, Follettie MT, Gallo MV, Chee MS, Mittmann M, Wang C, Kobayashi M, Horton H, Brown EL. Expression monitoring by hybridization to high-density oligonucleotide arrays. Nat Biotechnol 1996; 14:1675–1680.
103. Golub TR, Slonim DK, Tamayo P, Huard C, Gaasenbeek M, Mesirov JP, Coller H, Loh ML, Downing JR, Caligiuri MA, Bloomfield CD, Lander ES. Molecular classification of cancer: class discovery and class prediction by gene expression monitoring. Science 1999; 286:531–537.
104. Perou C, Sørlie T, Eisen M, Van De Rijn M, Jeffrey S, Rees C, Pollack J, Ross D, Johnsen H, Akslen L, Fluge Ø, Pergamenschikov A, Williams C, Zhu S, Lønning P, Børresen-Dale A-L, Brown P, Botstein D. Molecular portraits of human breast tumours. Nature 2000; 406:747–752.
105. Van 'T Veer L, Dai H, Van De Vijver M, He Y, Hart A, Mao M, Petersen H, Van Der Kooy K, Marton M, Witteveen A, Schreiber G, Kerkhoven R, Roberts C, Linsley P, Bernards R, Friend S. Gene expression profiling predicts clinical outcome of breast cancer. Nature 2002; 415:530–536.
106. van de Vijver M, He Y, van't Veer L, Dai H, Hart A, Voskuil D, Schreiber G, Peterse J, Roberts C, Marton M, Parrish M, Atsma D, Witteveen A, Glas A, Delahaye L, van der Velde T, Bartelink H, Rodenhuis S, Rutgers E, Friend S, Bernards R. A gene-expression signature as a predictor of survival in breast cancer. N Engl J Med 2002; 347:1999–2009.
107. Alizadeh A, Eisen M, Davis R, Ma C, Lossos I, Rosenwald A, Boldrick J, Sabet H, Tran T, Yu X, Powell J, Yang L, Marti G, Moore T, Hudson JJ, Lu L, Lewis D, Tibshirani R, Sherlock G, Chan W, Greiner T, Weisenburger D, Armitage J, Warnke R, Levy R, Wilson W, Grever M, Byrd J, Botstein D, Brown P, Staudt L. Distinct types of diffuse large B-cell lymphoma identified by gene expression profiling. Nature 2000; 403:503–511.
108. Hacia JG, Brody LC, Chee MS, Fodor SP, Collins FS. Detection of heterozygous mutations in BRCA1 using high density oligonucleotide arrays and two-colour fluorescence analysis. Nat Genet 1996; 14:441–447.
109. Cutler DJ, Zwick ME, Carrasquillo M, Yohn CT, Tobin K, Kashuk C, Mathews DJ, Shah NA, Eichler EE, Warrington JA, Chakravarti A. High-throughput variation detection and genotyping using microarrays. Genome Res 2001; 11:1913–1925.
110. Cho RJ, Mindrinos M, Richards DR, Sapolsky RJ, Anderson M, Drenkard E, Dewdney J, Reuber TL, Stammers M, Federspiel N, Theologis A, Yang WH, Hubbell E, Au M, Chung EY, Lashkari D, Lemieux B, Dean C, Lipshutz R, Ausubel F, Davis RW, Oefner PJ. Genome-wide mapping with biallelic markers in *Arabidopsis thaliana*. Nat Genet 1999; 23:203–207.
111. Pollack JR, Perou CM, Alizadeh AA, Eisen MB, Pergamenschikov A, Williams CF, Jeffrey SS, Botstein D, Brown PO. Genome-wide analysis of DNA copy-number changes using cDNA microarrays. Nat Genet 1999; 23:41–46.
112. Jain K. Applications of biochip and microarray systems in pharmacogenomics. Pharmacogenomics 2000; 1:289–307.
113. Monni O, Bärlund M, Mousses S, Kononen J, Sauter G, Heiskanen M, Paavola P, Avela K, Chen Y, Bittner ML, Kallioniemi A. Comprehensive copy number and gene expression profiling of the 17q23 amplicon in human breast cancer. Proc Natl Acad Sci USA 2001; 98: 5711–5716.
114. Hyman E, Kauraniemi P, Hautaniemi S, Wolf M, Mousses S, Rozenblum E, Ringner M, Sauter G, Monni O, Elkahloun A, Kallioniemi OP, Kallioniemi A. Impact of DNA amplification on gene expression patterns in breast cancer. Cancer Res 2002; 62:6240–6245.
115. Zhu H, Bilgin M, Bangham R, Hall D, Casamayor A, Bertone P, Lan N, Jansen R, Bidlingmaier S, Houfek T, Mitchell T, Miller P, Dean R, Gerstein M, Snyder M. Global analysis of protein activities using proteome chips. Science 2001; 293:2101–2105.
116. Zhu H, Snyder M. Protein arrays and microarrays. Curr Opin Chem Biol 2001; 5:40–45.
117. Rosenwald A, Wright G, Chan W, Connors J, Campo E, Fisher R, Gascoyne R, Muller-Hermelink H, Smeland E, Staudt L. The use of molecular profiling to predict survivial after chemotherapy for diffuse large B-cell lymphoma. N Engl J Med 2002; 346:1937–1947.

118. Sotiriou C, Powles TJ, Dowsett M, Jazaeri AA, Feldman AL, Assersohn L, Gadisetti C, Libutti SK, Liu ET. Gene expression profiles derived from fine needle aspiration correlate with response to systemic chemotherapy in breast cancer. Breast Cancer Res 2002; 4:R3.
119. Bamberger C, Bamberger A, de Castro M, Chrousos G. Glucocorticoid receptor, a potential endogenous inhibitor of glucocorticoid action in humans. J Clin Invest 1995; 95:2435–2441.
120. Lane S. Pathogenesis of steroid-resistant asthma. Br J Hosp Med 1997; 57:394–398.
121. Sousa A, Lane S, Cidlowski J, Staynov D, Lee T. Glucocorticoid resistance in asthma is associated with elevated in vivo expression of the glucocorticoid receptor—isoform. J Allergy Clin Immunol 2000; 105:943–950.
122. Sher E, Leung D, Surs W, Kam J, Zieg G, Kamada A, Szefler S. Steroid-resistant asthma: cellular mechanisms contributing to inadequate responses to glucocorticoid therapy. J Clin Invest 1994; 93:33–39.
123. Woolcock A. Steroid resistant asthma: what is the clinical definition? Eur Respir J 1993; 6:743–747.
124. Hakonarson H, Bjornsdottir US, Halapi E, Bradfield J, Zink F, Mouy M, Helgadottir H, Gudmundsdottir AS, Andrason H, Adalsteinsdottir AE, Kristjansson K, Birkisson I, Arnason T, Andresdottir M, Gislason D, Gislanson T, Gulcher JR, Stefansson K. Profiling of genes expressed in peripheral blood mononuclear cells predicts glucocorticoid sensitivity in asthma patients. Proc Natl Acad Sci USA 2005; 102:14789–14794.
125. Hakonarson H, Bjornsdottir U, Halapi E, Palsson S, Adalsteinsdottir E, Gislason D, Finnbogason G, Gislason T, Kristjansson K, Arnason T, Birkisson I, Frigge ML, Kong A, Gulcher JR, Stefansson K. A major susceptibility gene for asthma maps to chromosome 14q24. Am J Hum Genet 2002; 71:483–491.
126. Oestreicher JL, Walters IB, Kikuchi T, Gilleaudeau P, Surette J, Schwertschlag U, Dorner AJ, Krueger J, Trepicchio W. Molecular classification of psoriasis disease-associated genes through pharmacogenomic expression profiling. Pharmacogenomics J 2001; 1:272–287.
127. Ewart S, Kuperman D, Schadt E, Tankersley C, Grupe A, Shubitowski D, Peltz G, Wills-Karp M. Quantitative trait loci controlling allergen-induced airway hyperresponsiveness in inbred mice. Am J Respir Cell Mol Biol 2000; 23:537–545.
128. Karp CL, Grupe A, Schadt E, Ewart SL, Keane-Moore M, Cuomo PJ, Kohl J, Wahl L, Kuperman D, Germer S, Aud D, Peltz G, Wills-Karp M. Identification of complement factor 5 as a susceptibility locus for experimental allergic asthma. Nat Immunol 2000; 1:221–226.
129. Cox LA, Birnbaum S, VandeBerg JL. Identification of candidate genes regulating HDL cholesterol using a chromosomal region expression array. Genome Res 2002; 12:1693–1702.
130. Lock C, Hermans G, Pedotti R, Brendolan A, Schadt E, Garren H, Langer-Gould A, Strober S, Cannella B, Allard J, Klonowski P, Austin A, Lad N, Kaminski N, Galli SJ, Oksenberg JR, Raine CS, Heller R, Steinman L. Gene-microarray analysis of multiple sclerosis lesions yields new targets validated in autoimmune encephalomyelitis. Nat Med 2002; 8:500–508.

2
Methods of Genotyping

Matthias Wjst
Gruppe Molekulare Epidemiologie, GSF—Forschungszentrum für Umwelt und Gesundheit, Neuherberg/Munich, Germany

Monika Werner
GSK Glaxo Smith Kline Beecham, Munich, Germany

INTRODUCTION

Human genetic variation is most frequently seen as single-nucleotide polymorphism (SNP). Many of these have been discovered more or less by chance when comparing sequence trace files of overlapping contigs from different individuals. A more systematic approach by comparative sequencing in a defined group of individuals by the SNP consortium has now greatly improved our understanding of genetic variation. SNP coverage across the human genome is not random and may be completely absent in highly conserved regions or highly abundant in other regions where genetic diversity is biologically important. Large-scale association studies by genotyping many individuals by many single SNPs are considered to be the most promising method to identify the cause of complex diseases. In addition, it will also improve the understanding of the individual response to drugs, also termed pharmacogenetics.

The technical possibilities to genotype SNPs in individuals has exploded in the past few years with more than 20 different methods available today. Although traditional sequencing by the Sanger method is still the standard for assessing smaller insertions and deletions in DNA sequence, numerous new methods have been developed during the past 10 years for scoring SNPs (1). With an estimated count of more than 5 million SNPs in the human genome, SNP genotyping requires high-throughput (HT) methods. Only a few methods are suitable for HT cutting-edge genotyping (>5.000 genotypes/day/lab) or ultra HT (>100.000 genotypes/day/lab) requirements, which is caused by the recent shift from monogenic to complex diseases. Due to much weaker genetic effects in these traits, much higher sample numbers are required. An average case-control study will comprise more than 2000 samples. Genotyping of a single gene with 50 SNPs alone will result in 100,000 single-plex genotyping reactions, which is a daunting task for a traditional laboratory.

HIGH-THROUGHPUT GENOTYPING METHODS

Traditional genotyping methods like endonuclease cleavage assays are not suitable for HT genotyping. Even if liquid handling can be optimized, the manual scoring of the cleaved fragments on the gel will remain a major bottleneck. The first major requirement for HT genotyping is therefore the automation of sample preparation until the readout of the genotype. Liquid handling formats used at the moment are 96-well, 384- or 1536-well plates, where genotyping is usually done in large batches.

A second requirement is the availability of sufficient DNA template. Nearly all methods are based on PCR except the invader assay. Although being clearly an elegant assay, it turned out that due to the consumption of DNA in thousands of assays, amounts of source DNA for HT could be prohibitive. Non-PCR methods therefore seem to be a second choice for HT genotyping.

The third criteria for selecting the HT method is the accuracy and the time and effort needed with any given assay. A technician's time for individual optimization of the protocol may be a critical factor. Missing or incorrect genotypes, even in a minor ($<10\%$) number of samples, may double the time for genotyping. Either individual samples need to be rearrayed in a second step from original plates or—often faster—just repeated from the same source. Average set-up and process time for a single assay is therefore an important point to consider.

The fourth aspect relates to the costs of genotyping. A simple calculation of cent per genotype is of limited value as total costs are caused by buying and maintaining hardware devices for storage, liquid handling, thermocycling, and software for measuring genotypes. Some methods have relative low basic equipment costs of €50,000 (1 euro = $1.2 U.S., March 2006), high set-up costs for single assay (€100–500) with low genotyping costs (€0.20), whereas systems on the opposite site start with basic equipment costs of €500,000, have set-up costs less than €50 but costs per genotype of €0.40. Generally, assays using standard enzymes, nontoxic, nonradioactive reagents will facilitate the laboratory handling and are likely to have even lower prices in the near future.

TEST PRINCIPLES

Current methods (Table 1, Fig. 1) combine at least one of the four different principles of allelic discrimination (hybridization, primer extension, ligation, or restriction) with one of the four different detection techniques (chemoluminescence, fluorescence polarization, resonance energy transfer, and mass spectrometry). Assay formats range from (slab-)gel electrophoresis, plates, particles, fiber arrays and microchip arrays to semi- and homogenous assays that do not require any further sample separation or purification. Whereas homogeneous assays are flexible and probably not labor-intensive, the amount of multiplexing is usually limited. Solid-phase reactions can be carried out on glass slides, silicon chips, and magnetic beads. In other assay designs, defined oligonucleotides are attached to the solid phase, and samples interrogate the alleles being already printed on a chip. Discrimination in such assays is highly parallel and saves the time and efforts for setting up multiple individual reactions. A major drawback is that the custom design is not very flexible and can be done by the vendor only.

The different detection methods also have marked differences. Numerous labels are available, most of them with light-emitting properties that enable elegant assays. When the reaction product is separated from the initial reaction, usually only one label is necessary. Homogenous assays otherwise require two labels that change their property during the reaction. Fluorescence detection methods have higher set-up costs by the synthesis of

Table 1 High-Throughput Genotyping Methods

Principle	Method	Advantage	Reference
Hybridization	Microarrays	Highly parallel, fast	GeneChip® (Affymetrix)
	5′ exonuclease assay, allele-specific hybridization, real-time PCR	Simple assay	TaqMan® (Applied Biosystems)
	Molecular beacons	Versatile assay	
	Dynamic allele-specific hybridization	Inexpensive labeling	DASH® (Thermo Hybaid)
	Fiberoptic analysis of coded tags	Highly parallel, fast	Sentrex® (Illumina)
Primer extension	Minisequencing	Multiplexing capacity	Snapshot® (Applied Biosystems)
	Hapten-labeled nucleotides	Inexpensive, robust	SNPit® (Orchid)
	Chemoluminometric detection of pyrophosphate	Additional sequence information	Pyrosequencing™
	MALDI-TOF mass spectrometry	Fast set-up, accurate	Mass Extend® (Sequenom)
	Allele-specific PCR, FRET energy transfer	Specific reaction	Alpha Screen® (Packard Biosystems)
Ligation	Colorimetric OLA	Robust	
	Ligation and fiberoptic detection	Highly parallel	Illumina® (Bead Array)
Restriction	Upstream inserted oligonucleotide cleaved by flap endonuclease	No PCR necessary	Invader® (Third Wave)

Abbreviations: MALDI-TOF, matrix-assisted laser desorption/ionization time-of-light; PCR, polymerase chain reaction; FRET, fluorescence resonance energy transfer; OLA, oligonucleotide ligation assay; DASH, dynamic allele specific hybridization.

specific labeled primer, whereas no modified primers are necessary for mass spectrometry measurements. Although being the most direct and accurate approach, mass detection still has the disadvantage of a relatively expensive and a technically demanding equipment.

All systems are scalable from a few to many thousand genotypes per day. The limiting factor for HT genotyping probably lies more in general sample preparation than scoring of the genotypes. Typing more than 100,000 genotypes per day may even generate bottlenecks of the analysis and interpretation of the generated data.

The need of software organizing HT by assay and sample tracking is often underestimated. Thorough monitoring of the movement of all plates at all positions is critical for quality control in a HT genotyping laboratory. Most genotyping groups are using proprietary databases to manage this task. Usually client computer on freezer, liquid handlers, thermocyclers, and analysis devices are connected to a main database that monitors in-time the process flow. A single sample is identified by the address on a plate grid, which is linked back to the original sample. During assay set-up, every plate is linked to a particular assay, which by itself links to a genotype, making it possible to assign a genotype to an individual study participant.

From many assays available at the moment, we will now discuss in detail five methods that are most widely used. Additional methods may be found elsewhere (1–3).

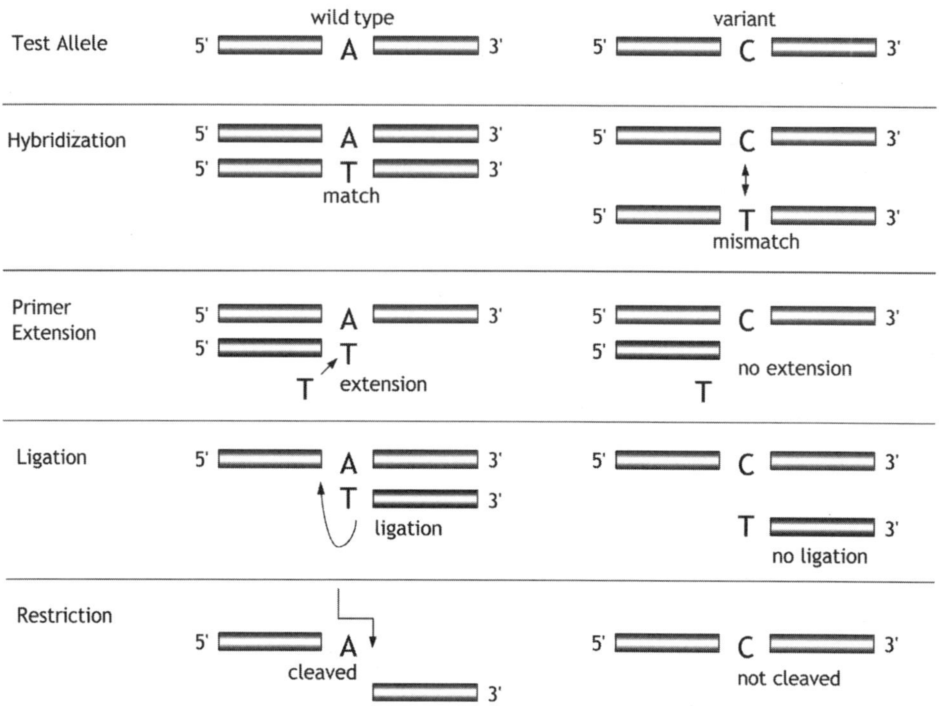

Figure 1 Assay principles.

Pyrosequencing

Pyrosequencing is an emerging genotyping method based on allele-specific primer extension (Fig. 2). This real-time sequencing technology comprises a cascade of four enzymatic reactions, yielding a luminometric signal that is proportional to incorporated nucleotides.

The pyrosequencing reaction is performed using a previously amplified target sequence. Prior to the allele-specific reaction, the PCR product should be purified from unincorporated nucleotides and PCR primers because they interfere with subsequent reactions. Generally, one of the PCR primers is biotinylated at the 5′-end to allow immobilization onto streptavidin-coated sepharose or magnetic beads. Following immobilization, the captured DNA template is purified from soluble PCR components and denaturated to obtain single-stranded DNA (ssDNA). Both the immobilized biotinylated and eluted strands can be used for pyrosequencing.

In the pyrosequencing reaction, a ssDNA template with a short annealed sequencing primer is incubated with DNA polymerase, adenosine triphosphate (ATP) sulfurylase, luciferase, and apyrase, and the substrates, adenosine 5′ phosphosulfate (APS) and luciferin. The four deoxynucleotide triphosphates (dNTPs) are added to the mixture in a defined order. If the added nucleotide is complementary to the base in the template strand, the DNA polymerase catalyzes the incorporation of the nucleotide, and pyrophosphate will be released. The new pyrophosphate will then be converted to ATP by an ATP sulfurylase. In the next step, luciferase mediates the conversion of luciferin to oxyluciferin using the previously generated ATP. The light emitted as a result of this reaction can be detected, where the signal corresponds to the number of nucleotides incorporated. The unincorporated dNTPs and excess ATP will be degraded by apyrase. If the added nucleotide is not complementary to the DNA template, it will not be incorporated, and no signal will be

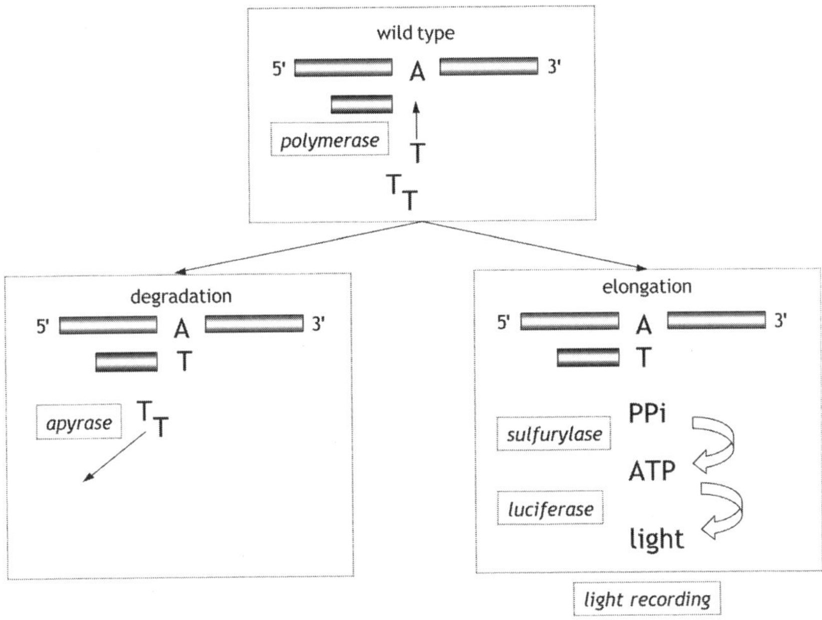

Figure 2 Pyrosequencing. *Abbreviations*: PPi, pyrophosphate; ATP, adenosine triphosphate.

generated. When degradation is complete, the primer strand is elongated by sequential addition of the different dNTPs, followed by degradation of excess nucleotides by apyrase.

Current available pyrosequencing instruments utilize 96-well and 384-well plate formats that facilitate analysis of between 5.000 and 50.000 SNPs per day. This technique offers high accuracy, flexibility in primer positioning, and real-time determination of more than 50 bp along the target sequence that allows analysis within 10 minutes. Contrary to other sequencing methods, it circumvents time-consuming electrophoresis and size separation. Sequencing also provides information on the adjacent nucleotides. Thus, one main advantage of this method is the detection of additional insertions and deletions and also novel polymorphisms across the DNA template.

One of the major drawbacks is the time-consuming template preparation due to immobilization and generation of ssDNA and also the use of target-specific biotinylated PCR primers. An enzymatic template preparation scheme has been developed that avoids labeled primers and the use of any solid support, thereby, reducing costs and simplifying automation of template preparation. Direct use of double-stranded DNA (dsDNA), instead of ssDNA, has simplified the template preparation step prior to performing an analysis using pyrosequencing. Recent developments enable single-step preparation of double-stranded templates using blocking PCR primers. Another challenge in pyrosequencing is the difficulty to determine the number of more than five incorporated identical nucleotides due to nonlinear light response and multiplex genotyping and pooling approaches to further reduce the cost of the analysis (see *Special Genotyping Applications*).

Mass Spectrometry

SNP genotyping by matrix-assisted laser desorption/ionization time-of-flight (MALDI-TOF) mass spectrometry (MS) takes advantage of mass differences between allele-specific primer extension products (Fig. 3). At present, three related assays are used, the PROBE

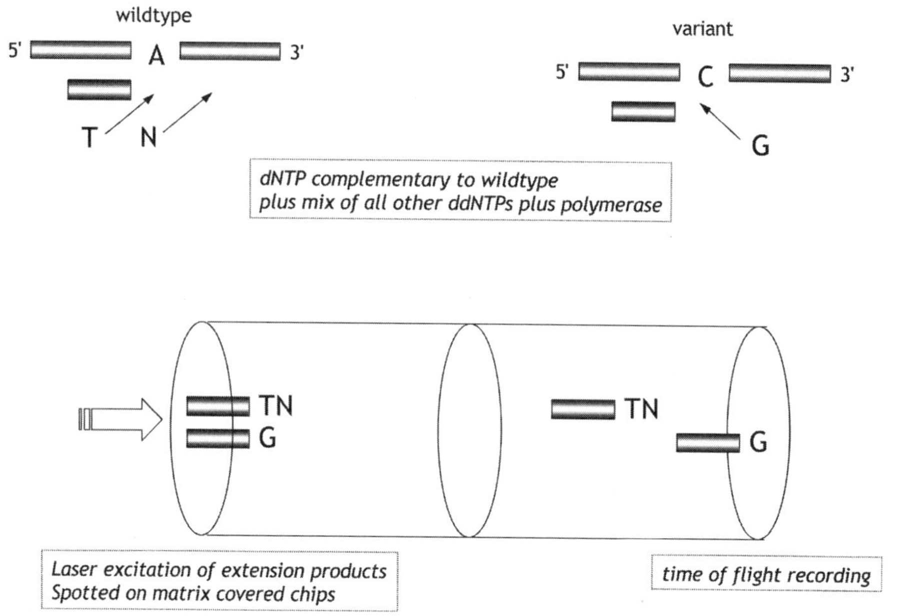

Figure 3 Primer extension and MALDI-TOF mass spectrometry. *Abbreviation*: MALDI-TOF, matrix-assisted laser desorption/ionization time-of-flight.

(primer oligobase extension assay further developed to the MassEXTEND® assay by Sequenom), the PinPoint, and the GOOD assay.

The PROBE assay involves annealing of a primer to previously generated PCR amplicon immediately up- or downstream of a SNP position. Prior to the primer extension reaction shrimp alkaline phosphatase (SAP) is added to the samples, which dephosphorylates any residual nucleotides, because the extension may be hampered by PCR components. The heat-labile SAP is then easily inactivated. A reaction cocktail containing the extension primer, a mix of dNTPs and ddNTPS, along with a thermostable DNA polymerase is added to the template. DNA polymerase adds the available nucleotides, which results in linear amplification of the extension primer. The reaction terminates if a single dideoxynucleotide is incorporated. The size of allele-specific extension products generated can then be used to identify the possible variants. After purification of the primer extension product, only a few nanoliters of products are transferred onto a matrix-loaded chip with a pintool spotting device. Chips can carry either 96 or 384 samples that are analyzed by high-resolution TOF MS. As the preparations are very small, there is little to no sample preparation heterogeneity.

The major strengths of mass spectrometric analysis are the accuracy of detection, automatic data accumulation, and HT capacity.

Recent commercially available fully automated systems allow up to 20,000 analytical reactions during 12 hours. Despite high initial set-up costs for instrumentation, the effort required for the assay development is low. Therefore, MS appears to be particularly suitable for analysis of a large number of markers. Apart from the genotyping capacity, MALDI-TOF MS provides the possibilities of multiplexing and quantification of allele frequencies in DNA.

A disadvantage of MALDI-TOF is the need for rigorous purification of extension products due to the higher sensitivity of the analysis to impurities than for other genotyping techniques. To circumvent this problem several strategies were established. The first available protocol (PROBE assay) included magnetic bead purification with a biotin-/streptavidin-binding system. The PinPoint assay uses reversed-phase tip purification, whereas the GOOD assay does not require purification due to the introduction of thiol groups into the 3′-region of the primer. For the MassExtend assay, a bead-free, homogeneous version of the MassExtend assay has now been developed, which allows a single-tube procedure with resin purification that can be used in automated sample preparation.

Microarray Analysis

Distinguishing alleles by hybridization takes advantage of the different thermal stabilities of a hybrid between an allele-specific probe and the SNP-containing sequence (Fig. 3). One approach to carry out allele-specific hybridization on microarrays is the GeneChip® assay introduced by Affymetrix.

On high-density microarrays thousands of allele-specific oligonucleotides complementary to a target sequence are attached to a solid surface. For each allele of a SNP, at least four oligomers are designed, differing only in the interrogating position. Additionally, in many cases a series of oligonucleotides walking over each variant of the SNP are used. The target sequence is amplified incorporating fluorescence-labeled nucleotides and hybridized to the array. Subsequently, the array is scanned to measure the fluorescence intensity for each hybrid. The reference sequence is expected to hybridize more efficiently to the corresponding probe and, therefore, gives stronger fluorescent signals than single base mismatches. These mismatch probes serve as control for cross-hybridization. The presence of homozygotes and heterozygotes give rise to different hybridization patterns with the probe complementary to the reference sequence showing the highest fluorescence intensity. In the presence of a sample with a substituted variant, the probe containing the complementary variant base will obtain the highest fluorescence intensity.

Hybridization-based genotyping can be an efficient method to monitor a large number of SNPs. The sophisticated technology of photolithography and solid-phase DNA synthesis allows construction of arrays carrying up to 260,000 features on a 1.28×1.28 cm array. Therefore, it seems to be feasible to rapidly screen thousands of SNPs using microarrays. The GeneChip HuSNP™ offers interrogation of nearly 1500 SNPs throughout the human genome. However, a drawback of the array format is the low flexibility in establishing an assay for a SNP. Due to high set-up costs of a project, it is difficult to add new SNPs or replace existing assays.

Another limitation is that the assays may fail to distinguish between homozygous and heterozygous, and deletions and insertions will not be detected as with pyrosequencing. A future challenge is to improve accuracy and decrease the false positive rate. The sensitivity of microarray-based hybridization is dramatically influenced by the target sequence, including inter- and intramolecular structures and also the presence of repetitive sequence elements. To allow more robust genotyping results dynamic allele-specific hybridization (DASH) monitoring duplex formation over a temperature gradient has been developed (1,2). Despite some disadvantages, future applications of microarray genotyping will be well established and custom-tailored medium density arrays for routine diagnostic screenings or pharmacogenetic studies.

5′ NUCLEASE ASSAY

A further currently used allele-specific hybridization method is performed in a homogenous, solution-phase reaction. In the 5′ nuclease, or TaqMan® assay introduced by

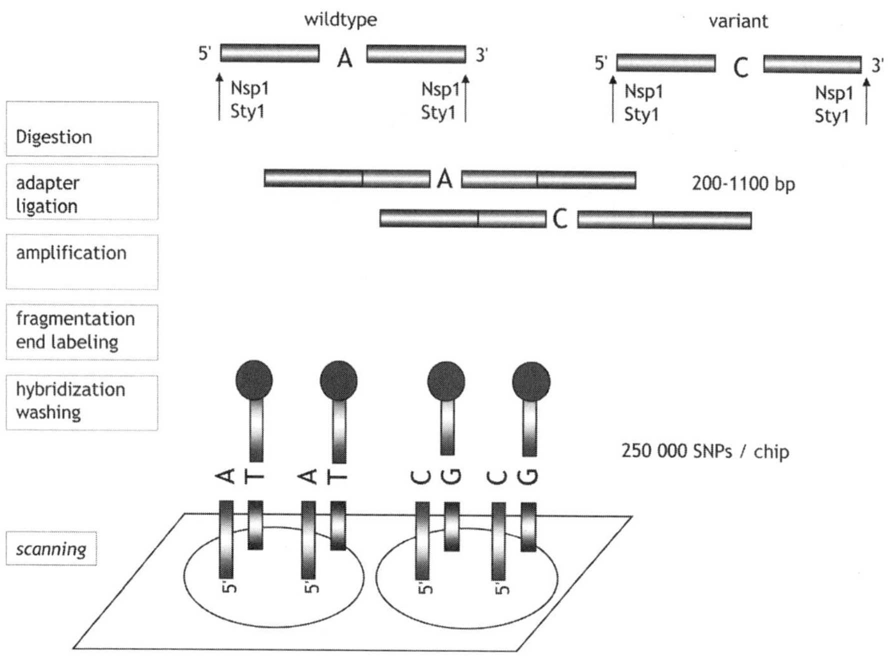

Figure 4 Primer extension using microarrays. *Abbreviations*: PCR, polymerase chain reaction; ddNTPs, dideoxy nucleotides.

Applied Biosystems, alleles are discriminated using the 5′ nuclease activity of Taq polymerase to detect a fluorescent reporter signal generated during PCR (Fig. 4).

In addition to PCR primers, one pair of TaqMan probes, consisting of an oligonucleotide labeled with both a 5′ fluorescent reporter dye, such as FAM, and a 3′ quencher dye, such as TAMRA, is included in a typical PCR. This is illustrated in Figure 5A. The TaqMan probes are designed to be complementary to the wild type and to the variant allele, which is located between the two PCR primers. During annealing of PCR primers, the probe hybridizes to the polymorphic template. Subsequent amplification of the probe-specific product causes cleavage of the probe by the 5′ nuclease activity of the Taq polymerase, generating an increase in reporter fluorescence because the reporter dye is liberated from the quenching activity of TAMRA. By using different reporter dyes, cleavage of allele-specific probes can be detected in a single tube. Each unique TaqMan probe binds preferentially to one of the alleles. As a consequence, binding of the TaqMan probe to the unmatched target sequence is highly reduced or even completely abrogated. Additionally, TaqMan probes modified with minor groove binder features provide better allelic discrimination. This modification allows shorter probes that enhance the affinity to the allele-specific target.

An alternative hybridization method for SNP genotyping uses wavelength shifting Molecular Beacon probes with a stem-loop structure. When not bound to the target, the hairpin stem keeps the fluorophore so close to the quencher that fluorescence does not occur. However, when the probe anneals to its target sequence, the fluorophore is separated from the quencher, and fluorescence restored. The increase in fluorescence during amplification can be monitored in real-time or at least after completion of the PCR. A sequence detection system (SDS) algorithm for allelic discrimination generates three clusters, and genotypes are inferred based on the fluorescence readout.

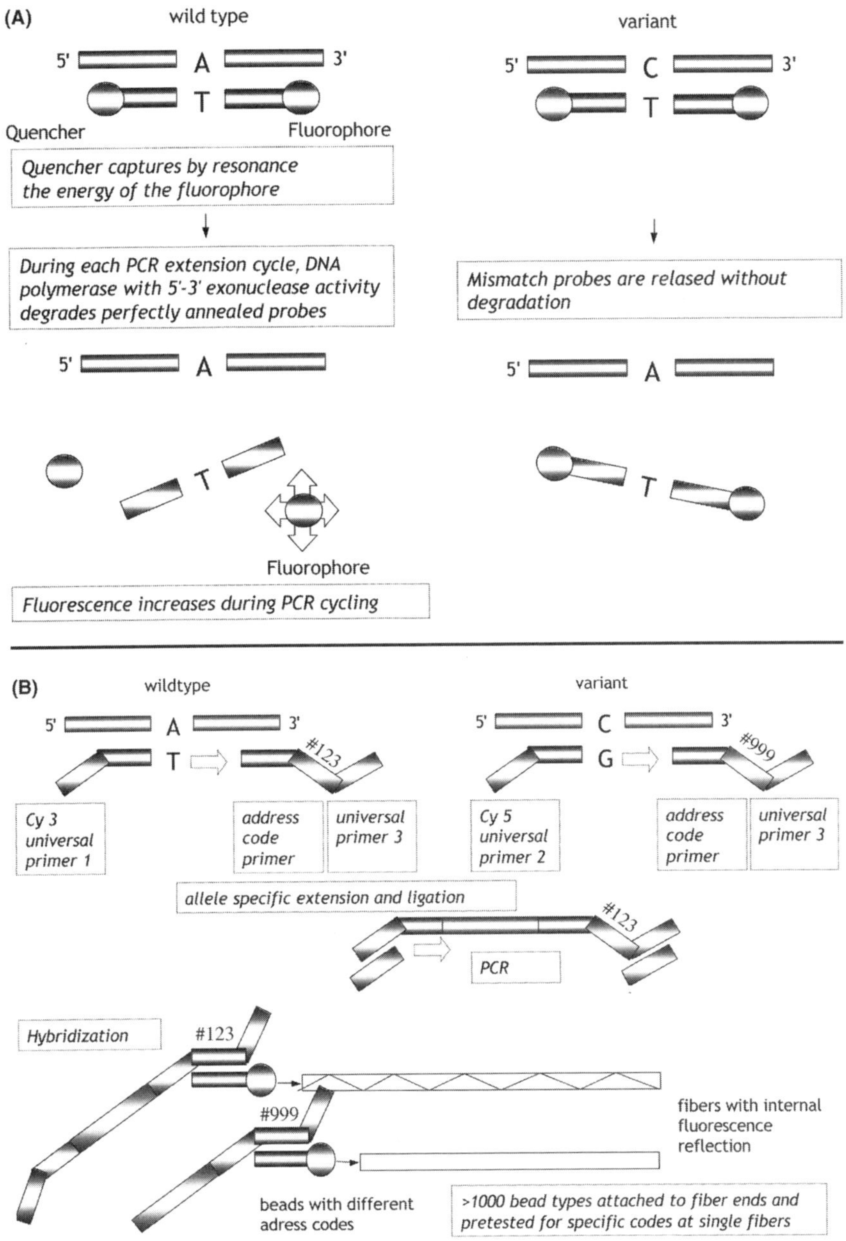

Figure 5 (**A**) 5′-Exonuclease assay (TaqMan®); (**B**) Bead array (Illumina®). *Abbreviation*: PCR, polymerase reaction chain.

Because costs of modified probes with fluorescent and quenching features is a limiting factor in application of the TaqMan approach this technology is most suitable for analyzing a limited number of SNPs in large samples. TaqMan assays can be performed in 96- or 384-well formats. Due to the incorporation of allele-specific probes in the PCR any post-PCR processing is avoided, thus, TaqMan technology is robust with low-error rates and has an user-friendly interface. Furthermore, the investment for instrumentation is relatively low compared with mass spectrometry.

The main disadvantage of TaqMan is that the design of probes and the establishment of assays require more labor. Accuracy is highly dependent on hybridization conditions influenced by buffer composition or primer concentrations. Therefore, the vendor offers assays on demand that provide design and validation of assays. Thus, TaqMan-based technology also makes HT assignment of genotypes feasible in daily routines.

Fiberoptic Bead Array

A new ultra HT method now used during the generation of the forthcoming haplotype map is an assay taking advantage of fiberoptic bead arrays developed by Illumina®. This technology takes advantage of fiberoptic array bundles and specifically prepared 3-μm sensor beads with specific DNA probe (address or ZIP code) sequences immobilized on the surface of each bead (Fig. 5B).

Up to 1520 different ZIP oligo sequences are pooled in one tube. Fibers are then introduced in bead pools, where beads self-assemble into pits at the fiber end. The assembly of beads is then checked by excitation of the fibers that transmit photons by internal reflection, where the photon either leaves the fiber end or is emitting fluorescence if hitting an attached bead. The bead that is self-assembled to a particular fiber is then tested by a defined series of hybridization and washing steps, making it possible to guess the present oligo ZIP code.

DNA template is prepared in the meantime by an allele-specific extension and ligation assay that builds a sequence consisting of a universal primer, 5′-primer, extended genomic region, 3′-primer, ZIP code oligo, and another universal primer. This initial step is then followed by a PCR using the two universal primers, leading to a molecule that can be probed with the fiber bundle for the presence of the ZIP code oligo.

The arrays are fabricated into microplate-compatible array matrices containing 16, 96, or 384 separate arrays. Illumina's 96-bundle array matrix can process up to 150,000 assays in parallel in a single experiment, making more than 1 million assays possible per day. Due to the probing of a predefined oligo, accuracy seems to be better than in assays that have to detect any variable genomic sequence.

SPECIAL GENOTYPING APPLICATIONS

To identify susceptibility genes for complex disorders, large-scale association studies have been considered as a powerful approach. Because numerous SNPs must be tested in large numbers of individuals for this purpose, intensive efforts have been undertaken to develop efficient HT tools to further reduce genotyping costs. One suitable way to address the requirement of cost and time-effectiveness is automated and accurate genotyping as the application of DNA pooling (4).

Any pooling strategy relies on the accurate measuring of SNP allele frequencies in pools of cases and controls. Several technologies allowing accurate and reliable estimates of allele frequencies have been developed so far. Current available pooling methods are based on allele-specific primer extension, allele-specific PCR, DHPLC, BAMPER, and SSCP analysis.

Although the potential of DNA pooling for large-scale genotyping is obvious, several practical and theoretical issues have to be taken into account. To ensure reliability of any genotyping method, each step must be quantitative. The first critical step is the construction of DNA pools containing equal amounts of DNA from each individual sample. Therefore, some protocols use DNA-specific fluorimetric methods for quantification. Furthermore, the reliability of assays depends on the DNA quality of samples. Another common problem is that all currently used SNP detection assays initially require a target amplification. Many SNPs show unequal representation of both alleles due to different amplification efficiency. The bias in allelic representation that is often observed might also be caused by differential incorporation of nucleotides (in primer extension assays), differential efficiency of hybridization (in hybridization-based assays), and differential detection efficiency of allele-specific products [e.g., in mass spectrometry (MS) detection]. To yield real allele frequencies the bias in allele representation must be corrected by the factor estimated from heterozygotes. Because heterozygous individuals have an equal number of copies of both alleles, the ratio of signal strengths of one allele to the other allele reflects the bias in allelic representation. Ignoring unequal allele representation can result in biased tests of allelic association (5).

In order to benefit from pooling designs, especially in the analysis of complex diseases, it is an essential prerequisite that allele frequency estimates are highly reproducible. Several pooling designs have been proposed involving, either the number of replicate pools, the number of individuals pooled, or the number of distinct pools made of subsets of individuals. The effect of the pool size on the accuracy of frequency estimates appears to be negligible. Therefore, the use of larger pools and multiple replicates are recommended, reducing the amount of genotyping. Three to four replicates of each PCR and detection should be sufficient.

Comparing accuracy and reproducibility of SNP detection methods applied for pooling analysis primer extension-based strategies appear to achieve the most reliable results with standard deviations of 1% to 2% between replicates. Allele frequency estimates deviate from real frequencies by about 1% to 3%. In contrast, quantification of differences between case and control pools by allele-specific hybridization is hampered due to insufficient hybridization specificity. The common limiting factor of any available pooling method is that allele frequencies can consistently be detected in the range from 5% to 50%. Thus, pooling strategies are preferentially suitable for screening common variants that are thought to be the causative variants in complex diseases.

Considering the preferred application of pooling strategies to screen a genomic region with large numbers of SNPs, but rather small samples of pooled DNA, genotyping technologies with low assay set-up costs are favored. Even with highly accurate and reproducible methodologies, frequency estimation from DNA pools is prone to some kind of errors and loss of individual information. Therefore, the most effective use of DNA pooling might be a two-stage approach in which a dense set of markers should be tested first in pooled samples, followed by individual genotyping restricted to the most promising SNPs. In this way, DNA pooling designs can considerably reduce the amount of genotyping required, and hence, can be an effective strategy for systematic association studies.

Multiplexing is another approach to significantly increase HT without significantly increasing the costs. It means that multiple SNPs can be assayed simultaneously. The differences in multiplexing capacity of the current genotyping technologies are substantial. Although mass spectrometric detection of allele-specific primer extension products has been demonstrated, the potential of stable fivefold multiplex assays multiplexing with pyrosequencing appears to be more difficult in this magnitude. Hybridization-based assays with fluorescence detection multiplexing can be achieved by use of different fluorescent dyes. However, these methods need labor for assay optimization, which makes multiplexing only suitable for frequently repeated assays.

FUTURE DEVELOPMENTS

There are numerous developments at all stages of genotyping. Examples include "genotype sorting" methods (microsphere sorting, Lynxgen) and also single molecule analysis of linear DNA strands (electromagnetic chips, U.S. Genomics).

The Lynxgen technology uses a library of approximately 16 million short synthetic DNA sequences, called "tags," and their complementary "antitags," to uniquely mark and process each DNA molecule in a sample. They are attached to 5 μm microbeads each of which carries multiple copies of a short antitag DNA sequence. The amplified tagged DNA molecules are then collected onto the microspheres through hybridization of the tags to the complementary antitags in a "a self-sorting process." Each microbead carries on its surface enough complementary antitags to collect approximately 100,000 identical copies of the corresponding tagged DNA molecule. Due to this process, each tagged DNA molecule in the original sample is converted into a microbead carrying about 100,000 copies of the same sequence. Therefore, in the complex mixture of a million or more identified DNA molecules substantially all the different DNA molecules present in a sample are represented in the final microbead collection, which can then be extracted, for example, by flow-cytometry methods.

A technology recently presented by U.S. Genomics relies on the direct and linear reading of large sections of single genomes. Linear analysis is powerful as there is no upper limit on the size of the DNA that is read. The biophysical rendering of the polymerase-DNA on an electromagnetic chip uses nanotechnology for positioning DNA and also fluorescent, electrical, and force-dependent detection technologies to allow for reading the sequence information.

These sophisticated techniques and instruments probably all require specialized instrumentation (1). Although a cutting-edge technology, many come still at a price too high for many laboratories. This may be overcome by the near future, either by further miniaturization ("lab-on-chip") or by commercial genotyping labs working in order and for account of academic laboratories. We will be facing a new era of studies involving the genotyping of thousands of SNPs every day, with an unprecedented number of samples wherein even genome-wide association studies will be possible. The planning and analysis of these studies will then cost more than the actual genotyping (7). Accurate genotyping and reporting, however, will always be a critical factor to find those associations ardently searched.

REFERENCES

1. Kwok P-Y. Methods for genotyping single nucleotide polymorphisms. Annu Rev Genomics Hum Gen 2001; 2:235–258.
2. Syvänen A-C. Accessing genetic variation: geneotyping single nucleotide polymorphisms. Nat Rev Genet 2001; 2:930–938.
3. Tsuchihashi Z, Dracopoli NC. Progress in high throughput SNP genotyping methods. Pharmacogen J 2002; 2:103–110.
4. Sham P, Bader J-S, Craig I, O'Donovan M, Owen M. DNA Pooling: a tool for large-scale association studies. Nat Rev Genet 2002; 3:862–871.
5. Le Hellard S, Ballereau SJ, Visscher PM, Torrance HS, Pinson J, Morris SW, Thomson ML, Semple CA, Muir WJ, Blackwood DH, Porteous DJ, Evans KL. SNP genotyping on pooled DNAs: comparison of genotyping technologies and a semi automated method for data storage and analysis. Nucleic Acids Res 2002; 30(15):e74.

6. Little J, Bradley L, Bray MS, Clyne M, Dorman J, Ellsworth DL, Hanson J, Khoury M, Lau J, O'Brien TR, Rothman N, Stroup D, Taioli E, Thomas D, Vainio H, Wacholder S, Weinberg C. Reporting, appraising, and integrating data on genotype prevalence and gene-disease associations. Am J Epidemiol 2002; 156:300–310.
7. Weiss KM, Buchanan AV. Evolution by phenotype. Perspect Biol Med 2003; 46:159–182.

3
Pharmacoproteomics

Alaisdair C. Stamps
UCB-Celltech, Slough, U.K.

Jonathan A. Terrett
Medarex, Inc., Milpitas, California, U.S.A.

INTRODUCTION

Pharmacoproteomics refers to the discovery and use of protein markers for disease diagnosis, toxicology, drug efficacy, and patient prognosis. Although these activities are by no means new to biomedical research, a number of developments have made possible the global analysis of proteins direct from diseased tissues or body fluids. These advances are predicted to yield unprecedented information about the effects of disease and pharmaceutical intervention on the entire set of naturally existing proteins, that is, the proteome, leading to the discovery of better indicators for disease treatment and drug development. The field of proteomics is currently undergoing rapid development and, although considerably less comprehensive and structured than, say, genomic microarray technology, nevertheless has significantly benefited from the advances in computer programming and data management applied to genomics. The coupling of these developments with the entire drug discovery process is now seen in most major pharmaceutical companies, many of which have large, dedicated pharmacogenomic and transcriptomic departments. Although proteomics is being used increasingly in drug discovery, lack of standardization and the need for greater efficiency means that it has not yet been incorporated to the same degree as the other "-omics" fields. In this chapter, the emerging field of pharmacoproteomics will be discussed in terms of the historical perspective of protein targets and markers, and, where current needs may be met by proteomics, followed by a description of existing and emerging protein discovery technologies.

HISTORICAL PERSPECTIVE

Because the activity of proteins controls all cellular functions, from metabolism to cellular architecture, signal responses, motility and replication, it could be argued that all pathologies stem from the dysfunction or inappropriate expression of proteins. This accepted, it follows that there must be a set of protein metrics to describe all forms of disease, a subset of which will be diagnostic, prognostic, or useful in monitoring disease status.

It is surprising, therefore, that at present diagnostic proteins for many common diseases, such as cancer, are almost nonexistent (Table 1). For cancer, this is in part due to lack of sensitivity but is largely through the heterogeneity of malignancies precluding the discovery of widely expressed markers. The estrogen receptor (ER) is currently the most reliable predictor of therapeutic response, based on hormone sensitivity in breast cancer (1). The epidermal growth factor receptor (EGFR) holds an equivalent but inverse prognostic value in conjunction with the ER status (2). Urokinase plasminogen activator (uPA), a serine protease causally involved in cancer invasion and metastasis, is also prognostic for poor outcome in breast cancer and other adenocarcinomas, such as gastric, colorectal, esophageal, renal, endometrial, and ovarian cancers (3). Carcinoembryonic antigen (CEA) is used in postoperative monitoring of colon carcinoma where preoperative levels are known (4). The increment of prostate-specific antigen (PSA) due to proliferation of cancerous prostatic epithelial cells is considered a useful marker of disease; indeed, the serine protease family of kallikreins (of which PSA is a member) have been implicated in the progression of endocrine tumors (5,6). Nevertheless, normal variation in PSA levels and its elevation in benign hypertrophy can confuse diagnosis, and more reliable markers are needed. More recently, prostate-specific membrane antigen (PSMA) and prostate stem cell antigen (PSCA) have been studied as clinical markers of prostate cancer, although neither of these proteins is entirely specific to prostate (7,8).

A major drawback in attempting to define a single marker for any particular cancer is the propensity for tumors to stop expressing proteins that have become deleterious. Thus the development of such markers as therapeutic targets, for example, c-erbB2 in a proportion of breast cancers, bcr/abl kinase in chronic myeloid leukemia (CML), is a logical step but the therapies themselves produce a selective pressure for mutations that no longer respond. These may take the form of nonexpressers (ER) or polymorphisms of the original marker (abl kinase); close monitoring of long-term treatments is required to detect resurgent disease. Both disease heterogeneity and mutability point to the need for a set of markers to be used in the monitoring and prognosis of long-term cancer. But the discovery of new markers is either serendipitous or through protracted effort, for example, extensive genotyping or subtractive analysis of antigens or cDNA collections. The ability to analyze proteins en masse in comparative disease versus normal studies would be a significant advantage in this respect.

To take another example, in Alzheimer's disease, diagnosis still remains within the domain of cognitive impairment analysis; there are no serum markers. In cerebrospinal fluid (CSF), elevated tau and decreased amyloid beta 42 have been correlated with marked deterioration in the disease and are potentially diagnostic (9). In a small subset of patients, genetic testing can suggest susceptibility to the disease; in particular, Apo E4 variant (10), mutations in presenilin-1 and -2 and beta-amyloid precursor polymorphisms (reviewed in Refs. 11,12), but there remains no proteomic prognostic markers for Alzheimer's disease.

The use of markers of toxicology is vital for clinical testing of new drugs. Measures of organ function in liver, kidney, and heart are routinely used in the toxicological evaluation of any new compound. Predictive markers of adverse events are highly desirable both in terms of patient safety and in reducing trial costs, and proteomic profiling enables comparison of new compounds with drugs that have established mechanisms of toxicity. Defining a toxicological profile may also enable targeting of the mechanism of toxicity in order to develop protective drugs. Serum and CSF are already collected in quantities containing sufficient protein, and these sources are proven to be amenable to proteomic analysis (13). Studies on serum are already established, and, because the aim would be to develop rapid readouts of early toxicity, a strong opportunity exists in this field.

The field of efficacy markers is also amenable to proteomics. The majority of drugs act by altering the activity of protein targets, for example, imatinib (Glivec) (14) acts by inhibiting the kinase activity of bcr-abl. This protein overphosphorylates proto-oncogene Crk-like protein (CRKL) in the disease state, and the efficacy of the inhibitor can be evaluated by measuring phosphorylation of this marker. Drug resistance is associated with mutation of the target kinase such that the inhibitor is no longer effective (15). Although relatively straightforward in the case of a circulating tumor, such as CML, in which blood extracts may be tested, monitoring of solid tumors is less reliable as, for instance, postoperative relapse is frequently at a remote and unpredictable site. The discovery of easily accessible, that is, circulating or excreted, protein markers altered by successful treatment of disease would provide a useful tool in molecular monitoring of drug efficacy. In the treatment of Gaucher disease the level of serum chitotriosidase is a significant marker of efficacy in both oral (miglustat) and enzyme replacement (Cerezyme) therapies (16,17), although measurement of this enzyme is also used to monitor beta-thalassemia (18). The use of single protein markers often proves inconclusive: Comprehensive comparative analyses of secreted or serum proteins can be used to define the efficacy of specific sets of markers or disease status, enabling more accurate monitoring of treatments.

Elucidation of the interactions and biochemical pathways mediated by proteins in vivo presents the next great challenge to biology and will have a revolutionizing effect on drug discovery. Genomics-driven target discovery has thrown up well-characterized genes, which await therapeutic drugs, for example, *B-raf* (19) and the breast cancer susceptibility genes, *BrCa1* (20) and *BrCa2* (21). Mutations in other genes, such as *ras* and tumor suppressor *p53*, induce constitutive activities affecting cell cycle and have well-documented roles in the process of carcinogenesis (22). The attractiveness of these proteins as targets is muted by their intractability in drug screens or chemical optimization; nevertheless, the cellular enzymatic and signaling pathways through which they effect abnormal replicative responses may prove amenable to modulatory therapy.

Heterozygosity, or polymorphic functional compromise of key enzymes or metabolite transporters in biochemical pathways, causes inherited errors of metabolism. In these cases the choice is either to replace the defective enzyme or to inhibit the build-up of metabolites caused by biochemical bottleneck by inhibiting another enzyme in the pathway. Thus, miglustat, an inhibitor of ceramide glucosyltransferase, has been shown to reduce the accumulation of glycosphingolipids caused by impairment of glucocerebrosidase activity in Gaucher disease (23). Proteomics offers a new means of discovering such enzymes either as targets or biomarkers. Metabolic and signaling proteins frequently form functional complexes on the surfaces of membranes or within organelles carrying out specific cellular activities: sensitive detection and microsequencing of these proteins is now achievable with the relatively small quantities of protein complexes enriched by affinity techniques. The discovery of well-characterized proteins in previously unknown settings can open the way to novel therapeutics.

Another aspect of genomic discovery has been the cataloging of gene families related to known drug targets. Indeed, such terminology as "druggable proteins" has been freely applied to homologous classes, such as G-protein coupled receptors (GPCRs), protein kinases, and ligand-activating proteases. Genomic (microarray) identification of these potential targets is rapid and relatively inexpensive; demonstrating protein expression and localization in disease tissues considerably less so. As a result, many proteins are suitable for pharmaceutical intervention, which have not yet been associated with disease. Proteomic analysis can provide a rapid route to validation of protein expression in the context of disease and therapeutic accessibility.

Therapeutic antibodies have recently risen in popularity within the pharmaceutical industry, which is attracted by their very high specificity, ease of synthesis, rapid lead selection, and (in the case of fully human antibodies) lack of toxicity relative to other

Table 1 Examples of Disease Biomarkers

Disease	Marker	Diagnostic	Prognostic	Disease monitoring	Prescription
Breast cancer	Her2neu	✓	✓	✓	✓
Breast cancer	ER	—	✓	✓	✓
Breast cancer	EGFR	—	✓	✓	✓
Breast cancer	BrCa1, BrCa2	✓	✓	—	—
GI, renal, ovarian, endometrial cancer	uPA	—	✓	—	—
Colon cancer	CEA	—	—	✓	—
Prostate cancer	PSA	—	—	✓	—
CML	CRKL	—	—	✓	—
CML	Bcr-abl	✓	—	✓	✓
Alzheimer's	Tau, amyloid β42	✓	—	✓	—
Alzheimer's	Apo E4 variant	✓	✓	—	—
Gaucher's	Chitotriosidase	—	—	✓	—
Gaucher's	Glucocerebrosidase	✓	—	—	—

Abbreviations: ER, estrogen receptor; EGFR, epidermal growth factor receptor; CEA, carcinoembryonic antigen; PSA, prostate-specific antigen; CML, chronic myeloid leukemia; GI, gastrointestinal; CRKL, proto-oncogene Crk-like protein.

biomolecule therapies. Success in bringing a number of antibodies to the clinic for cancer and immune disorders has led to a recent switching of resources on the part of many pharma and biotech companies onto the discovery and development of these new medicines (24). Although antibodies only bind effectively to cell surface proteins, they are somewhat less constrained by the need to target a cellular function and can be used to "mop-up" soluble ligands or to direct immune-mediated destruction of cancer cells and other dysplastic tissues. Proteomic discovery has been used to generate datasets enriched for plasma-membrane proteins, using subcellular fractionation techniques and high throughput annotation, from which targets may be selected and rapidly validated for clinical relevance (25–27).

PROTEOMIC TECHNIQUES

To date, the most widely utilized format for proteomics has been two-dimensional (2D) electrophoresis, a technique that has been used for the separation of charged biomolecules since the 1970s. The "-omics" suffix was only coined in 1993 (Wilkins) when informatic and technological advances in the form of large biological databases and peptide mass spectrometry (MS) were combined to generate protein annotation on a large scale. The potential was immediately clear: this new discipline could be employed to directly detect variations in expression, modification, or isoform of proteins when comparing normal versus diseased or treated samples. Other formats have also been explored, including "lab-on-a-chip" quantitative microarrays through to straightforward data-acquisition techniques, which preclude sample comparison in favor of higher throughput.

Comparative Proteomics: 2D Gel Technology

The principles of 2D electrophoresis as applied to proteomics are as follows: solubilized, denatured whole proteins are separated in a first dimension by their isolectric properties, then in a second dimension by their molecular weight. Thus, at the end of the process each protein would be expected to occupy a point within the 2D space, the position of which depends on its isolectric point (the combination of ionic charges on all of its side chains and modifications) and its molecular weight. In most cases this combination is unique, theoretically allowing the separation and concentration of all proteins if sample and gel size are unlimited. Even without knowing the identity of a single protein, the potential of this technology to profile the effects of diseases and therapeutics at the level of active proteins is obvious. Because fully translated and modified proteins may be analyzed directly from the patient, information is gained on which is additional to that and which is accessible through genomic microarrays.

In practice, a number of challenges are presented by 2D proteomics. Not least is the acquisition of samples. In contrast to genomic microarrays, relatively large samples are required in order to produce a detectable "spot" of protein, and although it may be routine to remove such tissues as tumors or such fluids as CSF in sufficient bulk from patients, willing "normal" donors are naturally very scarce. Once samples have been obtained, it is vital to preserve the proteins they contain as quickly as possible and in a state suitable for both long-term storage and future 2D analysis. For the analysis itself, the major hurdles are the conversion from one chromatographic medium to another within the same apparatus and reproducibility of the final protein display.

Sample Preparation

Proteins destined for isolectric focusing and molecular weight fractionation must be fully denatured in order to obtain accurate and reproducible data. Thus, lysis buffers are used, which combine strong reducing agents to break cysteine sulfhydryl bonds, and chaotropic mixtures, which disrupt the ionic and hydrogen bonds and hydrophobic partitioning of folded proteins. Other covalent modifications of proteins are preserved by these buffers, enabling observation of their effects on protein mobility in both the electrophoretic dimensions. Protein concentration needs to be high when the sample is applied to the system, necessitating maximal solute concentrations in lysis buffers. Many protein degrading and modifying enzymes continue to act even under harsh conditions, and so chemical inhibitors of these are included in the buffer in order to "freeze" the exact state of proteins at the point of extraction. The amounts of different proteins in biological samples varies to an extraordinary degree, to the extent that up to 90% of the protein content may be dominated by the products of just a few genes. Serum in particular contains large quantities of such proteins as albumins and immunoglobulins, and other proteins can be obscured even after 2D separation, or their relative concentration is too low to be detected in a standard protein loading. Depletion of these major components prior to analysis can be highly advantageous in revealing new serum markers, although further reproducibility problems can be introduced by this step.

2D Electrophoresis

The development of industrialized proteomics has led to some standardization in 2D gel technology, so that apparatus and reagents are now supplied commercially (e.g., Biorad, Hercules, California, U.S.A. GE Healthcare, Little Chalfont, U.K.). Batch production and quality control are essential for reproducibility, but it is mostly in sample quality and loading and in downstream data processing that the greatest gains are to be made. Proteins are resolved in solution in the first dimension, migrating within an immobilized pH gradient (IPG) until their individual isoelectric point is reached. The fractionated proteins are then coated with anionic detergent; when the current is switched by 90°, the proteins move into a thin polyacrylamide gel and are separated according to their molecular weight. After electrophoresis the proteins are stained and the images of the gels are recorded. Both methods represented here have a robust history in protein analysis, in the form of isolectric focusing (IEF) gels and SDS-polyacrylamide gel electrophoresis (SDS-PAGE). The integration of the two provides a very powerful analytical tool, but there are caveats and technical challenges involved at each stage. First, there is the problem of hydrophobic proteins. Traditionally, these are fractionated in gels by solubilization in ionic detergent, usually SDS, which produces an overall negative charge on every protein. This abrogates the natural isoelectric point (pI) of the protein, however, and so cannot be used for IEF. As a result, 2D gels tend to underrepresent hydrophobic species, such as integral membrane proteins. Second, the process of dimension switching can only be successful if the proteins are fully ionized by detergent infusion and with effective transfer from IPG to PAGE, enabling each protein to move in the second dimension as a discrete spot within the gel. Next, imaging of the fractionated proteins must be optimum. After electrophoresis, proteins are prevented from diffusing by fixing in weak acid to partially precipitate and attach them to the gel matrix. However, the gel itself is a very weak structure, which is not self-supporting. Torsions induced by polymerization cause the gel to change shape on release from the glass plates that are used to support it during electrophoresis. This problem can be overcome by binding the gel to one of the plates, preventing any movement of the electrophoretic matrix. Parallel to this advance in enhancing reproducibility has been an increase in the sensitivity of protein detection using fluorescent dyes with extensive linear dynamic ranges and detection limits extending into the femtomole range. Despite the caveats of 2D gel analysis, the result of these developments is that an excess of 2000 proteins can now be detected in a single sample using standard commercially available apparatus. By measuring the intensity of fluorescence, each protein spot (or "feature") can be accurately quantified relative to the total amount of protein in the gel. Finally, there is the challenge of mining the information provided by the gels. Slight fluctuations inevitably occur in gel composition and running conditions, with the result that for almost every protein there is always a slight positional variation between gels. This factor alone would have doomed 2D electrophoresis as a comparative tool had it not been for the development of software to manipulate gel images postacquisition, moving protein features relative to a set of trigonometric markers in order to produce a virtual, composite image. The accumulation of protein features by running sample replicates and adding to sample (patient) numbers is used to generate an electronic "master gel" comprising many thousands of protein features, all identifiable and quantifiable on the original, stored gels. This kind of image manipulation was pioneered by such proteomics companies as Oxford GlycoSciences and are now produced by leading proteomics suppliers, for example, GE Healthcare, U.K. (Ettan Progenesis™). The generation of such a large number of data points has itself necessitated additional software to mine and interpret the information. For example, the Swiss Institute of Bioinformatics (Geneva, Switzerland) developed the Melanie series of software programs; proteomics companies have developed sophisticated image analysis platform, such as Rosetta™ (OGS), Kepler™ (LSB), and ImageMaster™ (GE Healthcare), which aim to compare feature presence and intensity from different gels and samples using a variety of statistical parameters. Although these programs are essentially designed to manage large volumes of data, they also provide an important link with the next stage of the proteomic process—protein annotation—by identifying features that are interesting by virtue of statistically validated alteration in disease. Another approach has been to reduce sample requirements by employing direct comparison using differential staining of proteins prior to gel chromatography. GE Healthcare's two-color system, Ettan DIGE, aims to overcome gel–gel variation by running comparative samples on the same gel after prestaining each with a dye that fluoresces at a different emission wavelength. This system also employs an internal pooled standard so that different gels can be compared. A major source of error can be overcome using this approach, but the problem of consistent protein loading remains due to the viscosity of high concentration protein lysates required for detection of whole proteomes. Protein subfractions are much easier to standardize for gel loading, but the fractionation process itself can introduce broad variability.

Protein Identification

The application of the mass spectrometer to the study of proteins is fundamentally in the generation of precise mass measurements of ionized peptides. Indeed, molecular weight measurement of whole proteins as a screening process has been utilized in some proteomic platforms (e.g., SELDI, see section "Other Proteomic Technologies"). But it is in the area of peptide fragmentation, both enzymatic and via ionization, that MS has revolutionized protein identification. Precise measurements of tryptic peptides can be used to identify a protein from within a mixture, but the sequence of amino acids within these peptides can also be elucidated by secondary fragmentation of selected peptide ions in a tandem mass spectrometer (MS/MS). Measurements of ionized fragments produced by MS/MS can be reconstructed into subsets of possible amino acid sequences, which are then compared with theoretical tryptic fragments of electronic translations of real and predicted messenger RNA sequences found in genomic databases. From the set of candidate "hits" obtained in this way, the real peptide is identified by the comparison of the theoretical full fragmentation spectrum of each candidate with the original, real spectrum. Superposition of spectra identifies the peptide (and, therefore, the gene encoding it).

Automation of peptide ion sequencing process using such computer algorithms as Sequest (28) enabled extensive comparison of spectral analyses with genomic databases to elucidate protein sequence. This opened the possibility of high throughput protein annotation. Prior to this, researchers were dependent upon Edman degradation sequencing of proteins, requiring large quantities of purified protein. In contrast, MS/MS sequencing can accurately identify proteins in quantities close to the limit of detection of 2D gels, that is, in the femtomole range, from a starting material of less than 1 mg of the total protein. Rather than devoting an entire project to the purification of a protein of interest, this process can be completed for large numbers of different proteins from sample acquisition to protein sequence in a matter of days.

Semi-comparative and Continuous Data Acquisition Techniques

The low dynamic range of 2D gel electrophoresis, and its limitations with respect to druggable target discovery, have led some researchers to exclude the comparative step altogether. Instead, traditional one-dimensional (1D) Laemlli gels have been used to separate specifically enriched pools of proteins, which would not be resolved by 2D electrophoresis. The 1D gel is principally a deconvolution step to facilitate mass spec throughput, although additional information on the proteins can be inferred from molecular weight and the distribution and frequency of annotation, which provides semi-quantitative data comparable with expression patterns derived from cDNA libraries (e.g., TIGR expression profiles 29).

Protein Enrichment

In some cases, column chromatography is the only step used to fractionate proteins or peptides prior to mass spec analysis, for example, MudPIT analysis (30). Continuous data acquisition generates considerable lists of protein annotations and may be used to create nonquantitative expression profiles; otherwise its value in discovery is limited. Nevertheless, the discovery of proteins in unexpected contexts can be readily validated by more conventional techniques and is a powerful means of target identification, particularly if the protein in question is already well characterized. Enrichment of subcellular fractions, organelles, and protein functional complexes considerably improves the annotation efficiency. Recent publications have described large scale analyses of protein sequences from isolated spliceosome complexes (31,32), proteasomes (33), and yeast protein complexes binding to selected "bait" proteins (34). The expression by genetic engineering of affinity tags, which are exposed on the surface of protein complexes without disrupting normal protein function, has been exploited to enrich active complexes from living cells, in a process termed tandem affinity purification (35). Mass spectrometric sequencing of proteins captured in the complex reveals interaction pathways linking protein activities.

Thus, proteomics can be used to identify differentially expressed proteins en masse, considerably broadening the scope for biomarker discovery. The process in its current form is not yet sufficiently sensitive or rapid to replace clinical diagnostic technologies; what it provides is a rapid discovery platform yielding new potential diagnostic, prognostic, and pharmacologic indicators.

Other Proteomic Technologies

Despite the availability of rapid, convenient, and robust biomarker assays in these areas, considerable efforts are underway in the broadening arena of proteomics to develop new tools to serve the clinical market. Most developments have gone in the direction of miniaturization, taking advantage of the technological achievements of genomic platforms, for example, microarray spotting. Smaller apparatus means smaller sample quantities, and "lab-on-a-chip" technology suggests an ideal way to overcome the hurdle of sample size that limits conventional proteomics. Improvements in detection sensitivity through signal amplification and affinity capture, or a combination of both, have opened the way to true high-throughput proteomics requiring only tiny amounts of protein. Examples include random affinity capture of whole proteins, specific capture of proteins, and specific capture of peptides. SELDI (surface enhanced laser desorption ionization) generates mass spectra from samples of whole proteins, or trypsin-digested peptides, which are analyzed for statistically significant differences between diseased and normal samples (36,37). This technology has been coupled with laser capture microdissection (LCM), in which a few thousand diseased cells are separated from normal cells in order to produce a purified sample for comparison (38,39). LCM samples can also be applied to other miniaturized proteomic applications, such as those utilizing specific affinity capture. Other platforms have combined microfluidic technology, immobilization chemistries, and specific affinity reagents with high sensitivity optical or mass spectrometric detection to produce affinity capture arrays on a microscopic scale (40). Scrivener et al. (41) have developed an affinity array detection system based on peptide affinity capture, which can be adapted to both fluorescence-based detection and full MS/MS analysis of peptide sequence. In a "reverse proteomics" approach, SEREX (serological analysis of recombinantly expressed clones), cDNA libraries are expressed in an array format, and their resulting recombinant proteins are reacted with sera from autologous patients (42,43). Antibodies or other serum proteins specific to disease state (to date, largely in cancer analyses, 44), identify their corresponding sets of antigens, which can define new diagnostic markers or therapeutic targets. The concept of recombinant protein arrays has been taken further by the Protein Expression group at the Max Planck Institute for Molecular Genetics (45), who propose to express 10,000 human proteins with the purpose of elucidating protein–protein, DNA–protein, and ligand–protein interactions and to profile and characterize antibody and sera–protein binding onto the array.

These new platforms have advantages over conventional 2D gel proteomics in terms of sample consumption—statistically significant analyses can be performed using quantities of protein that are orders of magnitude smaller. Their limitation lies in the number of proteins they can accurately identify. In the case of SELDI this may be inconsequential provided clear sets of markers can be identified independent of sample variation and noise. For protein "chips," specific affinity reagents need to be generated beforehand. Theoretically it would be possible to produce an affinity partner for almost every protein or peptide (a parallel to today's genomic microarrays), but in practice there is still a substantial lead time to manufacture such a comprehensive array. Nevertheless, as a research tool protein chips hold considerable promise.

CURRENT ACTIVITIES IN PHARMACOPROTEOMICS

Widespread interest and commercial development of proteomic technologies have led to a number of discoveries, notably in the field of protein markers and more particularly in the form of protein isoforms and broadly based expression patterns. This information is largely unavailable other than at the level of transcription, because most proteomic technologies have been focused on the manifestations of posttranslational processing. As such, pharmacoproteomics complements genomic microarray profiling by providing data on gene products that are inaccessible to the latter technology.

SELDI technology has been used to identify patterns of protein expression by analyzing the relative intensity of molecular weight peaks over a large range of native protein sizes. An extensive study by the Food and Drug Administration (FDA) to identify serum markers of ovarian cancer was successful in defining a molecular weight expression pattern entirely consistent with the occurrence of the disease (46). This collaboration went on to define a haptoglobin isoform that is elevated in ovarian cancer, giving 90% specificity and 71% sensitivity, a level of accuracy exceeding any other serum-based assay for the disease. In another collaboration, SELDI was used to identify the CD8+ antiviral factor (CAF) associated with CD8+ T-lymphocytes of HIV-positive individuals who belong to the subpopulation of long-term nonprogressors, that is, do not go on to develop AIDS. Tandem MS of the peaks identified by SELDI revealed that the differential proteins thus identified belonged to the alpha defensin family. These findings enabled further validation studies supporting the role of these proteins in the suppression of viral replication (47). This study neatly demonstrated how the focused application of proteomics yielded rapid results on an HIV intervention opportunity, which was first identified 16 years beforehand.

The identification of reliable sets of progression markers remains a Holy Grail in medical oncology. SELDI technology has also been applied to this area in order to comprehensively analyze changes associated with the malignant state. Invasive pancreatic adenocarcinoma is a rapidly fatal disease and early identification is vital to increase the chances of successful intervention. Rosty et al. (48) reported the identification of a differentially expressed protein, HIP/PAP-I, secreted at high levels into the pancreatic fluid in 67% patients with pancreatic adenocarcinoma. Another group used cell lines derived from head and neck squamous cell carcinomas to identify proteins differentially expressed in metastases versus the primary tumor (49). A considerable body of published and unpublished data generated by SEREX analyses has been compiled into a database of serological cancer antigens (50).

In contrast to the "whole proteome" analyses favored by the technology platforms, some groups have applied proteomic annotation techniques to established areas of research. In a study that focused on a central signal transduction pathway, Lewis et al. (51) combined functional proteomics with selective deregulation of mitogen-activated protein kinases (MKK1 and MKK2), identifying 25 targets of the MKK/extracellular signal-regulated kinase (ERK) cascade, 20 of which appeared to be novel effectors of this pathway. These diverse targets suggested novel roles for this signaling cascade in cellular processes of nuclear transport, nucleotide excision repair, nucleosome assembly, membrane trafficking, and cytoskeletal regulation. Applying proteomics to a clinical study, Chen et al. (52) conducted a comparative analysis of 93 lung adenocarcinomas with 10 normal lung samples, with the objective of examining the isoform status of Oncoprotein 18, a key regulator of microtubule dynamics that influences cell growth and differentiation. They observed an upregulation of the protein in lung carcinomas with an increased proportion of phosphorylated isoforms, which they verified through conventional mRNA quantification, Western blotting, and immunohistochemistry.

Others have adopted an almost hypothesis-free approach to target discovery. Accepting the limitations of primary tissue analysis and the 2D gel system, some have taken the view that MS throughput is now so great that simply enriching subcellular fractions extracted from cultured cell lines can yield a significant proportion of potential targets in the annotated output. Crude membrane fractions of the colon carcinoma cell line, LIM1215, yielded 284 different protein annotations, of which more than a third were known membrane proteins (27). A later study defined 615 proteins of the human heart mitochondrial proteome, using 1D gel fractionation and high throughput MS (26). Using refinements of the membrane preparation protocol to increase plasma membrane representation and pools of estrogen receptor-positive or -negative breast cancer cell lines, Adam et al. (25) identified 500 proteins, of which 31% were known to be associated with the plasma membrane. This group utilized a peptide selection strategy aimed at avoiding reannotation of proteins commonly observed in proteomic analyses, with the result that a high proportion of novel and uncharacterized proteins were identified. These proteins were then analyzed in the context of primary cancer samples using conventional techniques of mRNA quantification, fluorescent tagging, and IHC analysis, which can be applied to very small amounts of sample and which are much more accessible in the large numbers required for clinical validation (Figure 1). This group was able to identify three novel plasma membrane proteins with clinical relevance to breast cancer; subsequent studies demonstrated protein functions consistent with neoplastic growth in two of these previously uncharacterized proteins (53). Above all, this study demonstrated the way in which large-scale screening of proteins with disease association from subcellular fractions enriched for drug targets can accelerate the target discovery process. Novel sequences are given relevance if it can be demonstrated that they are both natural translation products and plasma membrane-associated—this proteomic filter considerably narrows the subset of uncharacterized proteins, making the subsequent task of validation more efficient. The accrual of large amounts of proteomic data of this kind, with disease/tissue and fractionation information, will also enable informatic filtering akin to "electronic northerns" so that large numbers of commonly

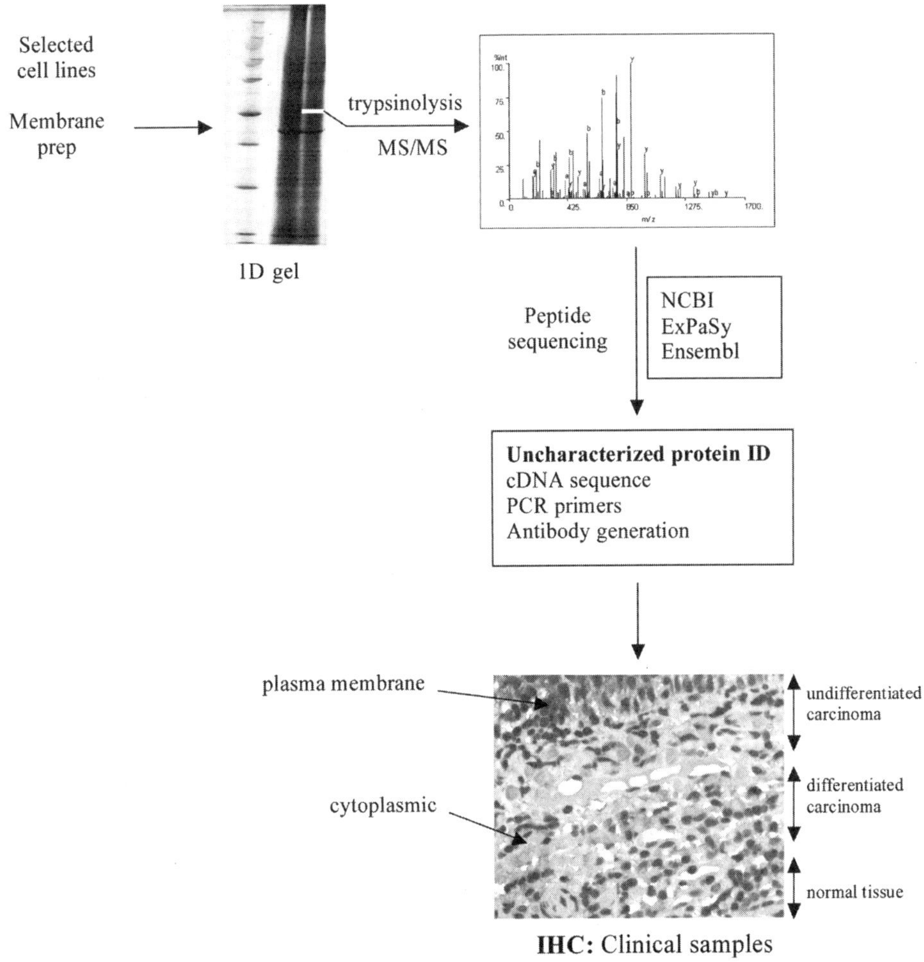

Figure 1 Cancer marker discovery by proteomics. Membrane protein fractions from selected cancer cell lines are separated on standard 1D polyacrylamide gels. Trypsinolysed peptides from thin slices of the gel are subjected to ion fragmentation MS/MS, and the resulting spectra compared with publicly available protein sequence databases, based on translations of cDNA and predicted gene sequences. Detection of uncharacterized proteins can be verified by conventional techniques, for example, mRNA quantification, IHC—shown here, a novel protein expressed predominantly in the cytoplasm of differentiated carcinoma but exclusively in the membrane of de-differentiated cells. *Abbreviations*: IHC, immunohistochemistry; MS/MS, tandem mass spectrometry; NCBI, National Center for Biotechnology Information; PCR, polymerase chain reaction.

expressed or nondruggable proteins can be excluded from outputs, further streamlining the process.

Proteomics in the Clinic—Rapid Diagnostics

Rapid detection of proteins for the purposes of diagnosis or monitoring is certainly nothing new: the Enzyme-linked immunosorbent assay (ELISA) test is a long-established feature of clinical laboratories, and portable kits based on this assay are regularly used in medical general practice and the home. Technologies for the development of protein detection kits are highly advanced and can precisely assay the level of diagnostic protein markers in minute samples of body fluids. Supporting matrices and miniaturized sensors are produced by a number of suppliers and the development of specific antibodies for protein capture has been fully industrialized. However, there are as yet relatively few point-of-care tests based on specific protein detection, and proteomics is therefore well placed to provide novel and multiple diagnostic proteins for validation in these formats. Biosite Inc has been successful in exploiting microdetection technology in the management of chronic heart failure. Excessive cardiac load causing distension of the ventricular walls induces release of B-type natriuretic peptide (BNP) from plasma membrane granules of the cells lining the ventricles (54). This hormone plays a role in fluid balance and blood pressure regulation and is a specific hormonal marker of chronic heart failure, which can be used diagnostically in preference to invasive or less accurate methods, such as echocardiogram or symptom assessment. The Biosite product assays BNP from a capillary of blood within 15 minutes using an antibody-based detection system, exemplifying the use of a protein to rapidly diagnose the disease. The advantage of this can be readily appreciated in terms of both appropriate patient triage and reduced costs through the avoidance of unnecessary tests and therapies. Biosite has utilized the same system to simultaneously measure myoglobin, troponin I, and creatinine kinase (CK-MB), to be used in ruling out myocardial infarction.

Toxicoproteomics

The opportunity to discover new markers of impending toxic side effects is ready to be exploited by existing proteomic technology (55). Some work has already been done in this area: Fountoulakis et al. (56) characterized the effects of xenobiotics on protein expression in rodent liver, in an attempt to define a liver proteomic toxicity database; a further study on hepatic protein changes associated with a number of drug treatments was carried out by Man et al. (57). Similar analyses have been carried out for specific compounds, such as the hepatotoxic effects of substituted pyrimidine derivatives (58) or nephrotoxicity in antimicrobial agents, such as gentamycin (59), and cyclosporin A (60). ICRF187, a cardio-protectant, has been shown to suppress a significant number of protein alterations in the serum of rats treated with cardiotoxic levels of doxorubicin (61), suggesting key protein markers of cardiotoxicity. The elucidation of markers affected by protective drugs may give functional hints as to the mechanism of protection, accelerating the development of more effective agents.

Proteomics in Pathogen Target Discovery

Like cultured cell lines, unicellular organisms offer the opportunity to study pathogenesis in a controlled and uniform laboratory environment, allowing for more precise measurements of protein/cell input and greater reproducibility in proteomic systems. In an attempt to characterize the adaptation of *Pseudomonas aeruginosa* to airway epithelia in cystic fibrosis, Guina et al. (62) carried out a full proteomic analysis of the organism using an in vitro model of the adaptive response, demonstrating the induction of an entire metabolic pathway affecting the homoserine lactone signaling pathway. The elucidation of the genomic structure and sequence of the malarial parasite *Plasmodium falciparum* paved the way for a thorough proteomic investigation of proteins expressed at each stage of its lifecycle. Using MudPIT, 2400 different proteins were annotated with correlation to the developmental stage and included some new findings relevant to pharmaceutical or immunological intervention (63). Cell surface interactions are considered to be important in pathogenicity, and proteomic studies have also focused on the identification of proteins extracted from in vitro biotinylated whole organisms, such as *Helicobacter pylori* (64).

Protein-based assays have been used for some time to detect pathogens. These can either be the direct detection of pathogen antigens or, in the case of many viral infections, detection of the antibodies naturally generated against them. The discovery of this type of antigen and antibody marker is well suited to proteomic studies because the induced protein profile changes can be absolute (i.e., presence versus absence of a particular protein), and the induction of an immune response could allow the use of such technologies as SEREX (42) to define pathogen antigens. These and many other studies indicate the potential to discover new markers for early identification of infections, or for the monitoring of infectious stages, through to novel antibiotic targets.

CONCLUSIONS

The current use of multiple protein assays in diagnosis, prognosis, efficacy, and toxicology suggests that these "markers" are discoverable through proteomics technologies. However, many of these assays performed on body fluids target proteins of abundances lower than is usually detectable in open system proteomics methods, such as 2D gels and the SELDI system. However, recent studies with these technologies demonstrate the potential of proteomics to examine the status of proteins in their naturally produced form and to discover changes relevant to pharmacoproteomics. As sensitivity is improved via protein chip, affinity, or more conventional separation technologies, it might be possible to identify relevant changes in low abundance proteins from a "blind" starting point. The construction of robust, quick, and cheap assays following the identification of protein markers has already been demonstrated in multiple settings, and so the challenge remains in the progression of technological developments that allow new protein discoveries.

REFERENCES

1. Duffy MJ. Clinical uses of tumor markers: a critical review. Crit Rev Clin Lab Sci 2001; 38:225–262.
2. Sinsbury JR, Farndon JR, Needham GK, Malcolm AJ, Harris AL. Epidermal-growth-factor receptor status as predictor of early recurrence of and death from breast cancer. Lancet 1987; 1:1398–1402.
3. Duffy MJ, Maguire TM, McDermott EW, O'Higgins N. Urokinase plasminogen activator: a prognostic marker in multiple types of cancer. J Surg Oncol 1999; 71:130–135.
4. Clinical practice guidelines for the use of tumor markers in breast and colorectal cancer. Adopted on May 17, 1996 by the American Society of Clinical Oncology. J Clin Oncol 1996; 14:2843–2877.
5. Bok RA, Small EJ. Bloodborne biomolecular markers in prostate cancer development and progression. Nat Rev Cancer 2002; 2:918 –926.
6. Yousef GM, Diamandis EP. Expanded human tissue kallikrein family—a novel panel of cancer biomarkers. Tumour Biol 2002; 23:185–192.
7. Gregorakis AK, Holmes EH, Murphy GP. Prostate-specific membrane antigen: current and future utility. Semin Urol Oncol 1998; 16:2–12.
8. Jalkut MW, Reiter RE. Role of prostate stem cell antigen in prostate cancer research. Curr Opin Urol 2002; 12:401–406.
9. Riemenschneider M, Lautenschlager N, Wagenpfeil S, Diehl J, Drzezga A, Kurz A. Cerebrospinal fluid tau and beta-amyloid 42 proteins identify Alzheimer disease in subjects with mild cognitive impairment. Arch Neurol 2002; 59:1729–1734.
10. Corder EH, Saunders AM, Strittmatter WJ, Schmechel DE, Gaskell PC, Small GW, Roses AD, Haines JL, Pericak-Vance MA. Gene dose of apolipoprotein E type 4 allele and the risk of Alzheimer's disease in late onset families. Science 1993; 261:921–923.

11. Kurz A, Riemenschneider M, Drzezga A, Lautenschlager N. The role of biological markers in the early and differential diagnosis of Alzheimer's disease. J Neural Transm Suppl 2002; 62:127–133.
12. Rogaeva E, Tandon A, St George-Hyslop PH. Genetic markers in the diagnosis of Alzheimer's disease. J Alzheimers Dis 2001; 3:293–304.
13. Anderson NL, Anderson NG. The human plasma proteome: history, character, and diagnostic prospects. Mol Cell Proteomics 2002; 1:845–867.
14. Capdeville R, Buchdunger E, Zimmermann J, Matter A. Gilvec (STI571, imatinib), a rationally developed, targeted anticancer drug. Nat Rev Drug Discov 2002; 1:493–502.
15. Gorre ME, Mohammed M, Ellwood K, Hsu N, Paquette R, Rao PN, Sawyers CL. Clinical resistance to STI-571 cancer therapy caused by BCR-ABL gene mutation or amplification. Science 2001; 293:876–880.
16. Guo Y, He W, Boer AM, Wevers RA, de Bruijn AM, Groener JE, Hollak CE, Aerts JM, Galjaard H, van Diggelen OP. Elevated plasma chitotriosidase activity in various lysosomal storage disorders. J Inherit Metab Dis 1995; 18:717–722.
17. Hollak CE, van Weely S, van Oers MH, Aerts JM. Marked elevation of plasma chitotriosidase activity. A novel hallmark of Gaucher disease. J Clin Invest 1994; 93:1288–1292.
18. Altarescu G, Rudensky B, Abrahamov A, Goldfarb A, Rund D, Zimran A, Elstein D. Plasma chitotriosidase activity in patients with beta-thalassemia. Am J Hematol 2002; 71:7–10.
19. Davies H, Bignell GR, Cox C, Stephens P, Edkins S, Clegg S, Teague J, Woffendin H, Garnett MJ, Bottomley W, Davis N, Dicks E, Ewing R, Floyd Y, Gray K, Hall S, Hawes R, Hughes J, Kosmidou V, Menzies A, Mould C, Parker A, Stevens C, Watt S, Hooper S, Wilson R, Jayatilake H, Gusterson BA, Cooper C, Shipley J, Hargrave D, Pritchard-Jones K, Maitland N, Chenevix-Trench G, Riggins GJ, Bigner DD, Palmieri G, Cossu A, Flanagan A, Nicholson A, Ho JW, Leung SY, Yuen ST, Weber BL, Seigler HF, Darrow TL, Paterson H, Marais R, Marshall CJ, Wooster R, Stratton MR, Futreal PA. Mutations of the BRAF gene in human cancer. Nature 2002; 417:949–954.
20. Miki Y, Swensen J, Shattuck-Eidens D, Futreal PA, Harshman K, Tavtigian S, Liu Q, Cochran C, Bennett LM, Ding W, et al. A strong candidate for the breast and ovarian cancer susceptibility gene BRCA1. Science 1994; 266:66–71.
21. Wooster R, Bignell G, Lancaster J, Swift S, Seal S, Mangion J, Collins N, Gregory S, Gumbs C, Micklem G, Barfoot R, Hamoudi R, Patel S, Rice C, Biggs P, Hashim Y, Smith A, Connor F, Arason A, Gudmundsson J, Ficenec D, Kelsell D, Ford D, Tonin P, Bishop DT, Spurr NK, Ponder BAJ, Eeles R, Peto J, Devilee P, Cornelisse C, Lynch H, Narod S, Lenoir G, Egilsson V, Barkadottir RB, Easton DF, Bentley DR, Futreal PA, Ashworth A, Stratton MR. Identification of the breast cancer susceptibility gene BRCA2. Nature 1995; 378:789–792.
22. Yuspa SH, Dlugosz AA, Cheng CK, Denning MF, Tennenbaum T, Glick AB, Weinberg WC. Role of oncogenes and tumor suppressor genes in multistage carcinogenesis. J Invest Dermatol 1994; 103(suppl 5):90S–95S.
23. Cox T, Lachmann R, Hollak C, Aerts J, van Weely S, Hrebicek M, Platt F, Butters T, Dwek R, Moyses C, Gow I, Elstein D, Zimran A. Novel oral treatment of Gaucher's disease with *N*-butyldeoxynojirimycin (OGT 918) to decrease substrate biosynthesis. Lancet 2000; 355:1481–1485.
24. Gura T. Therapeutic antibodies: magic bullets hit the target. Nature 2002; 417:584–586.
25. Adam PJ, Boyd R, Tyson KL, Fletcher GC, Stamps A, Hudson L, Poyser HR, Redpath N, Griffiths M, Steers G, Harris AL, Patel S, Berry J, Loader JA, Townsend RR, Daviet L, Legrain P, Parekh R, Terrett JA. Comprehensive proteomic analysis of breast cancer cell membranes reveals unique proteins with potential roles in clinical cancer. J Biol Chem 2003; 278:6482–6489.
26. Taylor SW, Fahy E, Zhang B, Glenn GM, Warnock DE, Wiley S, Murphy AN, Gaucher SP, Capaldi RA, Gibson BW, Ghosh SS. Characterization of the human heart mitochondrial proteome. Nat Biotechnol 2003; 21:281–286.
27. Simpson RJ, Connolly LM, Eddes JS, Pereira JJ, Moritz RL, Reid GE. Proteomic analysis of the human colon carcinoma cell line (LIM 1215): development of a membrane protein database. Electrophoresis 2000 May; 21:1707–1732.

28. Eng JK, McCormack AL, Yates JR III. An approach to correlate tandem mass spectral data of peptides with amino acid sequences in a protein database. J Am Soc Mass Spectrom 1994; 5:976–989.
29. http://www.tigr.org.
30. Washburn MP, Wolters D, Yates JR III. Large-scale analysis of the yeast proteome by multidimensional protein identification technology. Nat Biotechnol 2001; 19:242–247.
31. Rappsilber J, Ryder U, Lamond AI, Mann M. Large-scale proteomic analysis of the human spliceosome. Genome Res 2002; 12:1231–1245.
32. Zhou Z, Licklider LJ, Gygi SP, Reed R. Comprehensive proteomic analysis of the human spliceosome. Nature 2002; 419:182–185.
33. Leggett DS, Hanna J, Borodovsky A, Crosas B, Schmidt M, Baker RT, Walz T, Ploegh H, Finley D. Multiple associated proteins regulate proteasome structure and function. Mol Cell 2002; 10:495–507.
34. Ho Y, Gruhler A, Heilbut A, Bader GD, Moore L, Adams SL, Millar A, Taylor P, Bennett K, Boutilier K, Yang L, Wolting C, Donaldson I, Schandorff S, Shewnarane J, Vo M, Taggart J, Goudreault M, Muskat B, Alfarano C, Dewar D, Lin Z, Michalickova K, Willems AR, Sassi H, Nielsen PA, Rasmussen KJ, Andersen JR, Johansen LE, Hansen LH, Jespersen H, Podtelejnikov A, Nielsen E, Crawford J, Poulsen V, Sorensen BD, Matthiesen J, Hendrickson RC, Gleeson F, Pawson T, Moran MF, Durocher D, Mann M, Hogue CW, Figeys D, Tyers M. Systematic identification of protein complexes in Saccharomyces cerevisiae by mass spectrometry. Nature 2002; 415:180–183.
35. Rigaut G, Shevchenko A, Rutz B, Wilm M, Mann M, Seraphin B. A generic protein purification method for protein complex characterization and proteome exploration. Nat Biotechnol 1999; 17:1030–1032.
36. Merchant M, Weinberger SR. Recent advancements in surface-enhanced laser desorption/ionization time-of-flight mass spectrometry. Electrophoresis 2000; 21:1164–1177.
37. Rubin RB, Merchant M. A rapid protein profiling system that speeds study of cancer and other diseases. Am Clin Lab 2000; 19:28–29.
38. Emmert-Buck MR, Bonner RF, Smith PD, Chuaqui RF, Zhuang Z, Goldstein SR, Weiss RA, Liotta LA. Laser capture microdissection. Science 1996; 274:998–1001.
39. Banks RE, Dunn MJ, Forbes MA, Stanley A, Pappin D, Naven T, Gough M, Harnden P, Selby PJ. The potential use of laser capture microdissection to selectively obtain distinct populations of cells for proteomic analysis—preliminary findings. Electrophoresis 1999; 20:689–700.
40. Ruiz-Taylor LA, Martin TL, Zaugg FG, Witte K, Indermuhle P, Nock S, Wagner P. Monolayers of derivatized poly(L-lysine)-grafted poly(ethylene glycol) on metal oxides as a class of biomolecular interfaces. Proc Natl Acad Sci USA 2001; 98:852–857.
41. Scrivener E, Barry R, Platt A, Calvert R, Masih G, Hextall P, Soloviev M, Terrett J. Peptidomics: a new approach to affinity protein microarrays. Proteomics 2003; 3:122–128.
42. Sahin U, Türeci Ö, Schmitt H, Cochlovius B, Johannes T, Schmits R, Stenner F, Luo G, Schobert I, Pfreundschuh M. Human neoplasms elicit multiple specific immune responses in the autologous host. Proc Natl Acad Sci USA 1995; 92:11810–11813.
43. Türeci Ö, Sahin U, Pfreundschuh M. Serological analysis of human tumor antigens: molecular definition and implications, Mol Med Today 1997; 3:342.
44. http://www.licr.org/SEREX.html.
45. http://www.molgen.mpg.de/~proteingroup/ProjectsProtein2.html.
46. Petricoin EF, Ardekani AM, Hitt BA, Levine PJ, Fusaro VA, Steinberg SM, Mills GB, Simone C, Fishman DA, Kohn EC, Liotta LA. Use of proteomic patterns in serum to identify ovarian cancer. Lancet 2002; 359:572–577.
47. Zhang L, Yu W, He T, Yu J, Caffrey RE, Dalmasso EA, Fu S, Pham T, Mei J, Ho JJ, Zhang W, Lopez P, Ho DD. Contribution of human alpha-defensin 1, 2, and 3 to the anti-HIV-1 activity of CD8 antiviral factor. Science 2002; 298:995–1000.
48. Rosty C, Christa L, Kuzdzal S, Baldwin WM, Zahurak ML, Carnot F, Chan DW, Canto M, Lillemoe KD, Cameron JL, Yeo CJ, Hruban RH, Goggins M. Identification of

hepatocarcinoma-intestine-pancreas/pancreatitis-associated protein I as a biomarker for pancreatic ductal adenocarcinoma by protein biochip technology. Cancer Res 2002; 62:1868–1875.
49. Wu W, Tang X, Hu W, Lotan R, Hong WK, Mao L. Identification and validation of metastasis-associated proteins in head and neck cancer cell lines by two-dimensional electrophoresis and mass spectrometry. Clin Exp Metastasis 2002; 19:319–326.
50. http://www.licr.org/SEREX.html
51. Lewis TS, Hunt JB, Aveline LD, Jonscher KR, Louie DF, Yeh JM, Nahreini TS, Resing KA, Ahn NG. Identification of novel MAP kinase pathway signaling targets by functional proteomics and mass spectrometry. Mol Cell 2000; 6:1343–1354.
52. Chen G, Wang H, Gharib TG, Huang CC, Thomas DG, Shedden KA, Kuick R, Taylor JM, Kardia SL, Misek DE, Giordano TJ, Iannettoni MD, Orringer MB, Hanash SM, Beer DG. Overexpression of oncoprotein 18 correlates with poor differentiation in lung adenocarcinomas. Mol Cell Proteomics 2003; Feb. 12 (e-pub ahead of print).
53. Fletcher GC, Patel S, Tyson K, Adam PJ, Schenker M, Loader JA, Daviet L, Legrain P, Parekh R, Harris AL, Terrett JA. hAG-2 and hAG-3, human homologues of genes involved in differentiation, are associated with oestrogen receptor-positive breast tumours and interact with metastasis gene C4.4a and dystroglycan. Br J Cancer 2003; 88:579–585.
54. Bonow RO. New insights into the cardiac natriuretic peptides. Circulation 1996; 93:1946–1950.
55. Wilkins MR. What do we want from proteomics in the detection and avoidance of adverse drug reactions. Toxicol Lett 2002; 127:245–249.
56. Fountoulakis M, Berndt P, Boelsterli UA, Crameri F, Winter M, Albertini S, Suter L. Two-dimensional database of mouse liver proteins: changes in hepatic protein levels following treatment with acetaminophen or its nontoxic regioisomer 3-acetamidophenol. Electrophoresis 2000; 21:2148–2161.
57. Man WJ, White IR, Bryant D, Bugelski P, Camilleri P, Cutler P, Heald G, Lord PG, Wood J, Kramer K. Protein expression analysis of drug-mediated hepatotoxicity in the Sprague-Dawley rat. Proteomics 2002; 2:1577–1585.
58. Newsholme SJ, Maleeff BF, Steiner S, Anderson NL, Schwartz LW. Two-dimensional electrophoresis of liver proteins: characterization of a drug-induced hepatomegaly in rats. Electrophoresis 2000; 21:2122–2128.
59. Kennedy S. Proteomic profiling from human samples: the body fluid alternative. Toxicol Lett 2001; 120:379–384.
60. Aicher L, Wahl D, Arce A, Grenet O, Steiner S. New insights into cyclosporine A nephrotoxicity by proteome analysis. Electrophoresis 1998; 19:1998–2003.
61. Bandara LR, Kennedy S. Toxicoproteomics—a new preclinical tool. Drug Discov Today 2002; 7:411–418.
62. Guina T, Purvine SO, Yi EC, Eng J, Goodlett DR, Aebersold R, Miller SI. Quantitative proteomic analysis indicates increased synthesis of a quinolone by Pseudomonas aeruginosa isolates from cystic fibrosis airways. Proc Natl Acad Sci USA 2003; 100:2771–2776.
63. Florens L, Washburn MP, Raine JD, Anthony RM, Grainger M, Haynes JD, Moch JK, Muster N, Sacci JB, Tabb DL, Witney AA, Wolters D, Wu Y, Gardner MJ, Holder AA, Sinden RE, Yates JR, Carucci DJ. A proteomic view of the Plasmodium falciparum life cycle. Nature 2002; 419:520–526.
64. Sabarth N, Lamer S, Zimny-Arndt U, Jungblut PR, Meyer TF, Bumann D. Identification of surface proteins of Helicobacter pylori by selective biotinylation, affinity purification, and two-dimensional gel electrophoresis. J Biol Chem 2002; 277:27896–27902.

4

Potential Social, Ethical, and Legal Issues Raised by the Development of Pharmacogenetics

Paul Martin, Andrew Smart, and Robert Dingwall
Institute for the Study of Genetics, Biorisks and Society, University of Nottingham, Nottingham, U.K.

INTRODUCTION—ASSESSING THE POTENTIAL IMPACT OF PHARMACOGENETICS

Trying to assess the social, ethical, legal, and practice issues raised by a medical innovation is not easy, as great uncertainty often surrounds the technology, how it might be used in the clinic, and the responses of patients, professionals, and the public. Despite the difficulties of trying to achieve a meaningful and realistic appraisal, it is a vitally important task. If controversial new technologies are introduced into the clinic without careful consideration of the issues they raise and if appropriate governance mechanisms are not put in place in response, there is a real danger that public acceptance will be low, resulting in poor uptake and a loss of trust in the integrity of the profession.

Pharmacogenetics is at a very early stage of development, with few working examples established in routine clinical practice. The analysis presented here will therefore look at a series of possibilities or "options" for the application of the technology and explore the potential social, ethical, and legal problems that might be realistically associated with them. This list of options is not hypothetical but has been drawn up on the basis of detailed research on the commercial and clinical development of pharmacogenetic technology. It therefore represents the applications most likely to become a reality. However, it must be stressed that some applications may never be translated into practice, because they are contingent on technical feasibility, proven clinical utility, and commercial success. As a consequence, a number of the social and ethical problems that we described may remain only as possibilities.

This chapter starts with a brief outline of some of the well-established principles used to assess the ethics of medical research and practice. It sets out the limitations to an approach based purely on "principlism." The most realistic options for the development of pharmacogenetics technology will then be described. This will be followed by a discussion of the main social, ethical, and legal issues that are raised. In conclusion, we highlight the key points to have arisen from this analysis and suggest how public policy might provide an effective governance framework for this important new technology.

BIOETHICS AND ITS LIMITATIONS

The most influential approach to bioethics over the last 25 years has been "principlism," the idea that most issues in clinical and research ethics can be resolved by reference to a set of four basic principles: beneficence, respect for persons, justice, and nonmaleficence.

The first three principles were set out by the U.S. National Commission for the Protection of Human Subjects of Biomedical and Behavioral Research (1979) in *The Belmont Report: Ethical Principles and Guidelines for the Protection of Human Subjects of Research*. In many respects, however, they reassert the guidelines articulated in the Nuremberg Code, which forms part of the judgment on German doctors accused of crimes against humanity in their experiments on concentration camp inmates during World War II (1). The Allied Powers were slow to acknowledge that similar concerns could be raised about some of their research and clinical practices (2). In the United States and the United Kingdom, growing concern was expressed during the 1950s and 1960s about the way in which some patients were being treated (3–6). Some of this was reflected in the drafting of the Declaration of Helsinki in 1964 (1; current text can be found at (7), but a further set of U.S. scandals (8,9) provoked Congress to intervene by establishing the National Commission in 1974.

The *Belmont Report*'s principles will be considered together with the additional principle of nonmaleficence introduced by Beauchamp and Childress (10) in the first edition of their classic textbook.

Beneficence. An action should achieve some positive good rather than simply being carried out for its own sake. Research should not be carried out on human subjects merely to increase scientific knowledge. There must be a clear and identifiable potential benefit either to those taking part or to others similarly situated in the future. Similarly, patients should not be given a treatment that the clinician knows to be ineffective or futile. There is, of course, room to debate as to what constitutes a benefit, whether the benefit is proportional to the risks, how the future benefits can be weighed against present hazards, and so on.

Nonmaleficence. Beauchamp and Childress noted that it was often difficult in medicine to be certain of the benefits of a treatment or the outcomes of a trial. Indeed the element of uncertainty is part of the moral justification for research and experiment. If beneficence could not be demonstrated, they argued that the intervention at least should do no harm. Different bioethicists differ in how widely they define harm. Some concentrate on physical harms, whereas others include possible social harms. These might include being embarrassed or stigmatized by the public disclosure of private medical information.

Autonomy. Human beings in full possession of their faculties should be allowed to determine their own fate. Other people should not take decisions for them or restrict their decision-making. This principle is often used to criticize medical paternalism, where doctors limit the information and choices offered to patients in the belief that they, as experts, know better than the patients as to what actions are in their best interests. It also underlies the notion of informed consent, that people have a right to be aware of all the risks and benefits attached to a course of action and to decide for themselves whether to accept them. Bioethics often struggles to deal with the definition of "full possession of their faculties." Does autonomy apply to people with mental health problems? Does autonomy apply to people with Alzheimer's? Does autonomy apply to children? Who counts as a child for this purpose? A related issue is the position of people whose rights to self-determination may be compromised, such as prisoners. Can a convicted prisoner freely decide whether to take part in a risky medical experiment?

Justice. People who are equal in relevant respects should be treated equally. The difficulty here is often one of defining "relevant respects" and "equal treatment." The principle is intended to be one of nondiscrimination on medically relevant criteria. However, this leaves open the possibility of discrimination on social criteria, which comes to the same thing. For example, in the United States, it may not be acceptable to discriminate between people in need of health care on the grounds of race. However, it is entirely acceptable to discriminate on the grounds of income, which can have a similar effect. There is a comparable difficulty in deciding what is a medically relevant criterion. In the United Kingdom, some cardiac surgeons have refused to give coronary artery grafts on smokers the same priority as given for nonsmokers. Is this discrimination against an autonomous patient choice or on the basis of the different risk/benefit ratio of the intervention and a desire to focus resources on those most likely to benefit for longest? Similarly, should age be disregarded as a criterion in allocating organs for transplant, focusing purely on the prospective recipient's current health status, or should preference be given to the youngest recipient at a given health status on the basis that they are likely to survive longest post-transplant?

These principles have had a wide international influence and are often used almost as if they were a checklist for ethical decision-making. In recent years, however, they have come under increasing criticism: even Beauchamp and Childress (11) have conceded their limitations in the most recent (fifth) edition of their textbook. Much of the criticism is targeted on the way that they prioritize individual rights over collective welfare: when justice and autonomy conflict, autonomy almost always wins (12). Although this is understandable in the historical context, the results have been to ally bioethics to U.S. individualism in ways that are damaging to more collectively oriented health systems (13,14). There is now greater interest in developing ways of thinking about ethical issues that strike a different balance between autonomy and community, recognizing that there is sometimes a collective interest in limitations on individual choices of treatment or in actively encouraging participation in research.

A number of issues covered by these four principles are raised by the development of pharmacogenetics. However, the analysis presented here will also discuss several broader topics relating to the potential social impact of the technology on individuals, their families and particular social groups, and also legal issues about professional responsibility and corporate liability.

POSSIBLE APPLICATION OF PHARMACOGENETICS

A number of discrete technological options for the clinical and commercial application of pharmacogenetics can be identified. The most realistic of these are described briefly in the following.

Pharmacogenetics to Improve Drug Discovery

Pharmaceutical companies are increasingly using pharmacogenetic techniques and data to improve the drugs discovery process. There are two main ways in which this is being done.

Discovering New Drugs that Work Well in the Entire Population

Drug candidates can be screened for variable responses against the most common alleles of a particular genomic target. Only those candidates who show no significant variation in efficacy are then taken into drug development. This type of screening reduces the risk of candidates being rejected at a later stage and increases their likelihood of success. Drugs developed this way are more likely to work well in all patient groups.

Discovering New "Pharmacogenomic" Drugs Aimed at Genomic Subpopulations

A significant number of companies are developing strategies to create new drugs aimed at particular genomic subpopulations; this is widely known in the industry as "pharmocogenomics." In most cases the target groups will be individuals who are most likely to benefit from therapy, the so called "good responders." These drugs would probably have to be approved as safe in all groups but would be licensed and marketed for good responders. In principle, this might increase the chance of an effective drug being approved, but at the expense of it having a restricted market. If such drugs were developed, they would be more likely to be clinically effective in their target group.

Pharmacogenetics to Improve the Safety and Efficacy of Drug in Development

One of the main ways by which pharmacogenetics may have an impact on drug development is in the design and analysis of clinical trials, with a number of authors claiming that this will lead to smaller, smarter, and cheaper trials (15,16). Others have suggested that drugs causing adverse drug reactions (ADRs) in particular genomic groups could be "rescued" in late stage trials. A third possibility would be to target drug development at patients most likely to respond to a therapy. These two latter applications would most likely be used in a stepwise manner when there is a clear need to ensure a return on the very heavy costs of late stage drug development.

Preclinical Testing and the Redesign of Early Clinical Trials

In early, preclinical studies or prospectively in Phase I trials, genotyping might be used either to exclude or to include particular genomically defined groups in order to increase the chances of a drug being shown to be safe (17). However, this type of prescreening is likely to meet significant opposition from regulatory authorities, due to the risk of missing serious ADRs. It seems more likely that companies will actually use pharmacogenetics to ensure that sample populations are representative of the general population for particular alleles associated with drug metabolism (e.g., CYP2D6). This could greatly help to minimize the risk of trial bias, or reduce the risk of a drug failing at a later stage of development as a result of bias, and to improve the safety profile of the final product.

"Rescue" of Products in Late Stage Trials Due to ADRs

In later stage Phase II and III trials, pharmacogenetics may be used retrospectively to identify particular genomically defined groups who are at higher risk of ADRs. This might be particularly important in "rescuing" a therapy that was highly effective but was associated with a small number of serious genetically based ADRs. These groups could be identified and excluded from subsequent pivotal trials. A drug developed in this way would only be licensed for use in specific subpopulations and would need careful monitoring, because of the risk of it being given to the wrong patient group.

Consequently, it would have to be used in conjunction with a test for pre-prescription genotyping and have a restricted market. Regulators might license such a product solely for use in specialist secondary and tertiary settings, due to the higher risk of off label prescribing in primary care.

The Creation of New Drugs for Particular Subpopulations of "Good Responders"

In later stages of Phase II and III trials pharmacogenetics might be used in two ways to improve efficacy. First, prospective studies could test new drugs in subpopulations of patients believed to be good responders. This might significantly increase the chance of a drug reaching the market. Second, where the overall benefit of a drug across the whole population is shown to be marginal, pharmacogenetics might be used retrospectively to identify a genomic subgroup who are particularly good responders to the therapy. These groups could be specifically included in subsequent pivotal trials. In both cases this would lead to the development of new drugs licensed purely for use in a specific genomic group. The breast cancer therapy herceptin (trastuzumab) is an example of a very successful product developed for a genetically defined group of patients whose tumors overexpress the *HER-2* gene product. Although this drug is largely safe in all patients, it is only effective in this subpopulation.

Improving the Prescription of Licensed Drugs

Much attention has been given to the way in which pharmacogenetics might benefit the pharmaceutical industry in the discovery and development of new drugs. However, the technology offers significant advantages to clinicians, healthcare providers, patients, and companies by improving the purchase, prescription, use, marketing, and surveillance of licensed products. This might be achieved in a number of ways.

Extending the Use of Products Restricted by ADRs

A number of approved drugs already have restricted markets as a result of safety problems. For example, the HIV/AIDS drug Abacavir requires very close monitoring for the first few months of its use due to a severe hypersensitivity reaction in approximately 5% of the patients. This places limits on its clinical use. Trials are currently under way to identify the genomic subgroup who are most at risk of this ADR, so that prescreening can be used to exclude them from therapy. Such strategies might be used to extend the uses of drugs with practice and label restrictions and result both in therapy for a great number of patients and in increased product sales.

Preprescription Screening to Identify Patients at Risk of ADRs

One of the most widely publicized applications of pharmacogenetics is the development of "personalized medicine" in which patients are genotyped to enable physicians to give "the right drug to the right person." Attention has been focused particularly on the possibility of preprescription testing to identify patients at greatest risk of genetically based ADRs resulting from the use of a given drug. These patients could either be offered an alternative therapy or be closely monitored, if none exists. A number of laboratories and private companies in the United States already offer thiopurine methyltransferase (TPMT) genotyping to identify patients most at risk of severe adverse reactions as a result of their inability to metabolize the chemotherapy drug 6-mercaptopurine. This type of application of pharmacogenetics is attractive to doctors, patients, and health care providers, as it would lead to safer prescription and reduce the burden posed by serious ADRs.

Postmarketing Surveillance of Approved Drugs

Pharmacogenetics could also be incorporated into improved postmarketing surveillance of medicines. Patients who have suffered an ADR could be genotyped to see whether there was a genetic basis for their response (16). This might lead to the creation of a test to identify people at high risk of rare ADRs. Rather than leading to drug withdrawal, the introduction of this form of pharmacogenetic testing might also enable some products to remain on the market (18) or to be "rescued" after withdrawal (17). However, regulators have indicated that this latter option is unlikely to win much support.

Preprescription Screening to Identify "Good Responders"

In a similar fashion to preprescription patient safety testing, pharmacogenetics could be used to identify those most likely to respond positively to a specific drug. It is already well established that some patients fail to respond to such common prescription medicines as Prozac. Lichter and Kurth (19) claim that testing for nonresponders would be cost-effective for health care providers, as the expense of genotyping would be more than offset by savings from reducing ineffective prescription. In some cases this might lead to an overall reduction in healthcare costs (18). However, the use of pharmacogenetics by purchasers to reduce the overuse of ineffective drugs in groups of nonresponders clearly conflicts with the interests of the pharmaceutical industry as it is predicated on reduced drug sales (18).

Use of Efficacy Data in Drug Marketing

Pharmacogenetic information could also allow doctors to make a more informed choice about the use of one medicine compared with another in the same drug class. This might also provide some pharmaceutical companies with a powerful marketing tool if they could demonstrate that their medicine was more effective in a particular patient group than a rival product. Such a prospect would be particularly attractive to companies whose products are ranked lower in sales.

SOCIAL AND ETHICAL ISSUES

A number of general social, ethical, and legal problems are raised by the use of genetic testing in research, development, and clinical practice. These include the need to ensure informed consent for the use of DNA and genetic information (20), issues of confidentiality and privacy (15,21), the storage and use of personal genetic information by third parties, and the potential for discrimination and stigmatization (20,21). These have been extensively discussed by many authors and will not be covered in detail here. However, it must be stressed that they are of great public concern and have been a major focus of policy discussion in recent years, as shown by the reports of National Institutes of Health (NIH) Task Force on Genetic Testing in the United States (22) and the Human Genetics Commission in the United Kingdom (23).

In addition to these wider concerns about genetic testing, a number of social and ethical issues are raised by the applications described previously, which are specific to pharmacogenetics.

The Redesign of Clinical Trials

The exclusion of particular groups from clinical trials, such as women, elderly people, children, and ethnic minorities, has long been problematic (24). Exclusion on the basis of genotype raises similar difficulties about the loss of benefits from research participation and unfair representation in the trial and raises issues about the justice of such research (17). Moreover, major technical issues surround the reliability and validity of clinical trials designed and streamlined according to genomic criteria. These include statistical problems with small subdivided patient samples, reduced chances of detecting rare ADRs, sample bias, lack of consistency in controlling for pharmacogenetic variables in multicenter trials, and difficulty in replicating genetic association studies (17). As a consequence, regulatory authorities are taking a cautious approach to the redesign of trials, as this may increase the possibility of unsafe medicines reaching the market. The FDA has initially indicated that the pharmacogenetic arm of any pivotal trial will be additional to normal trial procedures. If trials ultimately contain an element of selection based on genotype, there may be a greater need for tight clinical governance and improved post-marketing surveillance.

Clinical Validity and Utility

Some of the most important issues surrounding the introduction of a new genetic test concern its validity and clinical utility. Clinicians and patients will need to be confident that a test gives meaningful and useful data that helps guide prescription and treatment, in order to ensure that there is a clear benefit from treatment. However, there have been major problems involved in reproducing a number of important genetic association studies, which form the basis for claims about the genetics of drug response (17). Even where this evidence exists, it is not always clear how it should guide practice (25). A solid evidence base needs to be created in support of a test before it is widely used. At present, many national regulatory authorities do not require evidence of a genetic test's clinical validity or utility before marketing, as their main concern has been about quality assurance to ensure reliability. There is a strong case for improved regulatory oversight in order to ensure patients' benefit and maintain confidence in pharmacogenetic tests. This point has already been endorsed in relation to diagnostic genetic testing in general by the U.S. NIH Task Force on Genetic Testing (22).

Exclusion from Therapy

Another consideration regarding pharmacogenetic testing is the problem that nearly all results will be a matter of probability. Although some genetic associations will be very strong, in other cases a significant number of patients identified as "at risk" will not in fact suffer an adverse event. They would be inappropriately excluded from treatment. Exclusion from treatment may also result from pharmacogenetic testing that identifies a patient as a "nonresponder." Here again, a number of these patients would actually be benefited from the therapy. In cases where the genetic association is not very strong and there is no therapeutic alternative, the ethical justification for exclusion from treatment, whether on the grounds of beneficence or nonmaleficence, is problematic. As a consequence, the case for denying a patient therapy on the basis of pharmacogenetic tests will often be a matter of professional judgment, involving the balancing of different factors, including the availability of alternative therapeutic options (18).

Others have argued that knowledge of a genetic association is insufficient to form the basis of clinical decision making:

> However, genotyping or haplotyping for a drug-metabolizing enzyme alone is not a substitute for a thorough patient history that includes a list of prescription and non-prescription drugs that the individual is taking . . . This clinical information must be integrated with the genotypic information to assess risk for ADEs. Furthermore, it will not be sufficient for the physician to merely understand drug–drug and drug–genotype interactions within their own specialty. Rather it will be also be necessary to understand predisposition to risk for ADEs involving other disease/organ systems (26).

It is imperative that exclusion from therapy is a decision based on clear evidence. Patients must be fully informed of the risks they are taking in cases when they still want a therapy despite having a genotype associated with serious adverse reactions to it. Similarly, clinicians will need to know the chances of response when giving a potentially ineffective medicine to patients identified as nonresponders.

Although exclusion from treatment raises a number of important ethical problems, it should be recognized that large numbers of patients are currently put at risk when given drugs that are in reality either harmful or ineffective in them. The introduction of pharmacogenetics offers the possibility of reducing the risks from these situations. These benefits are likely to significantly outweigh the problems outlined previously.

The Creation of New Orphan Patient Groups

In cases where either no effective therapy is available or existing therapy is inadequate, major ethical problems are raised if new drugs will only be developed either for the most common genotypes or for groups identified as good responders. In both cases, new products might not be developed for patients with the "wrong genotype" or for genomic groups that are too small in size to attract investment from the industry. This would create new therapeutic "orphan populations" that are economically unattractive to the pharmaceutical industry and have no access to new and more effective therapy (15,17). This problem might be exacerbated in the case of poor populations (as in developing countries) or in minority groups, who already have serious problems getting access to health care. Significant public sector investment in research, increased drug pricing, and new policies, similar to existing orphan drug legislation in the US and Europe might be required to provide the resources and financial incentives to encourage the private sectors to invest in these areas (18,27).

The High Cost of Pharmacogenetic Products

In addition to exclusion from treatment and the creation of new orphan populations, other significant justice issues about access to care are raised by the development of pharmacogenetic-based therapies. Although there may be important cost savings for the industry from improved drug discovery and development, it seems highly likely that pharmacogenetic- based drugs will have narrower and more restricted markets. This may mean that it is harder for these products to become blockbusters, with sales exceeding $1 billion a year. In an analysis of the economics of pharmacogenetics Danzon and Towse conclude.

> The problem of patient fragmentation that results from genetic testing is most appropriately addressed by adjusting prices to reflect higher benefits of targeted treatment. However, two potential problems remain: 1. Payers may be reluctant to adjust prices upwards for targeted treatments . . . Doing so requires companies and payers to use

economic evaluation to identify the higher value associated with such targeting. 2. If genetic testing reduces populations eligible for treatment, but does not significantly reduce the costs of R&D, and if prices are not adjusted, then an increasing number of potential treatments may be shelved for lack of commercial viability at normal payer thresholds (27).

This suggests that there will be significant pressure to increase the price of pharmacogenetic products. It is widely anticipated that new pharmacogenetic-based drugs will be expensive (15,17,18). Marketing strategies based on the use of efficacy data might also lead to the premium pricing of more effective new products and the creation of niche markets, where patients and providers pay more for improved therapy.

Several social issues arise from this. First, there is a need for cost-effectiveness and cost-benefit analysis of various pharmacogenetic applications to assess their potential impact on the costs of healthcare, and also on industry research and development (R&D) costs, pricing and incentives to innovate. Carefully balanced policies will have to be adopted to promote innovation and the creation of new medicines, while enabling healthcare payers and providers to reap the benefits. Without cost-benefit data there is a danger that providers may not be willing to purchase these more expensive products. Second, if pharmacogenetic products are significantly more expensive than conventional medicines, this will raise issues about the distribution of access to the better treatment they offer. The National Health Service (NHS) in the United Kingdom may be unable to afford to give all patients access to these new drugs. This may lead to rationing. In some cases these products may be only available to those who can afford to use private health providers. Similarly, on a global scale, developing countries may have little access to these improved therapies.

The Risk of Off-Label Prescribing

Where a pharmacogenetic drug has a restricted market due to the possibility of serious ADRs in a section of the patient population, the successful use of the drug will require careful control so that people with the wrong genotype are not given the product (18). In this context, the potential for inappropriate off-label or nonlabel use of medicines is of major concern. A small percentage of the U.K. doctors do not currently follow drug labels carefully enough. In the well-publicized case of the inappropriate long-term use of barbiturates, this has caused very serious problems for the patients involved, including addiction and chronic illness (28). Improved training, strong clinical governance, and improved drug labeling will be required to ensure that the prescribing of pharmacogenetic products to patients with the incorrect genotype does not occur when clinicians are unfamiliar with the technology. New forms of postmarketing surveillance may also be required to monitor the risks of this type of medication and its prescription in particular settings.

Standards of Care and Liability

Pharmacogenetic information may be an important consideration in the licensing of new medicines. Its management and disclosure during drug development and approval raises a number of important issues. For example, ADR data on one drug in a particular class may be highly relevant to the approval of another compound in the same class or active against the same target. However, it is generally not in the commercial interests of drug companies to disclose detailed findings from many of their unpublished clinical trials. This raises important questions about how to enable interfirm data sharing where it is in the public interest, while protecting proprietary information. Other issues are raised about company liabilities and responsibilities for the disclosure of pharmacogenetic data to regulators. This has been highlighted in a recent case where four individuals filed a class action against SmithKline Beecham alleging that the company failed to warn patients when it knew that some individuals would be genetically susceptible to arthritis when given the company's vaccine against Lyme disease (15).

The increased use of pharmacogenetic data may also have implications for the liabilities and responsibilities of health care providers and professionals. In particular, it is likely to change professional norms about the information used in diagnosis:

> By increasing the information available for consideration in drug therapy and the importance of matching the right drug to the right person, pharmacogenomics will raise the standard of care applicable to all involved in the safe prescription and distribution of pharmaceuticals (15).

This will have important consequences for the tort liability of doctors and pharmacists, as they may be expected to use pharmacogenetic testing increasingly in decision making.

The Social Consequences of Disease Stratification

Inherent in a number of applications of pharmacogenetics is the "stratification" of patient populations based on the subclassification of disease. For example, common conditions, such as asthma, diabetes, schizophrenia, and heart disease, are starting to be subdivided into different diagnostic categories according to their response to particular medicines. The profiling and stratification of patients based on the creation of new disease categories has many potential benefits. Diagnosis could be more precise and treatment more specific. However, one consequence may be that some individuals become categorized and are labeled as "good responders" and others as "non-responders" or "difficult to treat" (15). This might have a number of implications for patients:

> The social consequences that arise from new disease labels and their legitimisation would obviously involve interpersonal stigmatisation or identity issues. In addition, a wider range of possible societal concerns, such as those related to access to insurance, employment and health-care resources, will probably emerge (17).

If common diseases are increasingly "geneticized" in this way, family members related to affected individuals may also feel at increased risk of becoming ill and having fewer therapeutic options, even when the inherited risk has not been scientifically quantified.

The Link Between Pharmacogenetic Testing and Prognosis/Disease Susceptibility Testing

Pharmacogenetic-based disease stratification can also map onto differences in prognosis and the clinical development of disease (e.g., Alzheimer's, heart disease). For example, variations in the gene for the cholesteryl ester transfer protein (CETP) have been related to variations in response to the anti-cholesterol drug, prevastatin. The mutation associated with the greatest risk of heart attack (TaqIB) is also associated with the most positive response to treatment (29). This means that a pharmacogenetic test to decide on whether to prescribe prevastatin is also a prognostic test for the type and severity of the heart disease. In some cases, then, pharmacogenetic testing can act as a form of disease testing. This may have serious implications for both the patient and their family. In addition, some pharmacogenetic tests for one condition may actually give diagnostic information about another disease.

Some leading scientific advocates of pharmacogenetics acknowledge that the distinction between pharmacogenetics and disease genetic testing is difficult to maintain and therefore raises similar social, ethical, and legal concerns (30). However, this is in marked contrast to researchers who see pharmacogenetics more in terms of drug metabolism. For example, Allen Roses, a senior scientist at Glaxo SmithKline, stresses that "pharmacogenetics is not really about disease diagnosis" (31) and argues for the separation of the ethics of pharmacogenetics from disease testing: "Clear language and differentiation of respective ethical, legal, and societal issues are required to prevent inaccurate vernacular usage creating a confused public perception of 'genetic testing' "(16).

Ultimately, the debate on the status of pharmacogenetic knowledge will depend on the specific application and disease involved. In some cases, the information from a genetic test will not tell the doctor, the patient, or any third party anything about disease prognosis and progression. In this sense it will be similar in character to other nongenetic clinical diagnostics. However, as illustrated previously, there are well-established examples in which this is not the case and pharmacogenetic testing will raise all the ethical issues that have become associated with other forms of genetic diagnostics (consent, privacy, discrimination, and so on). In these cases, the knowledge created by the test can be seen as quite distinct from other forms of clinical diagnostics. The debate about the "exceptional nature" of genetic information is important, as this will have major consequences for how the technology is regulated by the state and governed by the medical profession (32,33). If pharmacogenetics is seen as posing serious social and ethical problems, it is likely to be tightly controlled, reducing its uptake and diffusion.

Pharmacogenetics and Race/Ethnicity

A number of studies have associated specific ethnic and racial groups with adverse or nonresponses to commonly used drugs because these populations have a greater frequency of a particular genetic allele. For example, Xie et al. (34) claim that "white patients require higher warfarin doses than Asians to attain a comparable anticoagulant effect" because of differences in the distribution of CYP2D6 alleles. Although some claim that racially based prescribing is "better than nothing" (35), there are important social risks involved in linking population groups to particular drug responses. First, it should be pointed out that the differences in the population frequency of deleterious alleles between these socially defined groups may be statistically significant but small in absolute size. Only a minority of a given group may carry these alleles. Problems arising from these claims include the danger of reinforcing discredited biological notions of race, which seek to explain social divisions and inequalities in crude genetic terms. Such ideas have historically formed the basis of discrimination and prejudice. Second, linking ethnic groups to particular diseases, such as Ashkenazi Jews to a higher incidence of hereditary breast cancer, may increase the stigmatization of the group as a whole and lead to discrimination in healthcare. Great care needs to be taken in basing prescription on crude markers of ethnicity, as the benefits of such an approach are still highly contentious.

CONCLUSION: THE SOCIAL AND ETHICAL ISSUES RAISED BY PHARMACOGENETICS—IMPLICATIONS FOR POLICY

This chapter has attempted to present realistic options for the development of pharmacogenetics and has highlighted the most important social and ethical problems that might result from their introduction. As stressed in the introduction, some of the problems may never arise, as they depend on the introduction of particular applications. Despite this there is a strong argument for considering each of these social and ethical issues seriously in advance of the introduction of pharmacogenetics. This would allow an assessment of the policies, regulation, and other measures that need to be put in place to ensure the greatest social benefit from the technology while minimizing the risk to public health and civil liberties. These can be outlined under three broad headings as follows.

Promoting the Safe Use of Pharmacogenetic Medicines

Considerations of beneficence and nonmaleficence direct us to the potential safety risks posed by the application of pharmacogenetics, including the reliability of safety testing based on the redesign of clinical trials, the harm that might be caused by the use of poorly validated testing, and the nonlabel and off-label use of pharmacogenetic drugs targeted at particular subpopulations. A number of measures could be adopted to address these concerns, including: the tight regulation of pharmacogenetics-based clinical development; regulatory guidelines to encourage interfirm data sharing; statutory oversight to ensure rigorous validation of new tests; better drug labeling and clinical governance measures to prevent off-label misuse; the training of doctors in pharmacogenetics; and improved postmarketing surveillance.

Promoting the (Cost-)Effective Use of Pharmacogenetic Medicines

Pharmacogenetics has the potential to significantly improve the effective use of medicines by prescribing more rational and evidence based. In particular, it offers a reduction in both genetically based ADRs and the use of drugs that are ineffective in specific patient groups. However, it must be recognized that while all parties involved in drug development and use have an interest in improving the safe use of medicines, the pharmaceutical industry has few commercial incentives to develop technology that will reduce its own sales. Issa (17) has suggested that "regulatory guidelines will need to be established to prevent companies from either 'trawling' for patents or avoiding offering genotyping that might limit their market for a particular drug." It will be left largely to health care providers and the public sector to carry out research on the efficacy of well-established prescription medicines in order to realize potential cost savings. The principle of justice requires public policy-makers and health care providers to investigate how they can fund clinical research on the application of pharmacogenetics to the prescription of the most widely used medicines. It will be particularly important to undertake careful evaluation and establish a strong evidence base, before expensive new pharmacogenetic tests are widely introduced into public health care systems so that tax payers are not asked to pay for inefficient or ineffective treatments.

Promoting the Just and Equitable Use of Pharmacogenetic Medicines

As discussed previously, the status of pharmacogenetic information is still being debated. However, it is clear that in some circumstances it raises many of the social and ethical issues associated with the use of diagnostic and presymptomatic genetic testing. The introduction of a robust regulatory framework to control the general use of genetic testing will be a prerequisite for the widespread use of pharmacogenetic technology in clinical practice. Moreover, pharmacogenetics raises a series of other social and ethical issues concerning access to care and discrimination, including: unfair participation in clinical trials; the stigmatization of "nonresponders" and its impact on other family members; the risk of discrimination in insurance and employment; exclusion from therapy and the creation of new orphan patient populations; access problems caused by the potentially high cost of pharmacogenetic-based treatment, especially in developing countries; and discrimination based on the unscientific use of ethnic and racial categories. In order to protect patients, their families, and the disadvantaged social groups, policies will need to be developed to promote equitable access to the technology. Antidiscrimination legislation may be required to prevent the misuse of personal genetic data and the stigmatization of particular groups. Public investment or incentives to the private sector might be required to prevent the creation of orphan patient groups. Finally, studies of the cost-effectiveness and cost-benefits of new medicines may also be required to ensure the fair pricing of pharmacogenetic products, which offers benefits to industry, providers, and patients.

The translation of pharmacogenetic research into clinical practice is likely to be technically demanding, slow, and expensive (25). At the same time it raises many ethical, social, and legal issues. These will need to be carefully considered by researchers, industry, and health care providers if the real promise of the technology to improve the discovery, development, and use of medicines is to be fully realized while maintaining public confidence in genetic technologies. This is a rapidly evolving situation and the critical use of the ethical principles outlined at the beginning of this chapter should help readers to formulate responses to the new challenges that will undoubtedly emerge in the years ahead.

REFERENCES

1. Annas GJ, Grodin MA, eds. Nazi Doctors and the Nuremberg Code: Rights in Human Experiments. Oxford: Oxford University Press, 1992.
2. Hazelgrove J. The old faith and new science: the Nuremberg Code and human experimentation ethics in Britain 1946–1973. Soc Hist Med 2001; 15(1):109–135.
3. Beecher H. Experimentation in man. J Am Med Assoc 1959; 169:461–478.
4. Beecher H. Ethics and clinical research. New Engl J Med 1966; 16:1354–1360.
5. Pappworth MH. Human guinea pigs: a warning. Twentieth Century 1962; 171:67–75.
6. Pappworth MH. Human Guinea Pigs: Experimentation on Man. London: Routledge & Kegan Paul, 1967.
7. http://www.wma.net/e/policy/17-c_e.html
8. Jones JH. Bad Blood: The Tuskegee Syphilis Experiment. New York: Free Press, 1981.
9. Rothman DJ. Strangers at the Bedside: A History of How Law and Bioethics Transformed Medical Decision Making. New York: Basic Books, 1993.
10. Beauchamp TL, Childress JF. Principles of Biomedical Ethics. 1st ed. New York: Oxford University Press, 1979.
11. Beauchamp TL, Childress JF. Principles of Biomedical Ethics. 5th ed. New York: Oxford University Press, 2001.
12. Wolpe PR. The triumph of autonomy in American bioethics: a sociological view. In: DeVries R, Subedi J, eds. Bioethics and Society: Constructing the Ethical Enterprise. Upper Saddle River, NJ: Prentice Hall, 1998:38–39.
13. Benatar SR. Just health care beyond individualism: challenges for North American bioethics. Cambridge Q Health Care Ethic 1997; 6:397–415.

14. Richards C, Dingwall R, Watson A. Should NHS patients be allowed to contribute extra money to their care? A debate from the Nottingham ethics of clinical practice committee. Brit Med J 2001; 323:563–565.
15. Rothstein MA, Epps PG. Ethical & legal implications of pharmacogenomics. Nat Rev Genet 2001; 2:228–231.
16. Roses AD. Pharmacogenetics and the practice of medicine. Nature 2000b; 405:857–865.
17. Issa AM. Ethical perspectives on pharmacogenomic profiling in the drug development process. Nat Rev: Drug Discov 2002; 1:300–308.
18. Robertson JA, Brody B, Buchannan A, Kahn J, McPherson E. Pharmacogenetic challenges for the health care system. Health Affairs 2002; 21(4):155–167.
19. Lichter JB, Kurth JH. The impact of pharmacogenomics on the future of healthcare. Curr Opin Biotechnol 1997; 8:692–695.
20. Clarke A, English V, Harris H, Wells F. Report on ethical considerations. Int J Pharmceut Med 2001; 15:89–94.
21. Robertson JA. Consent and privacy in pharmacogenetic testing. Nat Genet 2002; 28(3):207–209.
22. Holtzman NA, Watson MS. Promoting Safe and Effective Genetic Testing in the United States. The National Human Genome Research Institute, Bethesda, MD, 1997.
23. Human Genetics Commission. Inside information: balancing interests in the use of personal genetic information. London, Human Genetics Commission, 2002.
24. Mastroianni AC, Faden R, Federman D. Women and Health Research: Ethical and Legal Issues of Including Women in Clinical Studies. Institute of Medicine. Washington, DC: National Academy Press, 1994.
25. Goldstein DB. Pharmacogenetics in the laboratory and the clinic. N Engl J Med 2003; 348(6):553–556.
26. O'Kane DJ, Weinshilboum RM, Moyer TP. Pharmacogenomics and reducing the frequency of adverse drug events. Pharmacogenomics 2003; 4(1):1–4.
27. Danzon P, Towse A. The economics of gene therapy and of pharmacogenetics. Value in Health 2002; 5(1):5–13.
28. Medawar C. Power and Dependence: Social Audit on the Safety of Medicines. London: Social Audit, 1992.
29. Kuivenhoven J. The role of a common variant of the CETP gene in the progression of coronary arthersclerosis. N Engl J Med 1998; 338(2):86–93.
30. Lindpainter K, Foot E, Caulfield M, Hall I. Pharmacogenetics: focus on pharmacodynamics. Int J Pharmaceut Med 2001; 15:74–82.
31. Roses AD. Pharmacogenetics and future drug development and delivery. Lancet 2000a; 355:1358–1361.
32. Martin P, Frost R. Regulating the commercial development of genetic testing in the UK: problems, possibilities and practice. Crit Soc Policy 2003; 23(2):186–207.
33. Melzer D, Zimmern R. Genetics and medicalisation. Brit Med J 2002; 324(4):863–864.
34. Xie H-G, Kim RB, Wood AJJ, Stein CM. Ethnic differences in drugs disposition and response. Annu Rev Pharmacol Toxicol 2001; 41:815–850.
35. Satel S. I am a racially profiling doctor. New York Times Magazine. 5-5-2002.

5

Pharmacogenetics of Adverse Drug Reactions

Ana Alfirevic, B. Kevin Park, and Munir Pirmohamed
Department of Pharmacology and Therapeutics, University of Liverpool, Liverpool, U.K.

INTRODUCTION

Adverse drug reactions (ADRs) represent a major public health problem. A meta-analysis by Lazarou et al. (1), based mainly on studies conducted before 1990, showed that 6.7% of hospitalized patients developed serious ADRs, while 0.32% had a fatal ADR. Extrapolation of the fatality rate to the population of the United States suggested that ADRs killed more than 100,000 patients in the United States in 1994, making them between the fourth and sixth leading cause of death. In one of the largest prospective studies ever conducted, we have shown that even with present-day therapeutics, ADRs are responsible for 6.5% of all hospital admissions, accounting for 4% of the National Health Service (NHS) hospital bed occupancy at an annual cost approaching £0.5 billion (2). In children, the overall incidence of ADRs may be as high as 9.5% (3) although larger prospective studies are desperately needed in this area. The overall cost of drug-related morbidity and mortality in the United States (taking into account both primary and secondary care) has been estimated to be more than $76 billion (4). There are also cost implications for the pharmaceutical industry: the cost of bringing a drug to the market has been estimated to be up to $800 million (5). It has been estimated that up to 4% of the drugs marketed in the United Kingdom over a 20-year period were withdrawn because of safety issues (6).

Many factors contribute to the occurrence of ADRs. Prominent amidst this is poor prescribing behavior, for example, prescribing inappropriate doses in the presence of a contraindication or coprescribing of two drugs with a potential for interaction. However, even when such "environmental" factors are removed, a significant proportion of ADRs may occur because of genetic predisposition. Additionally, there may be an interaction between environmental and genetic factors that may also predispose to the development of an ADR. The overall contribution of host or genetic factors to the occurrence of ADRs is not clear. In order to address this issue, at least partially, a systematic review attempted to quantitate the role of polymorphisms in cytochrome P450 enzyme genes in predisposing to adverse drug reactions (7). Of the 27 drugs most frequently cited in ADR studies, 59% were metabolized by at least one enzyme with a variant allele associated with reduced activity, compared with 7% to 22% of the randomly selected drugs.

CYP1A2 and CYP2D6, which metabolize 5% and 25% of all prescribed drugs (8), respectively, were implicated in metabolizing 75% and 38% of the ADR drugs. This provides circumstantial evidence that dose alteration through knowledge of the patient's genotype may have prevented some of these ADRs. However, it is important to note that the design of the study (relating published ADR studies with review articles of drug metabolizing enzyme gene polymorphisms) shows an association and not causation, and it does not take into account the fact that ADRs can be polygenic and multifactorial in predisposition.

In this chapter, we review the evidence relating to the occurrence of ADRs to genetic factors, starting with a historical overview, and ending with socioeconomic perspectives.

DEFINITIONS AND CLASSIFICATION OF ADVERSE DRUG REACTIONS

An ADR can be defined as follows (9):

> An appreciably harmful or unpleasant reaction, resulting from an intervention related to the use of a medicinal product, which predicts hazard from future administration and warrants prevention or specific treatment, or alteration of the dosage regimen, or withdrawal of the product.

It is therefore important to note that patients who have taken overdoses, have misused drugs, and develop symptoms of disease recurrence as a result of poor compliance are excluded by this definition.

ADRs vary widely in their clinical manifestations and severity. ADRs can affect any organ system and can mimic any disease process, hence the importance of including drug-related disease in the differential diagnosis in every patient presenting with new symptoms (10). Fortunately, the majority of ADRs are mild and do not require specific therapy. However, a significant percentage, as indicated previously, can be serious and fatal. A serious adverse event has been defined by the International Conference on Harmonisation (11) as any untoward medical occurrence that at any dose:

1. Results in death,
2. Is life threatening,
3. Requires hospital admission or prolongation of stay in hospital,
4. Results in persistent or great disability, incapacity, or both,
5. Is a congenital anomaly, birth defect, or both.

There are many different classifications for ADRs; the simplest and most frequently used classification is that proposed by Rawlins and Thompson (12). ADRs are divided into two types: type A ("augmented") and type B ("bizarre") reactions. Type A ADRs are predictable from the known pharmacology of the drug, have a good dose–response relationship, and may improve on dose reduction. Type B, or idiosyncratic reactions, are uncommon (20% of all adverse reactions), cannot be related to the known pharmacological properties of the drug, do not show a simple dose–response relationship, and cannot be reproduced in animal models. A more recent classification has attempted to relate ADRs to the dose, timing of the ADR, and susceptibility (9).

HISTORICAL OVERVIEW

Perhaps the first example of an adverse reaction that has a pharmacogenetic basis was described in Southern Italy in 510 B.C. by Pythagoras, who reported that ingestion of fava beans can be harmful to some, but not all, individuals, leading to red cell hemolysis. This was also described with primaquine, an antimalarial drug, in 1956, and related to a deficiency of glucose-6-phosphate dehydrogenase (13). Another classic example reported in the 1950s was the occurrence of prolonged apnea after treatment with suxamethonium in patients with a deficiency of butyrylcholinesterase (14,15). In the 1960s, the occurrence of peripheral neuropathy associated with the intake of isoniazid was related to a deficiency of *N*-acetylation of the drug in the so-called slow acetylators (16). The first ADR with a P450 polymorphism, the occurrence of hypotension with debrisoquine (17), led to the discovery of CYP2D6 (at that time called debrisoquine hydroxylase). The same genetic defect was later associated with the development of hepatotoxicity and peripheral neuropathy in patients taking the antianginal perhexilene (18,19). Since then, the majority of pharmacogenetic studies of ADRs have concentrated on the role of drug metabolizing enzymes, but with the recent interest in active drug transport, there has also been increasing interest in drug disposition, which may not necessarily be metabolism related. However, it has long been recognized that genes other than those coding for proteins involved in drug disposition, may also predispose to ADRs. For instance, human leukocyte antigen (HLA) has been a focus of interest for many years, perhaps the best example of an association being the higher risk of hydralazine-induced lupus in patients who are HLA-DR4 positive (20,21). Hydralazine-induced lupus also provides an early example of the polygenic nature of the predisposition to ADRs because individuals who are both slow acetylators and HLA DR4-positive have a higher risk than those with one risk factor only (25 out of 26 patients with hydralazine-induced systemic lupus erythematosus (SLE) were slow acetylators) (22).

VARIABILITY IN DRUG HANDLING AND ADVERSE DRUG REACTIONS

ADRs can occur as a result of variability in either the pharmacokinetic and/or pharmacodynamic properties of drugs (Fig. 1). Some examples of how genetically determined variation in pharmacokinetics (absorption, distribution, metabolism, and excretion) can lead to ADRs are shown in Table 1. Genetically determined variation in pharmacodynamic properties of drugs leading to ADRs has been less well studied than pharmacokinetic variation and may in many cases represent a predominant risk factor (Table 2). With the completion of the human genome project and the identification of genetic variability in drug targets, this represents a fruitful area of research. Genetic factors leading to ADRs have been the subject of many reviews (7,23–32) to which the readers should refer and are also mentioned in other chapters in this book. In this chapter, we have concentrated on recent advances, pointing out where possible the strengths and weaknesses. We also cover the difficult area of what steps will be required before pharmacogenetics can be incorporated into clinical practice in order to reduce the burden of ADRs.

GENETIC VARIABILITY IN DRUG METABOLIZING ENZYMES

Polymorphisms have now been identified in more than 20 human drug metabolizing enzymes, often with diverse frequencies in various ethnic groups (33). These include both the Phase I (which are largely P450 enzymes) and Phase II (including glucuronyl transferases, *N*-acetyltransferases, sulfotransferases, and glutathione transferases) enzymes. Polymorphisms in the genes encoding these enzymes usually lead to a loss of

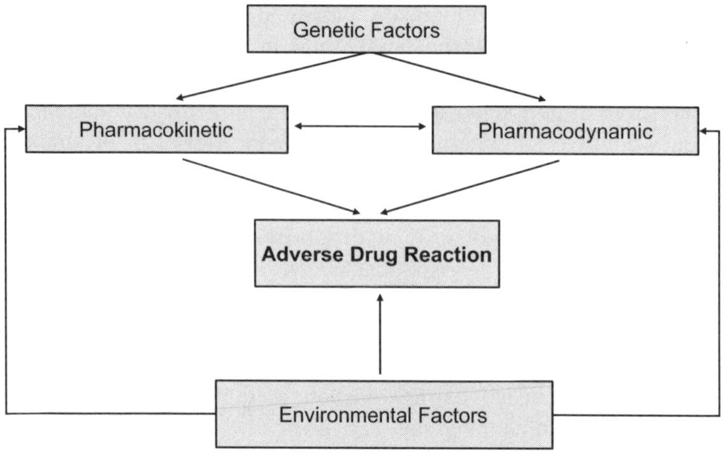

Figure 1 The interplay between genetic and environmental factors in the predisposition to adverse drug reactions.

Table 1 Examples of Adverse Drug Reactions Associated with Genetically Determined Variation in Drug Pharmacokinetics[a]

Gene symbol	Title	Drug	Adverse reaction
BCHE, CHE1	Butyrylcholinesterase	Succinylcholine	Prolonged apnea after anesthesia
	Butyrylcholinesterase	Cocaine	Increased toxicity
CYP2C9	Cytochrome P450 2C9	Warfarin	Bleeding
CYP1A2	Cytochrome P450 1A2	Phenacetin	Hypersensitivity
CYP2D6	Cytochrome P450 2D6	Codeine	Increased respiratory, psychomotor, and pupillary effects
GSTM1 and GSTT1	Glutathione-*S*-transferase	Tacrine	Transaminitis
GSTM1	Glutathione-*S*-transferase	Cisplatin	Ototoxicity
GSTM1 and GSTT1	Glutathione-*S*-transferase	Troglitazone	Hepatotoxicity
NAT-2	*N*-acetyltransferase	Sulfasalazine	Vomiting
	N-acetyltransferase	Isoniazid	Peripheral neuropathy
	N-acetyltransferase	Procainamide	SLE
UGT1A	Glucuronyltransferase	Tolcapone	Hepatotoxicity
	Glucuronyltransferase	Irinotecan	Neutropenia
	Glucuronyltransferase	Tranilast	Hyperbilirubinaemia
DIA1	Methemoglobin reductase	Nitrites, dapsone	Methaemoglobinemia, hemolysis
PBGD	Porphobilinogen deaminase	Barbiturates, anticonvulsants, sulfonamides	Acute porphyric crises
ACHE	Acetylcholinesterase	Pyridostigmine	Neurotoxicity

[a]Many of these associations have only been shown in single studies and/or may not have been replicated.
Abbreviation: SLE, systemic lupus erythematosus.

Table 2 Examples of Adverse Drug Reactions Associated with Genetically Determined Variation in the Pharmacodynamic Effects of Drugs[a]

Gene symbol	Name	Drug	Adverse reaction
HERG (KCNH2), KvLQT1 (KCNQ1), Mink (KCNE1), MiRP1 (KCNE2)	Potassium voltage-gated channels	Erythromycin, terfenadine, cisapride clarithromycin, quinidine, sulfamethoxazole	Increased risk of *torsade de pointes*, drug-induced long QT syndrome
RYR1	Ryanodine receptor	General anesthetics (halothane plus succinylcholine)	Malignant hyperthermia
OPRM1	Mu-opioid receptor	Morphine	Addiction
G6PD	Glucose-6-phosphate dehydrogenase	Primaquine, sulfonamides, dapsone	Hemolytic anemia
DRD3, HTR2A	Dopamine D3 receptor, Serotonin 5-HT-2A	Clozapine	Tardive dyskinesia
HTR2C	Serotonin 5-HT-2C receptor	Clozapine	Weight gain
ACE	Angiotensin I-converting enzyme	ACE inhibitors	Cough
BKR2	Bradykinin receptor B2	ACE inhibitors	Cough
F2 and F5	Prothrombin and Factor V	Oral contraceptives	Increased risk of deep vein and cerebral vein thrombosis
F9	Factor IX	Warfarin	Sensitivity, bleeding

[a]Many of these associations have only been shown in single studies and/or may not have been replicated.
Abbreviation: ACE, angiotensin-converting enzyme.

function, although occasionally, gain of function may occur. Alternatively, a polymorphism may lead to alteration in substrate specificity—this has been described for the P450 enzymes CYP2D6 and CYP2C9 (34–36). In general, variability in drug metabolism may lead to an ADR through one or more of the following mechanisms (25) (which are not mutually exclusive):

1. Increased concentration of the drug as a result of deficient metabolism leading to a dose-dependent ADR;
2. Deficient enzyme activity results in rerouting of metabolism leading to an ADR;
3. Exaggerated drug response as a result of increased metabolism when the drug effect is dependent on the active metabolite rather than the parent drug;
4. Variability in the formation of the reactive metabolite leading to idiosyncratic drug toxicity; and
5. Decreased bioinactivation of the reactive metabolite as a result of a deficiency in detoxication.

Deficient Metabolism Leading to Dose-Dependent Toxicity

The best example is the association of CYP2C9 polymorphisms with warfarin dose requirements and the risk of bleeding. Warfarin is widely used, perhaps the most common indication being the prevention of embolic complications in patients with atrial fibrillation. The major risk of warfarin treatment is hemorrhage; the incidence varies from 10 to 24 episodes per 100 patients for all bleeding complications and from 1.2 to 7.0 episodes per 100 patients for major bleeding complications (37). The risk of bleeding increases with the intensity of anticoagulation. Furthermore, there is about 10- to 50-fold interindividual variability in the dosage requirements necessary to maintain the international normalized ratio (INR) within a target range (most commonly between 2 and 3). Warfarin is administered as a racemate, with S-warfarin being three times more potent than R-warfarin (38,39). S-warfarin is metabolized by the P450 isoform CYP2C9; allelic variants of this isoform with reduced catalytic activity (between 5% and 12% of the activity of wild-type alleles), and in some cases, altered substrate specificity have been identified (40). Both the variants CYP2C9*2 and CYP2C9*3 show decreased clearance of warfarin in vitro and in vivo (compared with the wild-type CYP2C9*1). In accordance with this, individuals with these allelic variants require low doses of warfarin to achieve anticoagulation (41–44). Control of warfarin therapy on commencement is also more difficult in these patients, and they are also more liable to bleed while on warfarin (41). Despite the consistent data on the effect of CYP2C9 allelic variants on warfarin dosage and the risk of hemorrhage, it may be premature to advise routine pre-prescription genotyping for three main reasons. First, a great deal of interindividual variability exists even within the same genotype group (45), such that the predictive accuracy of CYP2C9 genotyping is likely to be too low to make it clinically useful. Second, polymorphisms in other genes in the warfarin pathway may also be important determinants in dosage, and their inclusion may improve the predictability of dose requirement. The utility of this has recently been shown by study of the vitamin K epoxide reductase gene (VKORC1), the target for the action of warfarin, which acts as a major determinant of daily warfarin dose requirements (46). Third, the interaction between these polymorphisms and environmental factors such as vitamin K intake has not been adequately defined. The importance of considering both genetic and environmental factors in determining daily warfarin dose requirements has recently been demonstrated by Sconce et al. (47). They were able to show that by combining age, height and *CYP2C9* (**2* and **3*) and the *VKORC1* (−1639G > A) single nucleotide polymorphisms, 55% of the variance in warfarin dose requirements could be accounted for.

Similar considerations also apply to Phase II enzymes. For example, slow acetylation has been associated with a number of adverse effects, including vomiting with sulfasalazine (48), peripheral neuropathy with isoniazid (49,50), and SLE with procainamide (51). More recently, a large number of functionally relevant polymorphisms have been identified in the various glucuronosyl transferase isoforms (52). A pharmacogenetic study of 12 candidate genes in patients who had developed hepatotoxicity with the anti-Parkinsonian drug tolcapone (53) showed an association only with the Ala181 and Ser184 variants in the UGT1A gene complex. This is in accordance with the fact that glucuronidation is the main metabolic route of tolcapone elimination. However, it is important to note that the authors used an elevation in transaminase levels of 1.5 times the upper limit of normal as a definition of hepatotoxicity, which may inadvertently have included some elderly patients who did not have true tolcapone-mediated liver damage. Perhaps, more convincing is the association between UGT1A polymorphisms and haplotypes and the risk of toxicity (including neutropenia) with irinotecan, an anticancer agent used in bowel cancer (54). More recently, a striking association was shown between tranilast-induced hyperbilirubnemia and the UGT1A1 promoter region polymorphism. Tranilast, a drug designed to prevent restenosis following coronary angioplasty, leads to increased bilirubin levels in 12% of the patients. The TA_7/TA_7 genotype in UGT1A1, which predisposes some individuals to Gilbert's syndrome, was present in 39% of the 127 hyperbilirubinemic patients, compared with 7% of the 909 controls ($P = 2 \times 10^{-22}$) (55,56). The mechanism of this association however remains unclear.

Deficient Enzyme Activity Leading to Rerouting of Metabolism

If a metabolic pathway that is responsible for the detoxification of a drug is deficient in an individual, the drug may be rerouted via another pathway that may lead to the formation of a toxic metabolite. This has been suggested for phenacetin, an analgesic that was withdrawn from the United Kingdom because of its potential to cause nephrotoxicity, carcinogenicity, and methaemoglobinemia (57–59). The first step in phenacetin metabolism is *O*-de-ethylation by cytochrome P450 1A2 (CYP1A2), which results in the formation of paracetamol. Further metabolism involves conjugation with glucuronide, sulfate, or glutathione that enables urinary excretion of the products. CYP1A2 metabolism has been implicated in toxicity of phenacetin (60,61). Numerous polymorphisms have been shown in the *CYP1A2* gene, some of which are capable of altering the metabolic capacity of the enzyme (62–64). Low catalytic activity of CYP1A2*11 allelic variant leads to reduced phenacetin *O*-de-ethylation (64). Peters et al. (65) examined the role of CYP1A2 in the toxicity and carcinogenicity of phenacetin in CYP1A2 knockout mice. They found that metabolism of phenacetin by CYP1A2 reduces its toxicity in the liver, kidney, and spleen, indicating that metabolism with CYP1A2 may protect against toxicity. It is therefore possible that in the absence of CYP1A2, other metabolic pathways may be enhanced leading to increased toxicity and carcinogenicity of phenacetin (65–68).

Gain-of-Function Polymorphisms Leading to an ADR

This is liable to be important when the drug itself is inactive but has an active metabolite responsible for its pharmacological and toxicological activities. An example is codeine, which is frequently used for the treatment of pain. About 10% of codeine undergoes *O*-demethylation to morphine, which is responsible for the analgesia. This biotransformation is performed by CYP2D6. Thus, poor metabolizers experience no pain relief from using codeine, whereas in ultrarapid metabolizers, which constitute between 1% and 30% of the population depending on ethnicity (69,70), the rate of conversion to the active metabolite may be greater leading potentially to increased respiratory, psychomotor, and pupillary effects (71,72). However, whether this is true in reality needs specific studies in ultrarapid metabolizers.

Variability in the Formation of the Toxic Metabolite

For many forms of idiosyncratic drug toxicity, the adverse reaction is thought to be caused not by the parent drugs but by its toxic or chemically reactive metabolite, which can be formed through metabolism in the body, a process termed bioactivation. Such toxic metabolites can be readily detoxified in the majority of individuals, a process termed bioinactivation. However, if there is an imbalance between bioactivation and bioinactivation, which may in some cases be genetically determined, it can lead to binding of the toxic metabolites to essential proteins in the body leading to various forms of toxicity, including carcinogenicity, teratogenicity, necrosis, and hypersensitivity (10,73,74).

One of the best examples of drugs causing ADRs through this mechanism is sulfamethoxazole (SMX), which is given in combination with trimethoprim. It is used in a variety of infections, including urinary tract infections, and in immunosuppressed patients for the treatment of pneumocystis pneumonia (10,74,75). SMX undergoes extensive metabolism in vivo, the main routes of metabolism being *N*-acetylation, glucuronidation, *N*-hydroxylation, and 5-hydroxylation. Although the formation of the hydroxylamine and subsequent oxidation to the nitroso metabolite represents a minor metabolic pathway (catalyzed by CYP2C9), it has been implicated in pathogenesis of SMX hypersensitivity (76–78). It has been also shown in HIV-negative individuals that slow acetylator phenotype is a risk factor for the development for hypersensitivity (76), the implication being that reduced *N*-acetylation allows a greater proportion of the drug to undergo metabolism via the toxication pathway, that is, through the formation of the hydroxylamine. Although this has not been shown in practice, it is a reasonable hypothesis because measurable quantities of the hydroxylamine in urine may not accurately reflect the total intracellular formation of the toxic metabolite. Interestingly, the frequency of SMX hypersensitivity is 10 to 30 times more common in HIV-positive patients; this seems to be a reflection of a disease-mediated change in the balance between these competing pathways, because it has been shown that neither slow acetylator genotype nor phenotype seems to predispose to SMX hypersensitivity (79–81).

Decreased Detoxification of the Reactive or Toxic Metabolite

Bioinactivation of toxic metabolites can be nonenzymatic, for example, conjugation with glutathione. However, in many cases, detoxification may be catalyzed by a number of enzymes. In this respect, the glutathione-*S*-transferases (GST) have attracted a great deal of interest, in particular in the field of cancer, where deficient detoxification of environmentally derived carcinogens, for example, from smoking, has been implicated in the pathogenesis of cancer (82,83). However, the GST superfamily, many members of which are polymorphically expressed (84), is also important in the detoxification of drugs, and thereby in the pathogenesis of ADRs. There are three examples where GST polymorphisms have been shown to play a possible role:

1. Cisplatin is an agent widely used in the treatment of epithelial malignancies. Cisplatin ototoxicity is an important ADR that may be due to oxidative stress. In a study of 20 patients with cisplatin ototoxicity, analysis of polymorphisms in five GST genes, showed that the carriage of the GSTM3*B allele may be protective (85).
2. Tacrine, an anticholinesterase used in Alzheimer's disease, caused transaminitis in up to 50% of the patients. Analysis of the GSTM1 and GSTT1 polymorphisms in a French cohort showed that individuals who had deficiencies of both GSTM1 and GSTT1 were more susceptible to tacrine hepatotoxicity (86). However, this was not replicated in a North American cohort (87,88).
3. Troglitazone was the first of a new class of antidiabetic agents, which was withdrawn from the market because of its potential to cause severe, and sometimes, fatal hepatotoxicity. In a study of 110 Japanese patients who had been prescribed troglitazone, an evaluation of 68 polymorphic sites in 51 candidate genes involved in drug metabolism, apoptosis, production, and elimination of reactive oxygen species, PPARγ2 and insulin, showed that a strong correlation

with transaminase elevations was observed only in patients with the combined glutathione-*S*-transferase *GSTT1-GSTM1* null genotype (89).

GENETIC VARIABILITY IN DRUG TRANSPORTERS AND ADVERSE DRUG REACTIONS

Transport proteins that actively mediate the influx and efflux of drugs across cell membranes have an important role in regulating the absorption, distribution, and excretion of many medicines. Many different influx and efflux transporters have now been described (90), and polymorphisms have been described in many of the genes encoding for these proteins (91,92). In general, an efflux pump may mediate toxicity via the following possible pathways:

- Reduced activity of the efflux pump may increase the oral bioavailabilty of the drug and reduce renal and biliary excretion leading to increased plasma levels for a given dose and possible dose-dependent adverse effects. Overactivity would thus have the opposite effect and may lead to the need for increased dosage requirements.
- Reduced activity at the level of the cell membrane may increase intracellular levels because of reduced efflux and lead to toxicity of drugs, where the mode of toxicity depends on intracellular accumulation, for example, anti-cancer agents.

Influx pumps and variability in their activities would have effects opposite of those outlined here but have not been adequately studied.

The most extensively studied of the transporters is *P*-glycoprotein, a member of the adenosine triphosphate (ATP) binding cassette family, which is encoded by the human *MDR1* (or *ABCB1*) gene. Many drugs including anticancer drugs, cardiac glycosides, immunosuppressive agents, glucocorticoids, and antiretrovirals are known substrates for *MDR1* (93–95). A single nucleotide polymorphism (C3435T) in exon 26 of the *MDR1* gene has attracted most attention, although subsequent studies have produced contradictory results as to the effects of this polymorphism on both the function of the transporter and its association with disease (96,97). This may be a reflection of the complicated pattern of linkage disequilibrium within this gene, and its variability in individuals of different ethnicity (98–100). Various ADRs have been related to this and other polymorphisms within the *MDR1* gene (Table 3), but none of these studies have been replicated, and the true significance of the findings remains unclear, given the uncertain functional nature of the polymorphisms.

Table 3 Adverse Drug Reactions Associated with Polymorphisms in the *MDR1* Gene

Drug	Adverse reaction
Nortryptiline	Hypotension
Tacrolimus	Neurotoxicity
Cyclosporin	Cyclosporin toxicity
Ivermectin	Neurotoxicity
Digoxin	Digoxin toxicity
Phenytoin	Phenytoin toxicity
Indinavir	Insulin resistance

There have been few studies with regard to the other transporters, but this reflects an important area of research that is likely to uncover novel mechanisms of ADRs. For instance, mutations have been identified in the photoreceptor-specific ATP-binding cassette transporter gene (*ABCA4*) in patients with Stargardt disease and age-related macular degeneration, both of which are disorders of the retinal pigment epithelium and neural retina. Because of certain phenotypic similarities between these disorders and 4-aminoquinoline (chloroquine and hydroxychloroquine)-induced retinopathy, a disorder where the mechanism is unclear, Shroyer et al. (101) were able to show that in eight patients with retinopathy, two had *ABCA4* missense mutations while three others had missense polymorphisms. This clearly does need to be investigated in a larger number of patients, but nevertheless, these preliminary findings provide some insight into the possible pathogenesis and genetic predisposition.

IMMUNOGENETIC POLYMORPHISMS

Based on symptomatology, many ADRs are thought to be immune-mediated (102). In view of this, there has been a great deal of interest in the role of the major histocompatiblity complex on the short arm of chromosome 6 in predisposing to such ADRs. Initial studies were based on serological typing and focused on drugs, such as gold and penicillamine (103); contradictory findings, which probably arose because of the relative insensitivity of serological typing in distinguishing between different major histocompatibility complex (MHC) alleles, resulted in such findings being relegated to the specialist literature. However, with the completion of the human genome project, and sequencing of the MHC (104,105), we now have a much better understanding of the complexity of the MHC. Coupled with our ability to undertake high-resolution genotyping and an increased understanding of the pattern of linkage disequilibrium within the region (106,107), this has led to more detailed studies, which have already produced some striking findings.

The use of abacavir, a potent HIV-1 reverse transcriptase inhibitor, has been hampered by the occurrence of hypersensitivity reaction in about 5% of the patients (108). These reactions are characterized by skin rash and gastrointestinal and respiratory manifestations and can occasionally be fatal, particularly on rechallenge. In an extensive investigation of the MHC, Mallal et al. (109) found a strong association between abacavir hypersensitivity and the haplotype comprising HLA-B*5701, HLA-DR7, and HLA-DQ3 with an odds ratio of more than 100. Subsequent studies have shown that this haplotype resides on the ancestral haplotype 57.1, and that the combination of HLA B*5701 and polymorphism in HSP-Hom has greater predictive accuracy than HLA B*5701 by itself (110). This association has now been shown in two other cohorts by GSK, the manufacturer of the drug, and independently in a cohort of patients from the United Kingdom (111–113). However, the odds ratios in both studies were lower than those obtained by Mallal et al. (109). Furthermore, the same association has not been shown in an African American population presumably because of differences in linkage disequilibrium on the MHC (112). Mallal et al. (109) have proposed that in Caucasians genotyping for HLA B*5701 should be performed before prescription of abacavir, and indeed in their clinic, this has resulted in a reduction of the prevalence of abacavir hypersensitivity (110). An analysis of the predictive value of prospective HLA B*5701 genotyping prior to abacavir hypersensitivity based on a meta-analysis of three cohorts showed that to prevent one case of hypersensitivity, eight HLA B*5701-positive patients would be denied abacavir, and to identify them, 48 patients would require testing (113). Given the potential severity of abacavir hypersensitivity, it has been suggested that only a test that is 100% predictive in all populations would be clinically useful. However, it has to be conceded that even the current test characteristics are striking and exceed those of many other tests that are widely used today, and perhaps we may have to be more modest in our requirements to introduce pharmacogenetics into clinical practice (114).

Carbamazepine (CBZ) is a widely used anti-convulsant that can cause rashes in up to 10% of the patients, and in occasional cases, this may be the precursor to the development of a hypersensitivity syndrome characterized by systemic manifestations, such as fever and eosinophilia (115,116). Rarely, CBZ can induce blistering skin reactions, such as Stevens-Johnson syndrome (SJS) and toxic epidermal necrolysis, two conditions associated with a high fatality rate (117). It has previously been shown that severe CBZ hypersensitivity reactions were associated with the haplotype TNF2-DR3-DQ2 (118). More recently, a study in a Han Chinese population from Taiwan showed that HLA-B*1502 may act as a genetic marker for CBZ-induced SJS, with an odds ratio that was greater than 1000 (119). This is an extremely important finding that suggests that in the Han Chinese population, testing for HLA-B*1502 (where it has a prevalence of 7% compared with 2% in Caucasians) may be warranted prior to starting CBZ. However, this may not necessarily be true in Caucasians in view of the differences in the pattern of linkage disequilibrium. Indeed, in our population in Caucasians (including two patients with SJS), we have not shown an association with HLA-B*1502 (unpublished data), but the possibility of a predisposing gene in this region has been further strengthened by the finding of an association with the *HSP*-gene locus in the MHC class III region (110).

The association of the *MHC* genes with abacavir hypersensitivity and carbamazepine hypersensitivity is biologically plausible because drug-specific T-cells have been demonstrated in affected individuals confirming the immune nature of the reactions (120). However, an association with genes on the MHC should not necessarily imply that the adverse reaction is immune-mediated. This is because there is extensive linkage disequilibrium within the MHC, and at least 40% of the genes do not have an immune function (121). This is also exemplified by the iron-handling disorder hemochromatosis, which shows an association with various *HLA* genes (122), but in fact has been shown to be caused by mutations in the linked *HFE* gene (123,124). Two examples of ADRs may also fall into this category.

The first example is that of clozapine, an antipsychotic used for the treatment of drug-resistant schizophrenia, which induces agranulocytosis in about 1% of the patients (125). Clozapine-induced agranulocytosis (CA) has been associated with the HLA haplotypes DRB1*0402, DQB1*0302, and DQA1*0301, and HLA-DR*02, DQB1*0502, and DQA1*0102 in Jewish and non-Jewish populations, respectively (126). Differences in linkage disequilibrium in the two populations to a causal variant within the MHC region may be responsible for the different allelic associations. Later, two further candidate genes, *HSP-70* and *TNF-α*, were also found to be associated with CA in both ethnic groups (127,128). The association with HLA haplotypes has also been shown in a German population (129,130). However, despite these findings it is unclear whether the associated genes are the causal variants or whether they merely reflect linkage disequilibrium with an unidentified gene, which possibly has a nonimmune function. With regard to the latter, there is no convincing evidence, even from rechallenge data, that CA is an immune-mediated adverse reaction (131).

The second example is that of lipodystrophy associated with the use of highly active antiretroviral therapy (HAART). Although HAART has greatly increased patient survival and decreased morbidity in HIV disease (132), it has also led to appearance of novel adverse effects, such as lipodystrophy (133), a syndrome characterized by abnormal fat redistribution and metabolic abnormalities, such as insulin resistance and hyperlipidemia (134,135). In a small study with strict inclusion and exclusion criteria, Maher et al. (136) demonstrated that a single nucleotide polymorphism at the -238 position in the promoter region of the *TNF-α* gene occurred at a significantly greater frequency in patients with lipodystrophy than in HIV patients without lipodystrophy who had been on HAART for at least 12 months. These findings have been confirmed in an Australian cohort, which suggested that the presence of the -238 polymorphism accelerated the time to onset of the development of lipodystrophy (137). Although the *TNF* gene resides within the MHC, this syndrome is clearly not an immune-mediated adverse reaction, and the association with *TNF-α* reflects its numerous actions on adipocytes and muscles (138), which collectively favor the development of insulin resistance and its associated metabolic abnormalities.

RECEPTORS

Variation in drug receptor genes can have a profound effect on drug efficacy and toxicity. Most of the pharmacogenomic research on drug receptors has focused on central nervous system (CNS) diseases. Dopaminergic, serotoninergic, adrenergic, and histaminergic signaling systems have been extensively investigated for their involvement in drug response and toxic effects. Most of the research to date has focused on clozapine, which is associated with adverse effects, such as weight gain and tardive dyskinesia (TD), in addition to agranulocytosis (139). Weight gain and TD can undermine patient compliance and thereby lead to relapse of patients with resistant schizophrenia. Clozapine has the greatest potential to induce weight gain in comparison with the other atypical antipsychotics (140). However, only a proportion of patients gain weight, which is estimated to be between 13% and 85%. A genetic predisposition has been suggested by some researchers (141,142), although it is likely that weight gain is due to a combination of factors, including alterations in satiety control mechanisms, energy expenditure, metabolism, and lipogenesis. In their comprehensive review, Basile et al. (143) suggested that weight gain induced by atypical antipsychotics results from multiple neurotransmitter/receptor interactions. They speculated that clozapine and some other antipsychotics may disturb satiety processing in the hypothalamus by binding to receptors involved in weight regulation. Genetic differences in receptors that are known to have an affinity for clozapine and are expressed in hypothalamus can therefore be considered to be appropriate candidate genes. Of the nine genes investigated, the genes encoding the $5\text{-}HT_{2C}$, $\beta3$ (ADRB3) and *α1* receptor genes, and *TNF-α*, showed nonsignificant trends towards an association with clozapine-related weight gain (144). More recently, an association with a novel promoter region polymorphism (C759T) in the $5\text{-}HT_{2C}$ gene that may alter its expression was demonstrated but has not been replicated in another study (145).

TD is an important adverse effect of antipsychotics that has been investigated in a number of pharmacogenetic studies. It is a potentially irreversible disorder that presents as an involuntary movement of orofacial musculature and occasionally peripheral muscles (146). The mechanism of TD is not fully understood, but overactivity of dopaminergic receptors may play a role. Many candidate genes have been postulated to play a role in its pathophysiology with contradictory results. The most consistent finding to date has been with the dopamine *D3* receptor gene (143,147–149). Lerer et al. (150), in an analysis of all published data, found a strong association between TD and the *D3* receptor gene Ser9Gly polymorphism. This polymorphism may alter the affinity of the receptor for dopamine. However, it is likely that the *D3* receptor polymorphism represents only one predisposing factor of a polygenic predisposition. In accordance with this, associations with polymorphisms in the drug metabolizing enzymes CYP1A2 and 2D6 (151,152) and the serotonin *2A* and *2C* receptor genes (153,154) have also been demonstrated.

Receptor variation may also lead to unpredictable toxicities, as seen in the development of malignant hyperthermia after administration of general anesthetics, such as halothane (155,156). Mutations in the ryanodine receptor gene are thought to account for susceptibility to malignant hyperthermia in more than 50% of the cases (155). More than 60 mutations within the ryanodine receptor gene have been identified (157). The functional effects of only some of these mutations have so far been characterized. For example, a study of human myotubes derived from a carrier of mutations in exon 44 showed that the defect in the ryanodine receptor makes it more sensitive to lower concentrations of stimulators of the opening (158). This may result in enhanced rates of calcium release from the sarcoplasmic reticulum during anesthesia, which in turn leads to the sustained muscle contraction and glycolytic and aerobic metabolism characteristic of malignant hyperthermia. Preanesthetic prediction of susceptibility can be undertaken in patients with a family history using an invasive phenotypic test (caffeine–halothane contracture test) (159). The genetic heterogeneity together with variable penetrance and unidentified defects in 50% of the patients means that genetic testing for diagnosing the susceptibility is currently not available.

MISCELLANEOUS DRUG TARGETS

Pharmacogenetic variation in drug targets will lead to variation in drug pharmacodynamics, manifested as either variation in efficacy or susceptibility to toxicity. There has been much less investigation of drug targets compared with drug pharmacokinetics. Several examples are presented in the following.

Drug-Induced Long QT Syndrome

Mutations in genes coding for cardiac potassium or sodium channels may cause the long QT syndrome (LQTS) (160), which in some patients may lead to drug-induced *torsade de pointes* or polymorphic ventricular tachycardia. These patients are usually asymptomatic until administration of the drug. Drugs implicated include the antimalarials—mefloquine and halofantrine, the antiarrhythmics—quinidine and disopyramide and amiodarone, the antihistamines—terfenadine and oxatomide, and the antibiotics clarithromycin, erythromycin, and sulfamethoxazole (161–163).

To date, only small numbers of patients have been studied, a major problem being the inconsistencies in the phenotypic classification of these patients and also the relative rarity of patients with torsades, when compared with the LQTS. Three mutations have been associated with the acquired LQTS in the potassium and sodium channels (161,164). However, in more than 85% of the patients with the acquired LQTS, no ion channel mutations have been identified so far. At present, therefore, genetic testing is not warranted; there are several ongoing large-scale studies both in the United Kingdom and United States, and their results are anxiously awaited.

Oral Contraceptive–Induced Venous Thromboembolism

Mutations in the coagulation factor V and prothrombin genes are known to be risk factors for venous thromboembolism. The polymorphism in the factor V gene, which has been termed factor V Leiden, comprises a missense mutation (R506Q) due to a G/A transition (G1691A) in exon 10 of the gene (165). The frequency of the polymorphism varies from 2% to 15% in different populations (166). Patients taking oral contraceptives are at higher risk of venous thromboembolism if they are carriers of the factor V Leiden polymorphism (167). The issue of whether to screen women for factor V Leiden before prescribing oral contraceptives remains controversial (166) and is probably not cost-effective. For instance, one episode of venous thromboembolism per year might be prevented by the withdrawal of oral contraceptives from 400 asymptomatic carriers of the factor V Leiden mutation. To identify them, however, approximately 10,000 asymptomatic women need to be tested (168).

Methotrexate-Induced Toxicity

Low-dose methotrexate (MTX) is now widely used in the treatment of rheumatoid arthritis, psoriatic arthritis, systemic lupus erythematosus, and ankylosing spondylitis (169–172). Given the nature of the drug, however, long-term use carries the risk of toxicity to several organs, including mucosal membranes, bone marrow, and liver. Genetic variability in methylenetetrahydrofolate reductase (MTHFR) has been found to be associated with higher risk of developing adverse reactions with MTX (173). Of the many polymorphisms described in the *MTHFR* gene, the C677T and A1298C polymorphisms reduce enzyme activity (174,175). In addition, the C677T polymorphism also leads to an increase in plasma homocysteine levels, which has been implicated in pathogenesis of some of the adverse effects, in particular the gastrointestinal symptoms (175,176). A recent study (177) showed that overall MTX toxicity in patients with rheumatoid arthritis, which included an increase in transaminases, stomatitis, nausea, hair loss and rash, was more common in paients with the T-allele at position 677 of the *MTHFR* gene.

Angiotensin-Converting Enzyme Inhibitor–Induced Cough

Angiotensin-converting enzyme (ACE) inhibitors have been successfully used in the therapy of hypertension, congestive heart failure, and myocardial infarction (178). However, up to 30% of the treated patients experience a persistent cough, which limits the use of the drug (179,180). Several gene variants have been investigated in the genetic predisposition to ACE-inhibitor induced cough, including the *ACE* (181,182) and bradykinin B_2 receptor (183,184) genes. An insertion/deletion polymorphism in the *ACE* gene is known to control the plasma ACE level (185,186). However, to date no consistent associations have been identified between the occurrence of cough and polymorphisms in the *ACE*, bradykinin receptor, and chymase genes (187).

SUMMARY AND FUTURE DIRECTIONS

The occurrence of an ADR is clearly dependent on both genetic and environmental factors; the contribution of both will vary between drugs and individuals. Importantly, there may also be an interaction between the genetic and environmental factors, which has not been really studied to any great extent. The nature of the genetic predisposition is also likely to vary; for some there might be a major genetic predisposing factor (the so called "low-hanging fruit"), with minor contributions from other genes, whereas for other adverse reactions (perhaps the majority), the situation might be much more complex with multiple genetic factors, each contributing to a small extent, but none of which by itself is necessary nor sufficient to lead to the adverse reaction, that is, the situation is similar to a polygenic disease with many susceptibility genes.

The challenge for researchers and clinicians is to incorporate pharmacogenetics of drug safety into clinical practice. To date, only phenotyping (and genotyping in some centers) for thiopurine methyltransferase (TPMT) has had substantial (but not complete) clinical uptake. Approximately 10% of the population has low enzyme activity (heterozygous patients), while one in 300 patients have no detectable TPMT activity (188). These patients are likely to develop severe hemopoietic toxicity with conventional doses of drugs, such as 6-mercaptopurine and azathioprine, and particularly for the former, recommendations for dose modifications have been suggested (189). This is covered in greater detail in the other chapters in this book.

Many factors will determine whether a genotyping test is taken up into clinical practice, which will include patient and clinician acceptance. The value of a pharmacogenetic test in preventing ADRs is dependent on three criteria, as defined by Phillips et al. (7). These are medical needs, clinical utility, and ease of use. In order to fulfill medical needs, the incidence of the ADR, the prevalence of the variant allele, and the use of the drug have to be high enough to warrant the use of genetic information. However, if the prevalence of the ADR and/or the variant allele is low, a genetic test may still be warranted if the ADR has severe clinical consequences. The clinical utility of a test depends on whether there is sufficient evidence to link the variant allele to the drug response, and the test criteria, that is, sensitivity, specificity, positive, and negative predictive values. Finally, the assay has to be easy to use, relatively inexpensive and reliable, and most importantly, clinicians should be able to interpret the results and use the information appropriately. How the latter would be implemented and the format it would take is unclear at present and needs further research.

An important aspect to consider is whether pre-prescription genotyping will be cost-effective. Danzon et al. (190) examined the potential impact of pharmacogenetic testing from societal, payer, and company perspectives. They concluded that testing was worthwhile for the payer if the ratio of nonresponders to the total population exceeds the ratio of the price of the test to the price of the drug. From the perspective of a drug company, pretreatment genetic tests are likely to be developed if they can yield a net saving to the payer. This happens when the cost of testing the entire patient population is less than the savings from avoiding treatment of nonresponders plus any savings from averting harm. This has recently been tackled in relation to abacavir hypersensitivity (113). Using data from three cohorts, it was possible to develop test characteristics, and by applying them into a decision analysis framework, it was shown that the cost-effectiveness of a test was largely dictated not by the cost of the genotyping test but by the costs of the alternative treatments that would have to be used should the patient prove to be positive for HLA-B*5701, a genetic determinant of abacavir hypersensitivity. Perhaps, one also needs to put into perspective the overall impact that the ADRs have on the health service and on the economy as a whole. For instance, the cost of drug-related morbidity and mortality in the United States has been estimated to be $76.6 billion (4). Clearly, this is a huge burden and anything that can help in reducing this burden has to be seriously considered and investigated, and if the relevant criteria are met, implemented into clinical practice. This is the challenge facing researchers in this area as they attempt to reduce the burden of ADR on the patient, the health care system, and the economy.

REFERENCES

1. Lazarou J, Pomeranz BH, Corey PN. Incidence of adverse drug reactions in hospitalized patients: a meta-analysis of prospective studies. J Am Med Assoc; 1998; 279(15):1200–1205.
2. Pirmohamed M, James S, Meakin S, Green C, Scott AK, Walley TJ, et al. Adverse drug reactions as cause of admission to hospital: prospective analysis of 18820 patients. Brit Med J 2004; 329(7456):15–19.
3. Impicciatore P, Choonara I, Clarkson A, Provasi D, Pandolfini C, Bonati M. Incidence of adverse drug reactions in paediatric in/out-patients: a systematic review and meta-analysis of prospective studies. Br J Clin Pharmacol 2001; 52(1):77–83.
4. Johnson JA, Bootman JL. Drug-related morbidity and mortality. A cost-of-illness model. Arch Intern Med 1995; 155(18):1949–1956.
5. Anonymous. Tufts Centre for the study of Drug Development Pegs Cost of a New Prescription Medicine at $802 Million. In: Tufts University ed. Boston: Tufts Centre for the study of Drug Development, 2001.
6. Jefferys DB, Leakey D, Lewis JA, Payne S, Rawlins MD. New active substances authorized in the United Kingdom between 1972 and 1994. Br J Clin Pharmacol 1998; 45(2):151–156.
7. Phillips KA, Veenstra DL, Oren E, Lee JK, Sadee W. Potential role of pharmacogenomics in reducing adverse drug reactions: a systematic review. J Am Med Assoc 2001; 286(18):2270–2279.
8. Wolf CR, Smith G. Pharmacogenetics. Br Med Bull 1999; 55(2):366–386.
9. Edwards IR, Aronson JK. Adverse drug reactions: definitions, diagnosis, and management. Lancet 2000; 356(9237):1255–1259.
10. Pirmohamed M, Kitteringham NR, Park BK. The role of active metabolites in drug toxicity. Drug Saf 1994; 11(2):114–144.
11. International Conference on Harmonisation; guidance on S7A safety pharmacology studies for human pharmaceuticals; availability. Notice. Fed Regist 2001; 66(135):36791–36792.
12. Rawlins MD, Thompson JW. Mechanisms of adverse drug reactions. In: Davies DM, ed. Textbook of Adverse Drug Reactions. Oxford: Oxford University Press, 1991:18–45.
13. Alving AS, Carson PE, Flanagan CL, Ickes CE. Enzymatic deficiency in primaquine-sensitive erythrocytes. Science 1956; 124(3220):484–485.
14. Love SHS. Prolonged apnoea following scoline. Anaesthesia 1952; 7:113–114.
15. Kalow W, Gunn DR. The relation between dose of succinylcholine and duration of apnea in man. J Pharmacol Exp Ther 1957; 120(2):203–214.
16. Goedde HW, Schloot W. Investigations into the polymorphism of acetylation of isonicotinic acid hydrazid (INH). Med Welt 1968; 51:2812–2821.
17. Evans DA, Mahgoub A, Sloan TP, Idle JR, Smith RL. A family and population study of the genetic polymorphism of debrisoquine oxidation in a white British population. J Med Genet 1980; 17(2):102–105.
18. Lhermitte F, Fardeau M, Chedru F, Mallecourt J. Polyneuropathy after perhexiline maleate therapy. Br Med J 1976; 1(6020):1256.
19. Long JP, Fitzgerald O, Maurer BJ. Hepatotoxicity following treatment with perhexiline maleate. Ir Med J 1980; 73(7):275–276.
20. Alarcon-Segovia D, Wakim KG, Worthington JW, Ward LE. Clinical and experimental studies on the hydralazine syndrome and its relationship to systemic lupus erythematosus. Medicine (Baltimore) 1967; 46(1):1–33.
21. Russell GI, Bing RF, Jones JA, Thurston H, Swales JD. Hydralazine sensitivity: clinical features, autoantibody changes and HLA-DR phenotype. Q J Med 1987; 65(246):845–852.
22. Batchelor JR, Welsh KI, Tinoco RM, Dollery CT, Hughes GR, Bernstein R, et al. Hydralazine-induced systemic lupus erythematosus: influence of HLA-DR and sex on susceptibility. Lancet 1980; 1(8178):1107–1109.
23. Meyer UA. Pharmacogenetics and adverse drug reactions. Lancet 2000; 356(9242):1667–1671.

24. Meyer UA, Gut J. Genomics and the prediction of xenobiotic toxicity. Toxicology 2002; 181–182:463–466.
25. Pirmohamed M, Park BK. Cytochrome P450 enzyme polymorphisms and adverse drug reactions. Toxicology 2003; 192(1):23–32.
26. Pirmohamed M, Park BK. Genetic susceptibility to adverse drug reactions. Trends Pharmacol Sci 2001; 22(6):298–305.
27. Alvarado I, Wong ML, Licinio J. Advances in the pharmacogenomics of adverse drug reactions. Pharmacogenomics J 2002; 2(5):273.
28. Roden DM, George AL Jr. The genetic basis of variability in drug responses. Nat Rev Drug Discov 2002; 1(1):37–44.
29. Ingelman-Sundberg M. Pharmacogenetics: an opportunity for a safer and more efficient pharmacotherapy. J Intern Med 2001; 250(3):186–200.
30. Roses AD. Idiosyncratic reactions to drugs: can medicine response profiles provide a dynamic drug surveillance system? Clin Chem Lab Med 2000; 38(9):815–818.
31. Roses AD. Pharmacogenetics. Hum Mol Genet 2001; 10(20):2261–2267.
32. Nebert DW, Jorge-Nebert L, Vesell ES. Pharmacogenomics and "individualized drug therapy": high expectations and disappointing achievements. Am J Pharmacogenomics 2003; 3(6):361–370.
33. Burroughs VJ, Maxey RW, Levy RA. Racial and ethnic differences in response to medicines: towards individualized pharmaceutical treatment. J Natl Med Assoc 2002; 94(suppl 10):1–26.
34. Fukuda T, Nishida Y, Imaoka S, Hiroi T, Naohara M, Funae Y, et al. The decreased in vivo clearance of CYP2D6 substrates by CYP2D6*10 might be caused not only by the low-expression but also by low affinity of CYP2D6. Arch Biochem Biophys 2000; 380(2):303–308.
35. Haining RL, Hunter AP, Veronese ME, Trager WF, Rettie AE. Allelic variants of human cytochrome P450 2C9: baculovirus-mediated expression, purification, structural characterization, substrate stereoselectivity, and prochiral selectivity of the wild-type and I359L mutant forms. Arch Biochem Biophys 1996; 333(2):447–458.
36. Takanashi K, Tainaka H, Kobayashi K, Yasumori T, Hosakawa M, Chiba K. CYP2C9 Ile359 and Leu359 variants: enzyme kinetic study with seven substrates. Pharmacogenetics 2000; 10(2):95–104.
37. Schulman S. Clinical practice. Care of patients receiving long-term anticoagulant therapy. N Engl J Med 2003; 349(7):675–683.
38. Banfield C, O'Reilly R, Chan E, Rowland M. Phenylbutazone–warfarin interaction in man: further stereochemical and metabolic considerations. Br J Clin Pharmacol 1983; 16(6):669–675.
39. Breckenridge AM, Cholerton S, Hart JA, Park BK, Scott AK. A study of the relationship between the pharmacokinetics and the pharmacodynamics of the 4-hydroxycoumarin anticoagulants warfarin, difenacoum and brodifacoum in the rabbit. Br J Pharmacol 1985; 84(1):81–91.
40. Lee CR, Goldstein JA, Pieper JA. Cytochrome P450 2C9 polymorphisms: a comprehensive review of the in-vitro and human data. Pharmacogenetics 2002; 12(3):251–263.
41. Aithal GP, Day CP, Kesteven PJ, Daly AK. Association of polymorphisms in the cytochrome P450 CYP2C9 with warfarin dose requirement and risk of bleeding complications. Lancet 1999; 353(9154):717–719.
42. Margaglione M, Colaizzo D, D'Andrea G, Brancaccio V, Ciampa A, Grandone E, et al. Genetic modulation of oral anticoagulation with warfarin. Thromb Haemost 2000; 84(5):775–778.
43. Taube J, Halsall D, Baglin T. Influence of cytochrome P-450 CYP2C9 polymorphisms on warfarin sensitivity and risk of over-anticoagulation in patients on long-term treatment. Blood 2000; 96(5):1816–1819.
44. Higashi MK, Veenstra DL, Kondo LM, Wittkowsky AK, Srinouanprachanh SL, Farin FM, et al. Association between CYP2C9 genetic variants and anticoagulation-related outcomes during warfarin therapy. J Am Med Assoc 2002; 287(13):1690–1698.

45. Daly AK, King BP. Pharmacogenetics of oral anticoagulants. Pharmacogenetics 2003; 13(5):247–252.
46. Rieder MJ, Reiner AP, Gage BF, Nickerson DA, Eby CS, McLeod HL, Blough DK, Thummel KE, Veenstra DL, Rettie AE. Effect of VKORC1 haplotypes on transcriptional regulation and warfarin dose. New Engl J Med 2005; 352(22):2285–2293.
47. Sconce EA, Khan TI, Wynne HA, Avery P, Monkhouse L, King BP, Wood P, Kesteven P, Daly AK, Kamali F. The impact of CYP2C9 and VKORC1 genetic polymorphism and patient characteristics upon Warfarin dose requirements: proposal for a new dosing regimen. Blood 2005; 106(7):2329–2333.
48. Pullar T, Hunter JA, Capell HA. Effect of acetylator phenotype on efficacy and toxicity of sulphasalazine in rheumatoid arthritis. Ann Rheum Dis 1985; 44(12):831–837.
49. Yamamoto M, Sobue G, Mukoyama M, Matsuoka Y, Mitsuma T. Demonstration of slow acetylator genotype of N-acetyltransferase in isoniazid neuropathy using an archival hematoxylin and eosin section of a sural nerve biopsy specimen. J Neurol Sci 1996; 135(1):51–54.
50. Goel UC, Bajaj S, Gupta OP, Dwivedi NC, Dubey AL. Isoniazid induced neuropathy in slow versus rapid acetylators: an electrophysiological study. J Assoc Physicians India; 1992; 40(10):671–672.
51. Sonnhag C, Karlsson E, Hed J. Procainamide-induced lupus erythematosus-like syndrome in relation to acetylator phenotype and plasma levels of procainamide. Acta Med Scand 1979; 206(4):245–251.
52. Guillemette C. Pharmacogenomics of human UDP-glucuronosyltransferase enzymes. Pharmacogenomics J 2003; 3(3):136–158.
53. Acuna G, Foernzler D, Leong D, Rabbia M, Smit R, Dorflinger E, et al. Pharmacogenetic analysis of adverse drug effect reveals genetic variant for susceptibility to liver toxicity. Pharmacogenomics J 2002; 2(5):327–334.
54. Gagne JF, Montminy V, Belanger P, Journault K, Gaucher G, Guillemette C. Common human UGT1A polymorphisms and the altered metabolism of irinotecan active metabolite 7-ethyl-10-hydroxycamptothecin (SN-38). Mol Pharmacol 2002; 62(3):608–617.
55. Danoff TM, Campbell DA, McCarthy LC, Lewis KF, Repasch MH, Saunders AM, et al. A Gilbert's syndrome UGT1A1 variant confers susceptibility to tranilast-induced hyperbilirubinemia. Pharmacogenomics J 2004; 4(1):49–53.
56. Hosford DA, Lai EH, Riley JH, Xu CF, Danoff TM, Roses AD. Pharmacogenetics to predict drug-related adverse events. Toxicol Pathol 2004; 32(suppl 1):9–12.
57. Dubach UC, Rosner B, Pfister E. Epidemiologic study of abuse of analgesics containing phenacetin. Renal morbidity and mortality (1968–1979). N Engl J Med 1983; 308(7):357–362.
58. Johansson S, Angervall L, Bengtsson U, Wahlqvist L. Uroepithelial tumors of the renal pelvis associated with abuse of phenacetin-containing analgesics. Cancer 1974; 33(3):743–753.
59. Shahidi NT. Acetophenetidin-induced methemoglobinemia. Ann NY Acad Sci 1968; 151(2):822–832.
60. Nakayama N, Masuda Y. Suppression of phenacetin-induced methemoglobinemia by diethyldithiocarbamate and carbon disulfide and its relation to phenacetin metabolism in mice. J Pharmacobiodyn 1985; 8(10):868–876.
61. Sesardic D, Edwards RJ, Davies DS, Thomas PE, Levin W, Boobis AR. High affinity phenacetin O-deethylase is catalysed specifically by cytochrome P450d (P450IA2) in the liver of the rat. Biochem Pharmacol 1990; 39(3):489–498.
62. Chevalier D, Cauffiez C, Allorge D, Lo-Guidice JM, Lhermitte M, Lafitte JJ, et al. Five novel natural allelic variants-951A>C, 1042G>A (D348 N), 1156A>T (I386F), 1217G>A (C406Y) and 1291C>T (C431Y)-of the human CYP1A2 gene in a French Caucasian population. Hum Mutat 2001; 17(4):355–356.
63. Chida M, Yokoi T, Fukui T, Kinoshita M, Yokota J, Kamataki T. Detection of three genetic polymorphisms in the 5′-flanking region and intron 1 of human CYP1A2 in the Japanese population. Jpn J Cancer Res 1999; 90(9):899–902.
64. Murayama N, Soyama A, Saito Y, Nakajima Y, Komamura K, Ueno K, et al. Six novel nonsynonymous CYP1A2 gene polymorphisms: catalytic activities of the naturally occurring variant enzymes. J Pharmacol Exp Ther 2004; 308(1):300–306.

65. Peters JM, Morishima H, Ward JM, Coakley CJ, Kimura S, Gonzalez FJ. Role of CYP1A2 in the toxicity of long-term phenacetin feeding in mice. Toxicol Sci 1999; 50(1):82–89.
66. Calder IC, Goss DE, Williams PJ, Funder CC, Green CR, Ham KN, et al. Neoplasia in the rat induced by N-hydroxyphenacetin, a metabolite of phenacetin. Pathology 1976; 8(1):1–6.
67. Mulder GJ, Kadlubar FF, Mays JB, Hinson JA. Reaction of mutagenic phenacetin metabolites with glutathione and DNA. Possible implications for toxicity. Mol Pharmacol 1984; 26(2):342–347.
68. Wirth PJ, Alewood P, Calder I, Thorgeirsson SS. Mutagenicity of N-hydroxy-2-acetylamino-fluorene and N-hydroxy-phenacetin and their respective deacetylated metabolites in nitroreductase deficient Salmonella TA98FR and TA100FR. Carcinogenesis 1982; 3(2):167–170.
69. Gaedigk A, Bradford LD, Marcucci KA, Leeder JS. Unique CYP2D6 activity distribution and genotype-phenotype discordance in black Americans. Clin Pharmacol Ther 2002; 72(1):76–89.
70. Bradford LD. CYP2D6 allele frequency in European Caucasians, Asians, Africans and their descendants. Pharmacogenomics 2002; 3(2):229–243.
71. Sindrup SH, Brosen K. The pharmacogenetics of codeine hypoalgesia. Pharmacogenetics 1995; 5(6):335–346.
72. Fagerlund TH, Braaten O. No pain relief from codeine...? An introduction to pharmacogenomics. Acta Anaesthesiol Scand 2001; 45(2):140–149.
73. Pirmohamed M, Madden S, Park BK. Idiosyncratic drug reactions. Metabolic bioactivation as a pathogenic mechanism. Clin Pharmacokinet 1996; 31(3):215–230.
74. Park BK, Pirmohamed M, Kitteringham NR. Role of drug disposition in drug hypersensitivity: a chemical, molecular, and clinical perspective. Chem Res Toxicol 1998; 11(9):969–988.
75. Pirmohamed M, Breckenridge AM, Kitteringham NR, Park BK. Adverse drug reactions. Brit Med J 1998; 316(7140):1295–1298.
76. Rieder MJ, Uetrecht J, Shear NH, Cannon M, Miller M, Spielberg SP. Diagnosis of sulfonamide hypersensitivity reactions by in-vitro "rechallenge" with hydroxylamine metabolites. Ann Intern Med 1989; 110(4):286–289.
77. Cribb AE, Miller M, Leeder JS, Hill J, Spielberg SP. Reactions of the nitroso and hydroxylamine metabolites of sulfamethoxazole with reduced glutathione. Implications for idiosyncratic toxicity. Drug Metab Dispos 1991; 19(5):900–906.
78. Gill HJ, Hough SJ, Naisbitt DJ, Maggs JL, Kitteringham NR, Pirmohamed M, et al. The relationship between the disposition and immunogenicity of sulfamethoxazole in the rat. J Pharmacol Exp Ther 1997; 282(2):795–801.
79. Wolkenstein P, Loriot MA, Aractingi S, Cabelguenne A, Beaune P, Chosidow O. Prospective evaluation of detoxification pathways as markers of cutaneous adverse reactions to sulphonamides in AIDS. Pharmacogenetics 2000; 10(9):821–828.
80. Pirmohamed M, Alfirevic A, Vilar J, Stalford A, Wilkins EG, Sim E, et al. Association analysis of drug metabolizing enzyme gene polymorphisms in HIV-positive patients with co-trimoxazole hypersensitivity. Pharmacogenetics 2000; 10(8):705–713.
81. Alfirevic A, Stalford AC, Vilar FJ, Wilkins EG, Park BK, Pirmohamed M. Slow acetylator phenotype and genotype in HIV-positive patients with sulphamethoxazole hypersensitivity. Br J Clin Pharmacol 2003; 55(2):158–165.
82. Miller DP, De Vivo I, Neuberg D, Wain JC, Lynch TJ, Su L, et al. Association between self-reported environmental tobacco smoke exposure and lung cancer: modification by GSTP1 polymorphism. Int J Cancer 2003; 104(6):758–763.
83. Sorensen M, Autrup H, Tjonneland A, Overvad K, Raaschou-Nielsen O. Glutathione S-transferase T1 null-genotype is associated with an increased risk of lung cancer. Int J Cancer 2004; 110(2):219–224.
84. Strange RC, Jones PW, Fryer AA. Glutathione S-transferase: genetics and role in toxicology. Toxicol Lett 2000; 112–113:357–363.
85. Peters U, Preisler-Adams S, Hebeisen A, Hahn M, Seifert E, Lanvers C, et al. Glutathione S-transferase genetic polymorphisms and individual sensitivity to the ototoxic effect of cisplatin. Anticancer Drugs 2000; 11(8):639–643.

86. Simon T, Becquemont L, Mary-Krause M, de Waziers I, Beaune P, Funck-Brentano C, et al. Combined glutathione-S-transferase M1 and T1 genetic polymorphism and tacrine hepatotoxicity. Clin Pharmacol Ther 2000; 67(4):432–437.
87. Green VJ, Pirmohamed M, Kitteringham NR, Knapp MJ, Park BK. Glutathione S-transferase mu genotype (GSTM1*0) in Alzheimer's patients with tacrine transaminitis. Br J Clin Pharmacol 1995; 39(4):411–415.
88. De Sousa M, Pirmohamed M, Kitteringham NR, Woolf T, Park BK. No association between tacrine transaminitis and the glutathione transferase theta genotype in patients with Alzheimer's disease. Pharmacogenetics 1998; 8(4):353–355.
89. Watanabe I, Tomita A, Shimizu M, Sugawara M, Yasumo H, Koishi R, et al. A study to survey susceptible genetic factors responsible for troglitazone-associated hepatotoxicity in Japanese patients with type 2 diabetes mellitus. Clin Pharmacol Ther 2003; 73(5):435–455.
90. Tirona RG, Kim RB. Pharmacogenomics of drug transporters. In: Licinio J, Wong ML, eds. Pharmacogenomics: The Search for Individualized Therapies. Weinheim, Germany: Wiley-VCH, 2002.
91. Hoffmeyer S, Burk O, von Richter O, Arnold HP, Brockmoller J, Johne A, et al. Functional polymorphisms of the human multidrug-resistance gene: multiple sequence variations and correlation of one allele with P-glycoprotein expression and activity in vivo. Proc Natl Acad Sci USA 2000; 97(7):3473–3478.
92. Marzolini C, Paus E, Buclin T, Kim RB. Polymorphisms in human MDR1 (P-glycoprotein): recent advances and clinical relevance. Clin Pharmacol Ther 2004; 75(1):13–33.
93. Borst P, Evers R, Kool M, Wijnholds J. A family of drug transporters: the multidrug resistance-associated proteins. J Natl Cancer Inst 2000; 92(16):1295–1302.
94. Brinkmann U, Roots I, Eichelbaum M. Pharmacogenetics of the human drug-transporter gene MDR1: impact of polymorphisms on pharmacotherapy. Drug Discov Today 2001; 6(16):835–839.
95. Choo EF, Leake B, Wandel C, Imamura H, Wood AJ, Wilkinson GR, et al. Pharmacological inhibition of P-glycoprotein transport enhances the distribution of HIV-1 protease inhibitors into brain and testes. Drug Metab Dispos 2000; 28(6):655–660.
96. Drescher S, Schaeffeler E, Hitzl M, Hofmann U, Schwab M, Brinkmann U, et al. MDR1 gene polymorphisms and disposition of the P-glycoprotein substrate fexofenadine. Br J Clin Pharmacol 2002; 53(5):526–534.
97. Gerloff T, Schaefer M, Johne A, Oselin K, Meisel C, Cascorbi I, et al. MDR1 genotypes do not influence the absorption of a single oral dose of 1 mg digoxin in healthy white males. Br J Clin Pharmacol 2002; 54(6):610–616.
98. Horinouchi M, Sakaeda T, Nakamura T, Morita Y, Tamura T, Aoyama N, et al. Significant genetic linkage of MDR1 polymorphisms at positions 3435 and 2677: functional relevance to pharmacokinetics of digoxin. Pharm Res 2002; 19(10):1581–1585.
99. Chowbay B, Cumaraswamy S, Cheung YB, Zhou Q, Lee EJ. Genetic polymorphisms in MDR1 and CYP3A4 genes in Asians and the influence of MDR1 haplotypes on cyclosporin disposition in heart transplant recipients. Pharmacogenetics 2003; 13(2):89–95.
100. Ameyaw MM, Regateiro F, Li T, Liu X, Tariq M, Mobarek A, et al. MDR1 pharmacogenetics: frequency of the C3435T mutation in exon 26 is significantly influenced by ethnicity. Pharmacogenetics 2001; 11(3):217–221.
101. Shroyer NF, Lewis RA, Lupski JR. Analysis of the ABCR (ABCA4) gene in 4-aminoquinoline retinopathy: is retinal toxicity by chloroquine and hydroxychloroquine related to Stargardt disease? Am J Ophthalmol 2001; 131(6):761–766.
102. Knowles SR, Uetrecht J, Shear NH. Idiosyncratic drug reactions: the reactive metabolite syndromes. Lancet 2000; 356(9241):1587–1591.
103. Balazs T. Immunogenetically controlled autoimmune reactions induced by mercury, gold and D-penicillamine in laboratory animals: a review from the vantage point of premarketing safety studies. Toxicol Ind Health 1987; 3(3):331–336.
104. Lander ES, Linton LM, Birren B, Nusbaum C, Zody MC, Baldwin J, et al. Initial sequencing and analysis of the human genome. Nature 2001; 409(6822):860–921.

105. Venter JC, Adams MD, Myers EW, Li PW, Mural RJ, Sutton GG, et al. The sequence of the human genome. Science 2001; 291(5507):1304–1351.
106. Tsunoda T, Lathrop GM, Sekine A, Yamada R, Takahashi A, Ohnishi Y, et al. Variation of gene-based SNPs and linkage disequilibrium patterns in the human genome. Hum Mol Genet 2004; 13(15):1623–1632.
107. Walsh EC, Mather KA, Schaffner SF, Farwell L, Daly MJ, Patterson N, et al. An integrated haplotype map of the human major histocompatibility complex. Am J Hum Genet 2003; 73(3):580–590.
108. Hetherington S, McGuirk S, Powell G, Cutrell A, Naderer O, Spreen B, et al. Hypersensitivity reactions during therapy with the nucleoside reverse transcriptase inhibitor abacavir. Clin Ther 2001; 23(10):1603–1614.
109. Mallal S, Nolan D, Witt C, Masel G, Martin AM, Moore C, et al. Association between presence of HLA-B*5701, HLA-DR7, and HLA-DQ3 and hypersensitivity to HIV-1 reverse-transcriptase inhibitor abacavir. Lancet 2002; 359(9308):727–732.
110. Martin AM, Nolan D, Gaudieri S, Almeida CA, Nolan R, James I, et al. Predisposition to abacavir hypersensitivity conferred by HLA-B*5701 and a haplotypic Hsp70-Hom variant. Proc Natl Acad Sci USA 2004; 101(12):4180–4185.
111. Hetherington S, Hughes AR, Mosteller M, Shortino D, Baker KL, Spreen W, et al. Genetic variations in HLA-B region and hypersensitivity reactions to abacavir. Lancet 2002; 359(9312):1121–1122.
112. Hughes AR, Mosteller M, Bansal AT, Davies K, Haneline SA, Lai EH, et al. Association of genetic variations in HLA-B region with hypersensitivity to abacavir in some, but not all, populations. Pharmacogenomics 2004; 5(2):203–211.
113. Hughes DA, Vilar FJ, Ward CC, Alfirevic A, Park BK, Pirmohamed M. Cost-effectiveness analysis of HLA B*5701 genotyping in preventing abacavir hypersensitivity. Pharmacogenetics 2004; 14(6):335–342.
114. Lindpaintner K. The importance of being modest—reflections on the pharmacogenetics of abacavir. Pharmacogenomics 2002; 3(6):835–838.
115. Vittorio CC, Muglia JJ. Anticonvulsant hypersensitivity syndrome. Arch Intern Med 1995; 155(21):2285–2290.
116. Leeder JS. Mechanisms of idiosyncratic hypersensitivity reactions to antiepileptic drugs. Epilepsia 1998; 39(suppl 7):S8–S16.
117. Rzany B, Correia O, Kelly JP, Naldi L, Auquier A, Stern R. Risk of Stevens-Johnson syndrome and toxic epidermal necrolysis during first weeks of antiepileptic therapy: a case-control study. Study Group of the International Case Control Study on Severe Cutaneous Adverse Reactions. Lancet 1999; 353(9171):2190–2194.
118. Pirmohamed M, Lin K, Chadwick D, Park BK. TNFalpha promoter region gene polymorphisms in carbamazepine-hypersensitive patients. Neurology 2001; 56(7):890–896.
119. Chung WH, Hung SI, Hong HS, Hsih MS, Yang LC, Ho HC, et al. Medical genetics: a marker for Stevens-Johnson syndrome. Nature 2004; 428(6982):486.
120. Naisbitt DJ, Britschgi M, Wong G, Farrell J, Depta JP, Chadwick DW, et al. Hypersensitivity reactions to carbamazepine: characterization of the specificity, phenotype, and cytokine profile of drug-specific T cell clones. Mol Pharmacol 2003; 63(3):732–741.
121. Milner CM, Campbell RD. Genetic organization of the human MHC class III region. Front Biosci 2001; 6:D914–D926.
122. Pietrangelo A. Hereditary hemochromatosis—a new look at an old disease. N Engl J Med 2004; 350(23):2383–2397.
123. Cardoso CS, de Sousa M. HFE, the MHC and hemochromatosis: paradigm for an extended function for MHC class I. Tissue Antigens 2003; 61(4):263–275.
124. Feder JN. The hereditary hemochromatosis gene (HFE): a MHC class I-like gene that functions in the regulation of iron homeostasis. Immunol Res 1999; 20(2):175–185.
125. Alvir JM, Lieberman JA, Safferman AZ, Schwimmer JL, Schaaf JA. Clozapine-induced agranulocytosis. Incidence and risk factors in the United States. N Engl J Med 1993; 329(3):162–167.

126. Yunis JJ, Corzo D, Salazar M, Lieberman JA, Howard A, Yunis EJ. HLA associations in clozapine-induced agranulocytosis. Blood 1995; 86(3):1177–1183.
127. Corzo D, Yunis JJ, Yunis EJ, Howard A, Lieberman JA. HSP70-2 9.0 kb variant is in linkage disequilibrium with the HLA-B and DRB1* alleles associated with clozapine-induced agranulocytosis. J Clin Psychiatry 1994; 55(suppl B):149–152.
128. Corzo D, Yunis JJ, Salazar M, Lieberman JA, Howard A, Awdeh Z, et al. The major histocompatibility complex region marked by HSP70-1 and HSP70-2 variants is associated with clozapine-induced agranulocytosis in two different ethnic groups. Blood 1995; 86(10):3835–3840.
129. Dettling M, Schaub RT, Mueller-Oerlinghausen B, Roots I, Cascorbi I. Further evidence of human leukocyte antigen-encoded susceptibility to clozapine-induced agranulocytosis independent of ancestry. Pharmacogenetics 2001; 11(2):135–141.
130. Dettling M, Cascorbi I, Roots I, Mueller-Oerlinghausen B. Genetic determinants of clozapine-induced agranulocytosis: recent results of HLA subtyping in a non-jewish caucasian sample. Arch Gen Psychiatry 2001; 58(1):93–94.
131. Faber HJ, Smit AJ, van de Loosdrecht AA. Clozapine induced agranulocytosis: hypothesis on immune-mediated pathogenesis and the role of haematopoietic growth factors. Neth J Med 1999; 55(2):86–87.
132. Palella FJ Jr, Delaney KM, Moorman AC, Loveless MO, Fuhrer J, Satten GA, et al. Declining morbidity and mortality among patients with advanced human immunodeficiency virus infection. HIV Outpatient Study Investigators. N Engl J Med 1998; 338(13):853–860.
133. Carr A, Samaras K, Thorisdottir A, Kaufmann GR, Chisholm DJ, Cooper DA. Diagnosis, prediction, and natural course of HIV-1 protease-inhibitor-associated lipodystrophy, hyperlipidaemia, and diabetes mellitus: a cohort study. Lancet 1999; 353(9170):2093–2099.
134. Mallal SA, John M, Moore CB, James IR, McKinnon EJ. Contribution of nucleoside analogue reverse transcriptase inhibitors to subcutaneous fat wasting in patients with HIV infection. Aids 2000; 14(10):1309–1316.
135. Reus S, Arroyo E, Boix V, Portilla J. Lipodystrophy and hyperglycemia produced by protease inhibitors. An Med Interna 2000; 17(3):123–126.
136. Maher B, Alfirevic A, Vilar FJ, Wilkins EG, Park BK, Pirmohamed M. TNF-alpha promoter region gene polymorphisms in HIV-positive patients with lipodystrophy. Aids 2002; 16(15):2013–2018.
137. Nolan D, Moore C, Castley A, Sayer D, Mamotte C, John M, et al. Tumour necrosis factor-alpha gene -238G/A promoter polymorphism associated with a more rapid onset of lipodystrophy. Aids 2003; 17(1):121–123.
138. Ryden M, Arvidsson E, Blomqvist L, Perbeck L, Dicker A, Arner P. Targets for TNF-alpha-induced lipolysis in human adipocytes. Biochem Biophys Res Commun 2004; 318(1):168–175.
139. Adverse effects of the atypical antipsychotics. Collaborative Working Group on Clinical Trial Evaluations. J Clin Psychiatry 1998; 59(suppl 12):17–22.
140. Allison DB, Mentore JL, Heo M, Chandler LP, Cappelleri JC, Infante MC, et al. Antipsychotic-induced weight gain: a comprehensive research synthesis. Am J Psychiatry 1999; 156(11):1686–1696.
141. Umbricht DS, Pollack S, Kane JM. Clozapine and weight gain. J Clin Psychiatry 1994; 55(suppl B):157–160.
142. Meltzer HY. Role of serotonin in the action of atypical antipsychotic drugs. Clin Neurosci 1995; 3(2):64–75.
143. Basile VS, Masellis M, Badri F, Paterson AD, Meltzer HY, Lieberman JA, et al. Association of the MscI polymorphism of the dopamine D3 receptor gene with tardive dyskinesia in schizophrenia. Neuropsychopharmacology 1999; 21(1):17–27.
144. Basile VS, Masellis M, McIntyre RS, Meltzer HY, Lieberman JA, Kennedy JL. Genetic dissection of atypical antipsychotic-induced weight gain: novel preliminary data on the pharmacogenetic puzzle. J Clin Psychiatry 2001; 62(suppl 23):45–66.

145. Basile VS, Masellis M, De Luca V, Meltzer HY, Kennedy JL. 759C/T genetic variation of 5HT(2C) receptor and clozapine-induced weight gain. Lancet 2002; 360(9347):1790–1791.
146. Chouinard G. New nomenclature for drug-induced movement disorders including tardive dyskinesia. J Clin Psychiatry 2004; 65(suppl 9):9–15.
147. Liao DL, Yeh YC, Chen HM, Chen H, Hong CJ, Tsai SJ. Association between the Ser9Gly polymorphism of the dopamine D3 receptor gene and tardive dyskinesia in Chinese schizophrenic patients. Neuropsychobiology 2001; 44(2):95–98.
148. Lovlie R, Daly AK, Blennerhassett R, Ferrier N, Steen VM. Homozygosity for the Gly-9 variant of the dopamine D3 receptor and risk for tardive dyskinesia in schizophrenic patients. Int J Neuropsychopharmacol 2000; 3(1):61–65.
149. Steen VM, Lovlie R, MacEwan T, McCreadie RG. Dopamine D3-receptor gene variant and susceptibility to tardive dyskinesia in schizophrenic patients. Mol Psychiatry 1997; 2(2):139–145.
150. Lerer B, Segman RH, Fangerau H, Daly AK, Basile VS, Cavallaro R, et al. Pharmacogenetics of tardive dyskinesia: combined analysis of 780 patients supports association with dopamine D3 receptor gene Ser9Gly polymorphism. Neuropsychopharmacology 2002; 27(1):105–119.
151. Kapitany T, Meszaros K, Lenzinger E, Schindler SD, Barnas C, Fuchs K, et al. Genetic polymorphisms for drug metabolism (CYP2D6) and tardive dyskinesia in schizophrenia. Schizophr Res 1998; 32(2):101–106.
152. Basile VS, Ozdemir V, Masellis M, Walker ML, Meltzer HY, Lieberman JA, et al. A functional polymorphism of the cytochrome P450 1A2 (CYP1A2) gene: association with tardive dyskinesia in schizophrenia. Mol Psychiatry 2000; 5(4):410–417.
153. Tan EC, Chong SA, Mahendran R, Dong F, Tan CH. Susceptibility to neuroleptic-induced tardive dyskinesia and the T102C polymorphism in the serotonin type 2A receptor. Biol Psychiatry 2001; 50(2):144–147.
154. Segman RH, Heresco-Levy U, Finkel B, Goltser T, Shalem R, Schlafman M, et al. Association between the serotonin 2A receptor gene and tardive dyskinesia in chronic schizophrenia. Mol Psychiatry 2001; 6(2):225–229.
155. Gillard EF, Otsu K, Fujii J, Khanna VK, de Leon S, Derdemezi J, et al. A substitution of cysteine for arginine 614 in the ryanodine receptor is potentially causative of human malignant hyperthermia. Genomics 1991; 11(3):751–755.
156. Brandt A, Schleithoff L, Jurkat-Rott K, Klingler W, Baur C, Lehmann-Horn F. Screening of the ryanodine receptor gene in 105 malignant hyperthermia families: novel mutations and concordance with the in vitro contracture test. Hum Mol Genet 1999; 8(11):2055–2062.
157. McCarthy TV, Quane KA, Lynch PJ. Ryanodine receptor mutations in malignant hyperthermia and central core disease. Hum Mutat 2000; 15(5):410–417.
158. Wehner M, Rueffert H, Koenig F, Olthoff D. Functional characterization of malignant hyperthermia-associated RyR1 mutations in exon 44, using the human myotube model. Neuromuscul Disord 2004; 14(7):429–437.
159. Allen GC, Larach MG, Kunselman AR. The sensitivity and specificity of the caffeine-halothane contracture test: a report from the North American Malignant Hyperthermia Registry. The North American Malignant Hyperthermia Registry of MHAUS. Anesthesiology 1998; 88(3):579–588.
160. Wehrens XH, Vos MA, Doevendans PA, Wellens HJ. Novel insights in the congenital long QT syndrome. Ann Intern Med 2002; 137(12):981–992.
161. Donger C, Denjoy I, Berthet M, Neyroud N, Cruaud C, Bennaceur M, et al. KVLQT1 C-terminal missense mutation causes a forme fruste long-QT syndrome. Circulation 1997; 96(9):2778–2781.
162. Abbott GW, Sesti F, Splawski I, Buck ME, Lehmann MH, Timothy KW, et al. MiRP1 forms IKr potassium channels with HERG and is associated with cardiac arrhythmia. Cell 1999; 97(2):175–187.
163. Sesti F, Abbott GW, Wei J, Murray KT, Saksena S, Schwartz PJ, et al. A common polymorphism associated with antibiotic-induced cardiac arrhythmia. Proc Natl Acad Sci USA 2000; 97(19):10613–10618.

164. Piippo K, Swan H, Pasternack M, Chapman H, Paavonen K, Viitasalo M, et al. A founder mutation of the potassium channel KCNQ1 in long QT syndrome: implications for estimation of disease prevalence and molecular diagnostics. J Am Coll Cardiol 2001; 37(2):562–568.
165. Bertina RM, Koeleman BP, Koster T, Rosendaal FR, Dirven RJ, de Ronde H, et al. Mutation in blood coagulation factor V associated with resistance to activated protein C. Nature 1994; 369(6475):64–67.
166. Rees DC, Cox M, Clegg JB. World distribution of factor V Leiden. Lancet 1995; 346(8983):1133–1134.
167. Vandenbroucke JP, Koster T, Briet E, Reitsma PH, Bertina RM, Rosendaal FR. Increased risk of venous thrombosis in oral-contraceptive users who are carriers of factor V Leiden mutation. Lancet 1994; 344(8935):1453–1457.
168. Martinelli I, Battaglioli T, Mannucci PM. Pharmacogenetic aspects of the use of oral contraceptives and the risk of thrombosis. Pharmacogenetics 2003; 13(10):589–594.
169. Chladek J, Grim J, Martinkova J, Simkova M, Vaniekova J, Koudelkova V, et al. Pharmacokinetics and pharmacodynamics of low-dose methotrexate in the treatment of psoriasis. Br J Clin Pharmacol 2002; 54(2):147–156.
170. Carneiro JR, Sato EI. Double blind, randomized, placebo controlled clinical trial of methotrexate in systemic lupus erythematosus. J Rheumatol 1999; 26(6):1275–1279.
171. Sampaio-Barros PD, Costallat LT, Bertolo MB, Neto JF, Samara AM. Methotrexate in the treatment of ankylosing spondylitis. Scand J Rheumatol 2000; 29(3):160–162.
172. van Jaarsveld CH, Jahangier ZN, Jacobs JW, Blaauw AA, van Albada-Kuipers GA, ter Borg EJ, et al. Toxicity of anti-rheumatic drugs in a randomized clinical trial of early rheumatoid arthritis. Rheumatology (Oxford) 2000; 39(12):1374–1382.
173. Ulrich CM, Yasui Y, Storb R, Schubert MM, Wagner JL, Bigler J, et al. Pharmacogenetics of methotrexate: toxicity among marrow transplantation patients varies with the methylenetetrahydrofolate reductase C677T polymorphism. Blood 2001; 98(1):231–234.
174. Goyette P, Rozen R. The thermolabile variant 677C–>T can further reduce activity when expressed in cis with severe mutations for human methylenetetrahydrofolate reductase. Hum Mutat 2000; 16(2):132–138.
175. Weisberg I, Tran P, Christensen B, Sibani S, Rozen R. A second genetic polymorphism in methylenetetrahydrofolate reductase (MTHFR) associated with decreased enzyme activity. Mol Genet Metab 1998; 64(3):169–172.
176. Kang SS, Zhou J, Wong PW, Kowalisyn J, Strokosch G. Intermediate homocysteinemia: a thermolabile variant of methylenetetrahydrofolate reductase. Am J Hum Genet 1988; 43(4):414–421.
177. Urano W, Taniguchi A, Yamanaka H, Tanaka E, Nakajima H, Matsuda Y, et al. Polymorphisms in the methylenetetrahydrofolate reductase gene were associated with both the efficacy and the toxicity of methotrexate used for the treatment of rheumatoid arthritis, as evidenced by single locus and haplotype analyses. Pharmacogenetics 2002; 12(3):183–190.
178. Garg R, Yusuf S. Overview of randomized trials of angiotensin-converting enzyme inhibitors on mortality and morbidity in patients with heart failure. Collaborative Group on ACE Inhibitor Trials. J Am Med Assoc 1995; 273(18):1450–1456.
179. The SOLVD Investigators. Effect of enalapril on survival in patients with reduced left ventricular ejection fractions and congestive heart failure. N Engl J Med 1991; 325(5):293–302.
180. McEwan JR, Choudry N, Street R, Fuller RW. Change in cough reflex after treatment with enalapril and ramipril. Brit Med J 1989; 299(6690):13–16.
181. Furuya K, Yamaguchi E, Hirabayashi T, Itoh A, Hizawa N, Ohnuma N, et al. Angiotensin-I-converting enzyme gene polymorphism and susceptibility to cough. Lancet 1994; 343(8893):354.
182. Takahashi T, Yamaguchi E, Furuya K, Kawakami Y. The ACE gene polymorphism and cough threshold for capsaicin after cilazapril usage. Respir Med 2001; 95(2):130–135.
183. Mukae S, Aoki S, Itoh S, Iwata T, Ueda H, Katagiri T. Bradykinin B(2) receptor gene polymorphism is associated with angiotensin-converting enzyme inhibitor-related cough. Hypertension 2000; 36(1):127–131.

184. Mukae S, Itoh S, Aoki S, Iwata T, Nishio K, Sato R, et al. Association of polymorphisms of the renin–angiotensin system and bradykinin B2 receptor with ACE-inhibitor-related cough. J Hum Hypertens 2002; 16(12):857–863.
185. Tiret L, Rigat B, Visvikis S, Breda C, Corvol P, Cambien F, et al. Evidence, from combined segregation and linkage analysis, that a variant of the angiotensin I-converting enzyme (ACE) gene controls plasma ACE levels. Am J Hum Genet 1992; 51(1):197–205.
186. Rigat B, Hubert C, Alhenc-Gelas F, Cambien F, Corvol P, Soubrier F. An insertion/deletion polymorphism in the angiotensin I-converting enzyme gene accounting for half the variance of serum enzyme levels. J Clin Invest 1990; 86(4):1343–1346.
187. Zee RY, Rao VS, Paster RZ, Sweet CS, Lindpaintner K. Three candidate genes and angiotensin-converting enzyme inhibitor-related cough: a pharmacogenetic analysis. Hypertension 1998; 31(4):925–928.
188. Krynetski EY, Evans WE. Pharmacogenetics of cancer therapy: getting personal. Am J Hum Genet 1998; 63(1):11–16.
189. Evans WE. Pharmacogenetics of thiopurine S-methyltransferase and thiopurine therapy. Ther Drug Monit 2004; 26(2):186–191.
190. Danzon P, Towse A. The economics of gene therapy and of pharmacogenetics. Value Health 2002; 5(1):5–13.

6
Pharmacogenetics of Respiratory Disease

Ian P. Hall[a]
Division of Therapeutics and Molecular Medicine, University Hospital of Nottingham, Nottingham, U.K.

Stephen B. Liggett[b]
Departments of Medicine and Physiology, University of Maryland School of Medicine, Baltimore, Maryland, U.S.A.

INTRODUCTION

Respiratory disease pharmacogenetics has been one of the more widely studied disease areas, although almost all studies to date have been in asthma or examined bronchodilator responses in populations with airflow obstruction. Few drugs used in the management of respiratory disease have narrow therapeutic windows (theophylline being an obvious exception), and hence the majority of studies have concentrated on examining pharmacodynamic rather than pharmacokinetic variables. To date there have been no studies examining pharmacogenetic effects in the management of interstitial lung diseases, although with increasing use of pharmacogenomic approaches (e.g., expression profiling) in these conditions it is likely that genetic factors, which may predict treatment response will become available. Therefore, this chapter will deal predominantly with the potential role of genetic variability in the key respiratory drug targets used in the management of airflow obstruction in asthma and chronic obstructive pulmonary disease (COPD).

β_2 ADRENOCEPTOR POLYMORPHISM

In many ways, the β_2-adrenergic receptor gene (β_2AR) is an ideal candidate for the study of genetic variation, biological relevance, and clinical consequences of polymorphisms. The receptor is expressed on most cells, and agonists and antagonists are used in treatment of a number of diseases, such as asthma, COPD, hypertension, heart failure, preterm labor, glaucoma, and migraine. On the other hand, all these diseases are complex and multifactorial, and most have a substantial environmental component. As such, the influence of

[a]Ian P. Hall's research is supported by the Medical Research Council and Asthma U.K.

[b]Stephen B. Liggett is supported by the National Heart Lung and Blood Institute Pharmacogenetics Research Network grant U01-HL65899.

a β_2AR genetic variant on the disease itself, the response to specific therapy (i.e., β-agonists), the response to other therapies where there is interaction (i.e., corticosteroids), and gene–environment interactions all have to be considered. Thus, studies of the effects of β_2AR polymorphisms in asthma and asthma treatment have been somewhat of a "case-study" in the evolution of our understanding of how to study polymorphisms and complex traits.

β-agonists are utilized in asthma and COPD as acute interventions during bronchospasm and as preventative therapy. The responses to these agents, as assessed by a number of physiologic or clinical outcomes, show a high degree of interindividual variability. Estimates have indicated that >50% of this variability has a genetic basis (1). Epidemiologic studies have also revealed that "excessive" use of β-agonists is associated with loss of asthma control and also increased morbidity and mortality [see Refs. (2,3) for reviews]. Indeed, β-agonists may predispose to bronchoconstriction through cross talk between β_2ARs and other signaling pathways in the airway (4). In addition, there are other classes of drugs that also have therapeutic efficacy in asthma and COPD management. This significant interindividual variability in the response to β-agonists, the potential for adverse effects, and alternative treatments prompted the investigation of the β_2AR gene for polymorphisms and their relevance in clinical medicine, so as to tailor therapy based on genetic profiles.

In 1993, the existence of polymorphisms of the human β_2AR was published (5). Shown in Figure 1 are the locations within the coding region of those polymorphisms. Subsequent studies have failed to uncover additional, nonsynonymous, single-nucleotide polymorphisms (SNPs) in the coding region. By far the two most common polymorphisms (Table 1) are in the amino-terminus at amino acids 16 and 27 (nucleotides 46 and 79). At

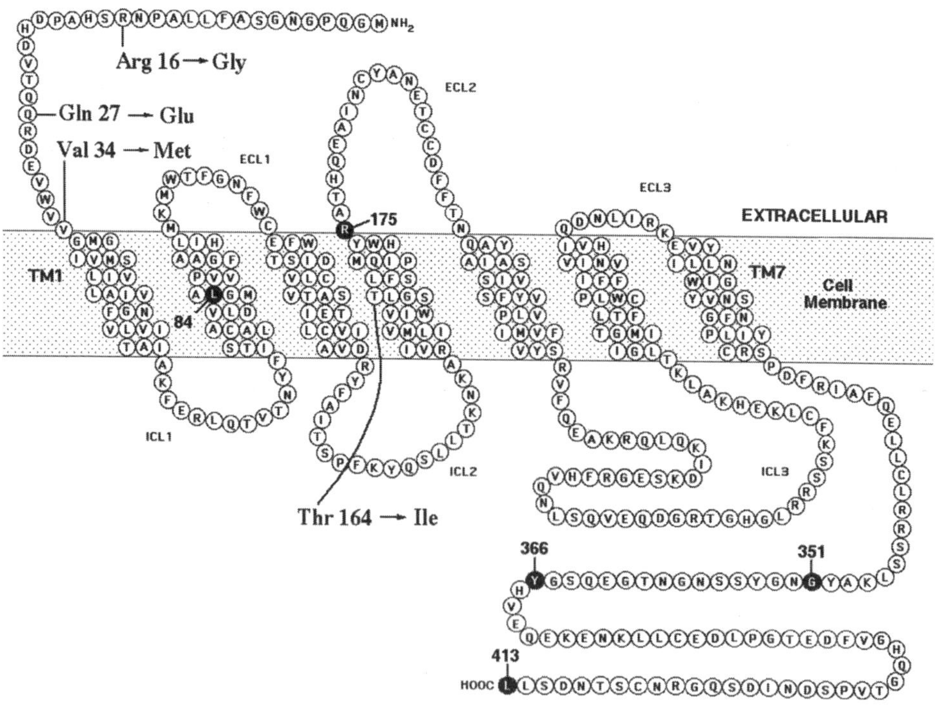

Figure 1 Schematic representation of the human β_2 adrenoceptor showing known coding region synonymous and nonsynonymous polymorphisms.

Table 1 Coding Region Variants of the Human β_2-Adrenergic Receptor

Nucleotide position	Nucleotides major/minor	Codon position	Amino acids major/minor
46	G/A	16	Gly/Arg
79	C/G	27	Gln/Glu
100	G/A	34	Val/Met
491	C/T	164	Thr/Ile
252	G/A	84	Leu (syn)
523	C/A	175	Arg (syn)
1053	G/C	351	Gly (syn)
1098	T/C	366	Leu (syn)
1239	G/A	413	Leu (syn)

Abbreviation: syn, synonymous.

amino acid 16, either Arg or Gly can be found, the former being the minor allele but for many years considered as the "wild type." At amino acid position 27 Gln or Glu can be found. A rare SNP, localized to a codon within the fourth transmembrane spanning domain, results in Thr or Ile at amino acid 164. An extremely rare variant has also been found at position 34 as shown. It is generally accepted that these β_2AR polymorphisms are not associated with risk for asthma, although there have been a few positive association studies (see next). The main emphasis has been on whether these polymorphisms modify asthma, such as defining certain clinical subsets, or alter the response to β-agonist therapy.

In order to have a better understanding of how each polymorphism affects the pharmacology of the receptor, a number of in vitro studies have been carried out (6–10). Initial work with the amino terminal polymorphisms was performed using transfected Chinese hamster fibroblasts, stably expressing each possible combination of the two polymorphisms (7). In membrane-based assays, all the variant receptors had similar functional coupling to adenylyl cyclase. In addition, radioligand-binding studies revealed no differences in agonist- or antagonist-binding affinities. Because the amino-terminus was known to be important in receptor trafficking and regulation by agonists, studies were carried out examining such short-term events as receptor internalization and long-term events, including receptor synthesis and agonist-promoted downregulation (loss of net receptor levels after 24 hours of exposure to agonists in culture). The most obvious phenotype, which arose from such studies, is summarized in Figure 2A. The Arg16/Gln27 receptor underwent $\sim$26% loss of receptor number under these conditions. The Gly16/Gln27 receptor had enhanced agonist-promoted downregulation ($\sim$41%), while the Arg16/Gln27 receptor showed very little downregulation. As discussed in the following, while the pharmacology of this latter variant is interesting, this combination (haplotype) is very uncommon. The Gly16/Glu27 receptor displayed enhanced downregulation similar to the Gly16/Gln27 receptor. Additional studies were subsequently performed with human airway smooth muscle cells, which were obtained from individuals without lung disease and grown in primary culture (8). The advantages of this system is that it is a cell type of interest, the endogenous promoter drives the expression of the receptor, and the levels of expression are "physiologic." However, there is no way to control the polymorphic variation of other genetic loci in genes associated with the signal transduction pathway of the β_2AR, and thus these cells have their limitations. Genotyping of positions 16 and 27 (but notably not in the promoter or untranslated regions) provided groups of cells to further examine the effects of polymorphisms at these two positions on

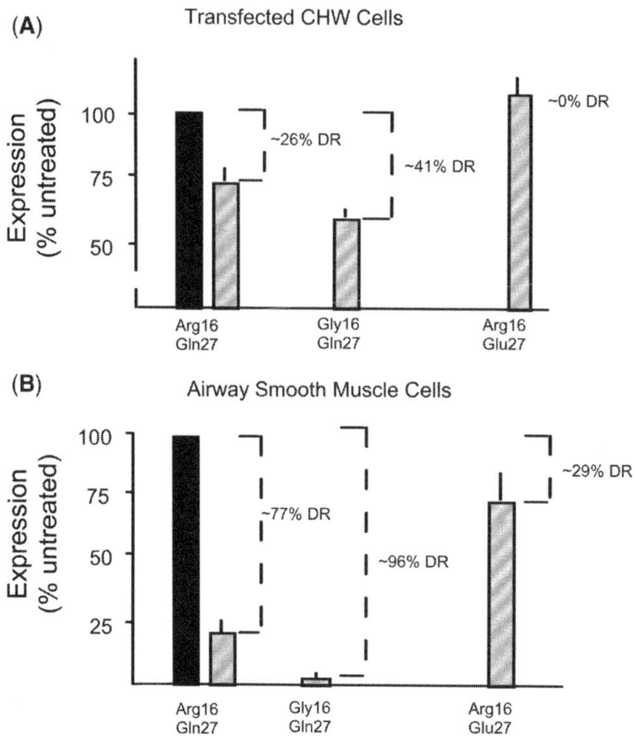

Figure 2 Downregulation profiles for different combinations of the codon 16 and 27 β_2 adrenoceptor polymorphisms following overnight exposure to isoproterenol (isoprenaline) in CHW cells (**A**) or primary cultures of human airway smooth muscle (**B**).

agonist-promoted downregulation. The results were qualitatively quite consistent with the transfected cell results, again showing the marked increase in downregulation of the Gly16 variant (Fig. 2B).

The SNP at position 164 has not been studied in asthma due to its low allele frequency (2–5% heterozygotes, no homozygous individual has been reported to date). However, its properties suggest that in the few patients who carry Ile164, the overall response to all the available β-agonists (such as bronchodilatation) and the duration of action to the agonist salmeterol may be reduced. In vitro, Ile164 is markedly uncoupled from stimulation of adenylyl cyclase (Fig. 3A) (6). In addition, salmeterol binding to the exosite in transmembrane spanning domain 4 is decreased, such that the duration of action [stimulation of cyclic AMP (cAMP)] is reduced by approximately 50% (Fig. 3B) (10).

As is discussed in the following, multiple studies have found correlations between one or more of the two major coding polymorphisms and an asthmatic phenotype. However, it became clear that there was some variability in a given trait (such as the bronchodilator response) even after stratification of patients by the polymorphisms at positions 16 and 27. This has prompted the examination of the promoter and 5′ UTR regions of the $\beta_2 AR$ gene for genetic variation (9,11). The gene is intronless, and the promoter has been characterized, to various extents, in several rodent genes as well as in the human (11–14). To address genetic variability, one group resequenced the $\beta_2 AR$ gene in multiple individuals from a reference repository composed of Caucasians, African Americans, Asians, and Hispanic Latinos (9). These results are shown in Table 2. Thirteen SNPs were noted from -1023 to $+523$. (of note, because further sequencing in the coding region had previously not revealed nonsynonymous SNPs, this region was not further

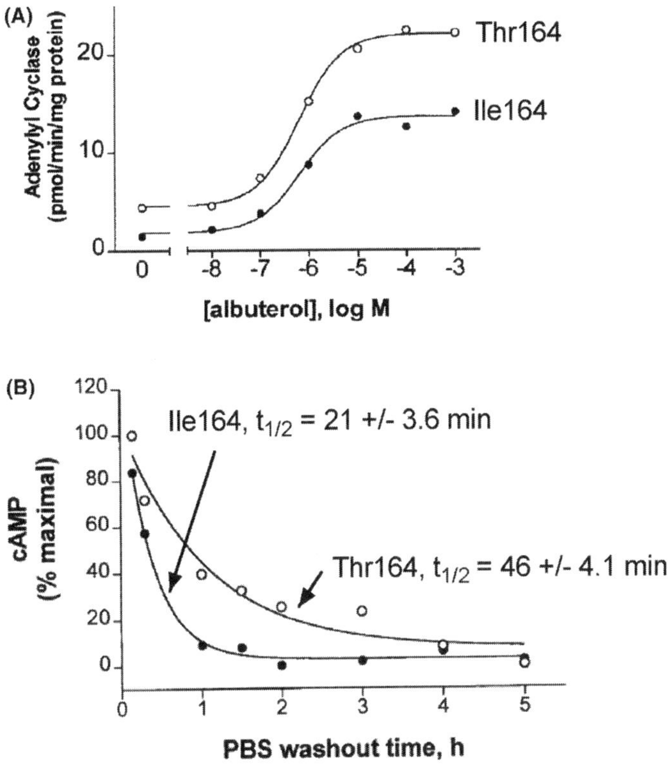

Figure 3 Effect of albuterol (salbutamol) on adenylyl cyclase activity (**A**) or cyclic AMP production time course (**B**) in cell lines expressing the Ile 164 and Thr 164 forms of the human β_2 adrenoceptor. *Abbreviations*: cAMP, cyclic AMP; PBS, phosphate buffered saline.

pursued. And, 3′ UTR sequencing was somewhat problematic, and so was not included in the analysis). Of the $2^{13} = 8192$ possible combinations of the 13 SNPs, only 12 haplotypes were detected. This, of course, does not exclude the possibility of additional SNPs, or haplotypes, that are present in the human population (or certain isolated populations). But, given the diversity of the population groups that were studied, we contend that any other SNPs/haplotypes found will be uncommon. It is interesting to note that the number of SNPs for this gene is approximately equal to the number of haplotypes (with frequencies $\geq 1\%$). This has turned out to be true for other G protein coupled receptor (GPCR) genes (15) and also for a large group of non-GPCR genes (16). So although one initially considers that the use of haplotypes could markedly expand the number of total possibilities, many of those combinations do not exist due to linkage disequilibrium between the various SNPs. With regards to the *β_2AR*, some of the haplotypes display significant differences in prevalence based on ethnicity. For example, haplotype 1 is ~40-fold more common in African Americans compared with the Caucasians. Other haplotypes are cosmopolitan, such as haplotypes 4, 6, and 2. Despite the relative short distances between these SNPs, the degree of linkage to disequilibrium is sufficiently low for certain positions (Fig. 4) that it is necessary to genotype multiple loci in order to obtain a sufficient amount of genetic information to assign the haplotype. Depending on whether one chooses to identify even the rare haplotypes, or to group certain rare haplotypes, the number of SNP positions that are required to be genotyped can vary. A grouping strategy requires genotyping about 4–6 SNP loci. In Caucasians, the most common homozygous haplotypes are haplotypes 2 and 4 (also referred to as haplotypes 2/2 and 4/4).

Table 2 Haplotypes of the Human β_2 Adrenergic Receptor

	Nucleotide													Frequency (%)			
Alleles	−1023 G/A	−709 C/A	−654 G/A	−468 C/G	−406 C/T	−367 T/C	−47 T/C	−20 T/C	46 G/A	79 C/G	252 G/A	491 C/T	523 C/A	Ca	A-A	As	H-L
Haplotype																	
1	A	C	G	C	C	T	T	T	A	C	G	C	C	0.7	25.0	12.5	10.0
2	A	C	G	G	C	C	C	C	G	G	G	C	C	48.3	6.3	10.0	26.7
3	G	A	A	C	C	T	T	T	A	C	G	C	C	0.7	0.0	0.0	0.0
4	G	C	A	C	C	T	T	T	A	C	G	C	C	33.0	29.7	45.0	40.0
5	G	C	A	C	C	T	T	T	G	C	G	C	C	1.4	0.0	0.0	0.0
6	G	C	G	C	C	T	T	T	G	C	A	C	A	13.2	31.3	30.0	13.3
7	G	C	G	C	C	T	T	T	G	C	A	T	A	1.0	1.6	0.0	3.3
8	G	C	A	C	C	T	T	T	A	C	A	C	A	0.7	0.0	0.0	0.0
9	A	C	G	C	T	T	T	T	A	C	G	C	C	0.0	4.7	0.0	0.0
10	G	C	G	C	C	T	T	T	G	C	A	C	C	0.7	0.0	0.0	3.3
11	G	C	G	C	C	T	T	T	G	C	G	C	C	0.3	0.0	2.5	0.0
12	A	C	G	G	C	T	T	T	A	C	G	C	C	0.0	1.6	0.0	3.3
Location	5′	5′	5′	5′	5′	5′	AA19 BUP Cys/Arg	5′	AA16 Gly/Arg	AA27 Gln/Glu	syn	AA164 Thr/Ile	syn				

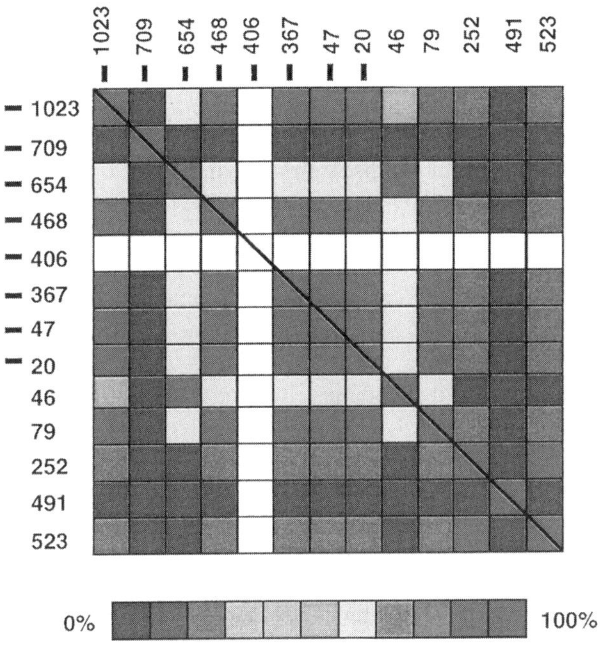

Figure 4 Linkage disequilibrium across the human β_2 adrenoceptor locus.

These genes were constructed exactly as they occur in nature, in a vector with no other promoters or enhancers. Transfection studies (9) were carried out in human embryonic kidney cells, which express a low level of β_2AR, and thus we presumed that there are transcription factors that regulate receptor expression. Haplotype 2 expression (both mRNA and protein) was greater than that of haplotype 4. Thus in this model system, there appears to be haplotype-specific directivity of receptor expression. There are a number of differences between haplotypes 2 and 4. In all, there are eight SNP positions, which differ between the two. These involve potential *cis*-acting elements in the 5′ region, including sites for AP-4, C/EBP, NF-1, and CP2, as well as the βAR upstream binding protein in the 5′ leader cistron. In addition, haplotypes 2 and 4 differ at the coding polymorphisms at amino acids 16 and 27.

Another group has constructed a large number of 5′ upstream haplotypes used to drive the expression of the luciferase gene, and only a few appeared to have an effect (17). Of note, the haplotypes that had the most dramatic changes in expression of the reporter are rare in the human population. In another study, the majority of the promoter activity for the β_2AR was found to be from −549 forward (11). Transfection of the two major haplotypes with a luciferase reporter construct into COS-7 cells showed differences in expression. The lower expression was obtained with a construct with a limited haplotype encompassed within haplotype 2 of Table 2. Another study analyzed receptor expression in peripheral blood mononuclear cells, which endogenously express β_2AR (18). Haplotypes were constructed based on positions −367, −47, +46, and +79. No differences in expression between the four possible β_2AR haplotypes were noted on these peripheral cells. The basis for the discrepancies in these various reports is not entirely clear but may lie in the fact that the methods utilized by each study are different. In addition, there may be a significant contribution of specific transcription factors found in the host cell, which ultimately sets the phenotype of a given polymorphic β_2AR gene.

CLINICAL CONSEQUENCES OF β_2AR POLYMORPHISMS

There have been many studies examining relationships between β_2AR SNPs, genotypic combinations, or haplotypes, and an asthmatic phenotype. Because the focus of this text is pharmacogenetics, the findings of studies specifically addressing this aspect will be primarily discussed. It should be noted, though, that a disease modifying effect of a β_2AR variant might act to alter the response to therapy through an indirect, or secondary, effect. For example, if a polymorphism alters severity, such that baseline lung function is affected, the clinical response from β-agonist could be altered. Similarly, if β_2AR polymorphisms alter bronchial hyperreactivity by cross talk with receptors, such as the M_3-muscarinic, bronchial hyperreactivity as assessed in methacholine challenge tests may be altered. So, any disease modifying effect of a variant needs to be taken into account when assessing results of pharmacogenetic studies. Indeed, there are reports of β_2AR polymorphisms associated with asthma severity (19,20), bronchial hyperresponsiveness (21,22), IgE levels (23), and the nocturnal phenotype (24).

The overall clinical response to β-agonist can be considered in several ways. One is the acute response to a standard dose of agonist [such as inhaled albuterol (salbutamol)]. Clinically, this corresponds to the response to agonist during an acute episode of bronchospasm. Another set of endpoints is the response to chronic β-agonist therapy. Here, both physiologic data as well as indices of long-term asthma control can be considered. The waning of responsiveness to agonist during continuous exposure is termed desensitization in vitro, or tachyphylaxis in vivo. In asthma, the loss of bronchodilatory responsiveness during chronic agonist treatment can be seen as strict tachyphylaxis, where there is a loss of the FEV_1 response, or as an increase in sensitivity to inhaled bronchoconstrictive agents, which has been termed as loss of the bronchoprotective effect. These two phenomena are interrelated and likely involve agonist-mediated regulation of the β_2AR itself and also other downstream or parallel pathways.

Although there are numerous studies specifically addressing response to therapy, only a few will be highlighted here. One of the first studies of β-agonist responsiveness in asthma examined the acute response to albuterol in 58 Japanese patients stratified by a BanI restriction fragment length polymorphism. Those with this restriction site (termed the 2.3-kb fragment) had a greater bronchodilator response than those without it. This polymorphic site was subsequently shown to be at nucleotide position 523, which is codon 175 (5). The polymorphism is synonymous (i.e., the encoded amino acid is not changed) but is in linkage disequilibrium with several SNPs, and indeed contributes to the unique sequence of haplotype cluster 6, 7, 8 compared to the other haplotypes (Table 2). Interestingly, this SNP-defined haplotype was shown in a study (9) several years later to also be associated with increased FEV_1 response to albuterol in Caucasian asthmatics when it appeared as the 2/6 or 4/6 haplotype pair. In this study, the acute bronchodilator response in 121 moderate Caucasian asthmatics was carried out by genotyping at all the SNP positions shown in Table 2 and haplotypes were assembled. There was no relationship between multiple clinical variables and SNPs or haplotypes. And no single SNP predicted bronchodilator response to albuterol. However, there was a relationship between haplotype and the bronchodilator response (change in FEV_1 percent predicted) as shown in Figure 5. Of the homozygous haplotypes, those with 2/2 had a greater response than those with 4/4. Interestingly, the 4/6 haplotype had the greatest response, but we were unable to ascertain the effects of 6/6 because there were no homozygous individuals in the cohort. The heterozygous 2/4 response was greater than the homozygous 4/4 and less than the 2/2 response, consistent with a gene–dose effect. In another Japanese cohort of 117 asthmatics, the polymorphisms at amino acid positions 16 and 27 were determined in order to assess potential relationships with

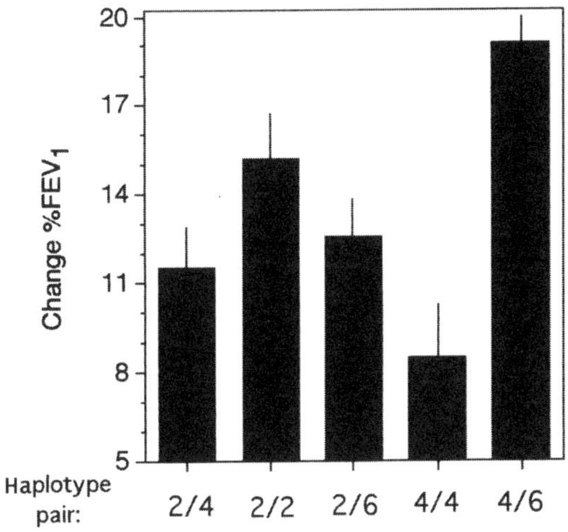

Figure 5 FEV_1 responses by haplotype at the human β_2 adrenoceptor locus (see text for details).

methacholine bronchoconstriction and albuterol bronchodilatation (25). The Gly16 polymorphism was associated with a decreased bronchodilator response to albuterol. Heterozygous individuals had an intermediate response. Neither the 16th or 27th position polymorphism was associated with the constrictive response to methacholine. It should be noted that the Gly16 allele is part of haplotype 2 (Table 2, nucleotide position 46) and is one of the SNPs that differentiates haplotype 2 from haplotype 4. And, in the study by Drysdale et al. (9), haplotype 2 subjects had the greater acute response to albuterol than those with haplotype 4. Lima et al. (26) also reported similar findings of SNPs at amino acid position 16 in adults, and Martinez et al. (27) reported in children. So, despite the various designs of these studies, a differential acute bronchodilator response to albuterol was observed with the same β_2AR genotype, or its analogous haplotype, in asthmatics. These collective data make the case for one of the genetic determinants for the acute response to β-agonists having been found. It should be noted, though, that some studies, which were designed to examine other outcomes or different dosing regimens, have provided data that could be analyzed for an association between the acute response and a β_2AR polymorphism [e.g., Refs. (28–30)]. In some cases no associations were found, but because this was not the primary outcome variable there may be issues of power or other factors that limit the interpretation.

Israel et al. (28) assessed the relationship between tachyphylaxis to the short-acting β-agonist albuterol and the β_2AR polymorphisms at amino acids 16 and 27 in 190 asthmatics. The study was originally designed to ascertain the effects of as needed, compared with regularly scheduled, albuterol in mild asthmatics. As a group, there was no evidence that regularly scheduled albuterol had undesirable physiologic or clinical sequelae (31). However, there was significant interindividual variability in these outcome measurements, which was postulated to be due to the β_2AR polymorphisms. Subsequently, genotyping was carried out on these patients, and the results were stratified by the genotype. The major findings are shown in Figure 6. Changes in peak expiratory flow rates were considered the primary outcome variable. As can be seen, patients who were homozygous for Arg16 and who were administered albuterol on a regular schedule (four times daily) had a progressive decrease in morning and evening peak expiratory flow rates over the course of the study, which continued during the withdrawal period. In contrast, no such changes were observed in the Arg16 homozygotes for patients who used albuterol on an as needed basis. Those with Gly16, even when on regularly scheduled

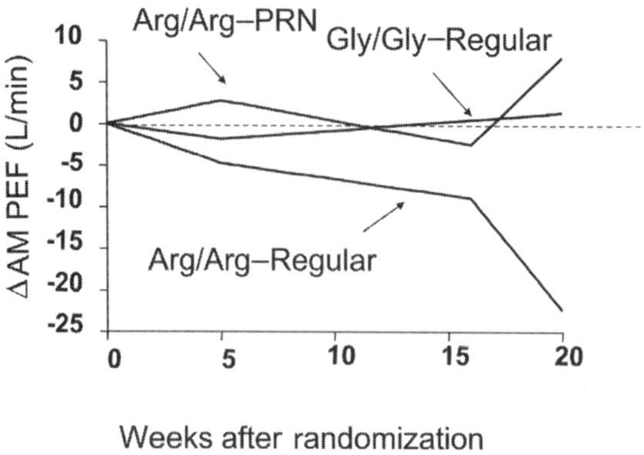

Figure 6 Change in morning peak expiratory flow rate (PEF) in asthmatic subjects homozygous for the human β_2 adrenoceptor Arg 16 or Gly 16 polymorphisms taking either regular or as required albuterol (salbutamol) (see text for details).

albuterol, had no evidence of tachyphylaxis. Taylor et al. (29) genotyped 115 patients for a retrospective study on regularly scheduled albuterol and salmeterol. As shown in Figure 7 the number of major and minor exacerbations was higher in patients on regular albuterol who were homozygous for Arg16 compared with those homozygous

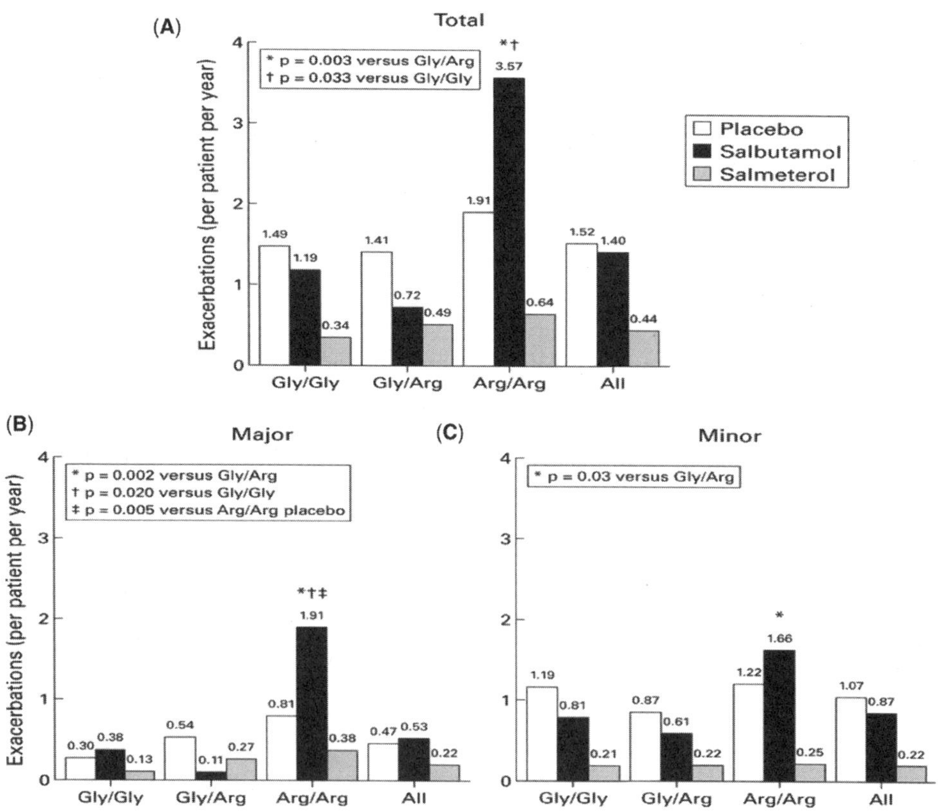

Figure 7 Exacerbations (total, **A**; major, **B**; minor, **C**) of asthma by genotype at codon 16 for the human β_2 adrenoceptor following treatment with placebo, salbutamols or salmeterol (see text for details).

for Gly16. These data are consistent with those of Israel et al. (28) and indicate that for short-acting, regularly administered β-agonists, the Arg16 genotype represents a risk for deleterious physiologic and clinical outcomes. It should be noted that the homozygous Arg16 genotype accounts for ~20% of the asthmatic population in the United States. The number of exacerbations in patients taking salmeterol in this latter study (29) was too low to assess a genotype association. Tan et al. (30) explored the relationship between β_2AR polymorphisms at amino acid position 16 and tachyphylaxis to the long-acting β-agonist, formoterol, in 22 moderately severe asthmatics. These results showed that bronchodilator tachyphylaxis was more prevalent in those with the Gly16 genotype compared with the Arg16 genotype. The discrepancies between this study and the aforementioned studies with albuterol (28,29) may be due to the different properties of the two agonists. Formoterol is a long-acting (~12 hours) near full agonist, whereas albuterol is a short-acting (four to six hours) partial agonist. In contrast to the association between β_2AR genotype and tachyphylaxis to the bronchodilating effects of formoterol, no association was found with the bronchoprotective effect of the agonist against methacholine challenge (32). This has led to the first reasonably sized prospective pharmacogenetic study addressing the potential importance of β_2AR genotype on treatment response (33). In this study Israel et al. (28) extended the observations made in the earlier study described previously by undertaking a prospective study stratified by genotype (the BARGE study): only Arg16 and Gly16 homozygotes were randomized to receive regular or as required albuterol. Again, as seen in the retrospective study, Arg16 homozygotes had worse outcome for all the major endpoints studied, including FEV_1, morning peak expiratory flow rate, relief medication usage, and symptom scores. Taken together, these studies suggest that individuals homozygous for Arg16, or a related haplotype, are less likely to respond as well to regular short-acting β_2AR agonists as the individuals homozygous for Gly16. The critical question regarding the responses of asthmatics with different genotypes at this locus to long-acting agents, such as salmeterol and formoterol, remains to be answered.

In considering the mechanism by which coding β_2AR variants may alter the clinical response to repetitive administration of short-acting agonists, we have considered several scenarios. One is that the SNP at amino acid 16 is in linkage disequilibrium with one or more SNPs in the 5′ or 3′ regions, which defines a haplotype. Although some progress has been made in defining these haplotypes, additional cell and clinical association studies are needed to establish a coherent mechanism. Indeed haplotypes may have unique expression or desensitization/downregulation properties that are yet to be explored in model cell-based systems, such as endogenously expressing human airway smooth muscle cells. It is also quite conceivable that the regulation of β_2AR is under tight dynamic control by both endogenous (epinephrine) and exogenous agonists, such as albuterol. As such, the cell-based downregulation studies, which did not utilize the endogenous promoter and showed that the Gly16 receptor downregulates to a greater extent, may not portray this more complex regulatory scheme. This is illustrated in Figure 8, where the two models, denoted as "static" and "dynamic" regulation, are depicted in a hypothetical physiologic system (34). In the static model, receptor expression is unaffected by circulating epinephrine, and tachyphylaxis is observed in subjects with Gly16 when an exogenous agonist is administered. In the dynamic model, the Gly16 receptor is already downregulated prior to exogenous agonist administration due to its greater propensity to downregulate to chronic epinephrine exposure. Potentially, then, further downregulation of Gly16 does not occur with the agonist, and so little tachyphylaxis is observed. In contrast, Arg16 is not readily downregulated by epinephrine, and so it is in a state to undergo such regulation by the relatively high doses of exogenous agonist administered to the lung. Although these are hypothetical, they do help to

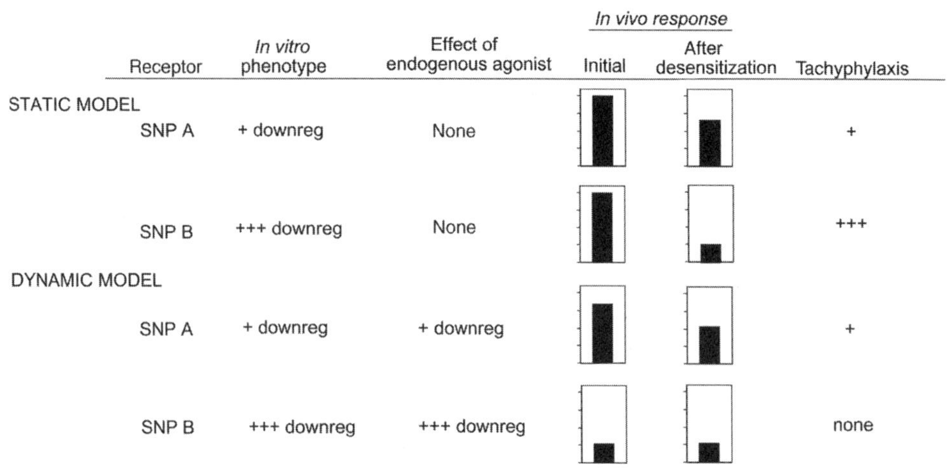

Figure 8 Models for β_2 adrenoceptor regulation by genotype. In the static model (e.g., cells in culture) apparent tachyphylaxis is greatest following agonist exposure for the downregulating genotype. However, in the dynamic model (e.g., in vivo, where tissue is exposed to endogenous catecholamines) apparent tachyphylaxis is greater for the resistant genotype (A). See text for further details.

emphasize the complexity in linking results from cell-based in vitro models to clinical outcome variables.

Taken together, the aforementioned studies suggest that $\beta_2 AR$ SNPs or haplotypes may act to modify drug responses in several ways. Indeed, it is possible that one variant controls one aspect of the response while another is involved in a different aspect. In the case of asthma, different SNPs/haplotypes may regulate baseline lung function, the acute response to short-acting β-agonist, the chronic response to repetitive short-acting β-agonist, and the chronic response to long-acting β-agonists. In addition, other drugs commonly coadministered in treating asthma, such as phosphodiesterase inhibitors, glucocorticoids, or leukotriene receptor antagonists, may further modify receptor expression or function through direct or indirect means by allele-specific mechanisms. Over the next few years these issues will be addressed, as there are numerous ongoing trials. Ultimately, then, a specific genetic $\beta_2 AR$ signature will be available to guide therapy with β-agonists and improve management through genetic testing.

PHARMACOGENETICS OF THEOPHYLLINE

β_2-agonists act by increasing the cAMP content of the cell; control of cAMP breakdown is by tissue phosphodiesterases. Theophylline has been used in the treatment of asthma and COPD for at least 70 years. Theophylline has both bronchodilator and anti-inflammatory properties. The bronchodilator component of the drug action is thought to be at least in part mediated by phosphodiesterase inhibition in airway smooth muscle cells, leading to elevated cAMP levels and hence smooth muscle relaxation. The phosphodiesterase (PDE) 4D subfamily is thought to be the critical family of phosphodiesterases involved in the hydrolysis of cAMP in airway smooth muscle cells and is probably the main target of theophylline. Polymorphism within the *PDE4D* gene could potentially influence theophylline efficacy, but to date no specific gene polymorphisms have been associated with theophylline efficacy or adverse effects in asthma. The development of selective PDE4 inhibitors for the treatment of COPD will lead to increased interest in this subject area.

CYS LEUKOTRIENE RECEPTOR PATHWAY POLYMORPHISM

With the increasing use of Cys leukotriene (LT1) receptor antagonists, such as montelukast, and the realization that not all individuals respond to this class of drugs, there has been considerable attention paid to the possibility that genetic factors may contribute to response to this class of drugs and also to other drugs active in leukotriene synthesis pathways, most notably 5-lipoxygenase (LO) inhibitors.

LTs are important mediators of airway narrowing in asthma. Their actions are mediated through two receptors, CLTR1 and CLTR2: Of these, CLTR1 is the major airway receptor and is responsible for mediating bronchoconstrictor effects. CLTR1 antagonists have been developed for the treatment of asthma, including montelukast and zafirlukast, and in addition there are leukotriene synthesis inhibitors, such as zileuton, which have also shown some clinical efficacy in trials. There are a number of regulatory steps, which control the expression of LTs in airway tissue and which are potentially subject to regulation at the genetic level, that might therefore be of pharmacogenetic interest. These are summarized in the following.

5-Lipoxygenase

5-LO catalyzes the conversion of arachidonic acid to LTA4 (see Fig. 9 for a summary of the LT synthesis pathway). The 5-LO gene (*ALOX5*) maps to chromosome 10q11.2, spans approximately 82 kb and is composed of 14 exons and 13 introns. Mutational analysis of the ALOX5 promoter identified two polymorphisms (−1708 G/A and −1761 G/A) and a

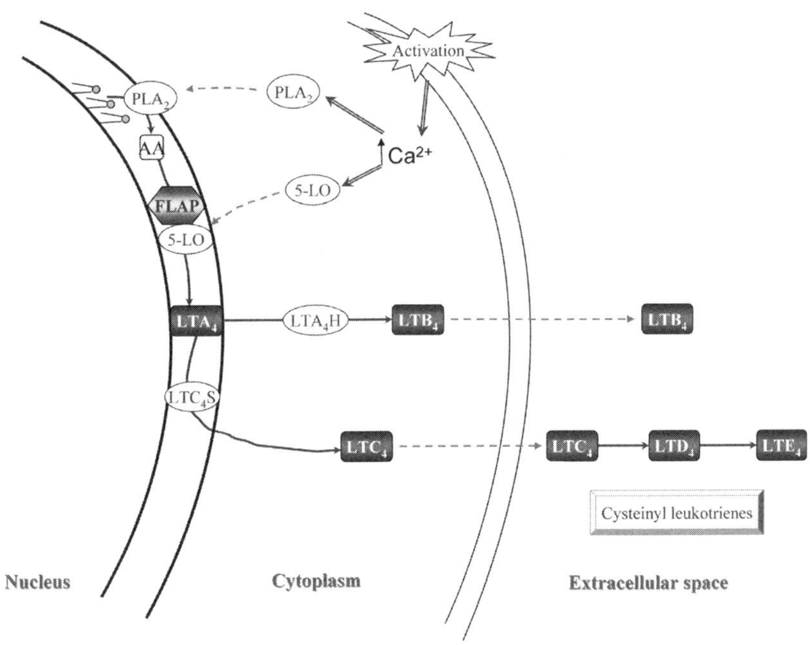

Figure 9 The Cys leukotriene synthesis pathway. Elevation of intracellular calcium activates phospholipase A2 (PLA2) and 5 lipoxygenase (5-LO) via a 5-lipoxygenase activating protein (FLAP) to convert arachidonic acid (AA) to LTA4. LTA4 can be converted via LTA4 hydrolase (LTA4H) to LTB4, or via LTC4 synthase (LTC4S) to LTC4 and hence LTD4 and LTE4. There are multiple potential pharmacogenetic variables which can influence LTD4 synthesis and action, including known SNPs in all the key regulatory enzymes and a promoter repeat sequence in the 5-LO (ALOX5) gene. See text for further details.

series of insertion or deletion mutations within the GC-rich transcription factor binding region at position −147 to −176 bp (35). Mutant alleles at this locus ($n <$ or >5) resulted in reduced Sp1/Erg1 binding and reporter gene transcription assessed by transient promoter-CAT transfections of HeLa cells (35). Subsequently a linear relationship was identified between the number of Sp1/Egr1 motifs and transcriptional activation using a Drosophilia SL2 co-transfection system (36).

Drazen et al. (37) undertook a retrospective analysis of a study involving 221 asthmatics and examined the pharmacogenetic significance of the Sp1/Egr1 polymorphism in determining the response to the novel 5-LO inhibitor ABT-761. In this study subjects possessing only mutant *ALOX5* alleles were relatively resistant to treatment (37). Mean FEV_1 improved by approximately $18.8 \pm 3.6\%$ ($n = 64$) for WT homozygotes and $23.3 \pm 6\%$ ($n = 40$) for heterozygotes, compared with $-1.2 \pm 2.9\%$ ($n = 10$) in individuals homozygous for non-wild-type alleles (37). These data provide proof of the principle that genetic variation in the pathways responsible for regulation of LT synthesis can influence the efficacy of therapeutics targeting the pathway. Subsequently, the role of the Sp1/Egr1 polymorphism in determining responses to the leukotriene receptor antagonists (LTRAs), montelukast, and zafirlukast was evaluated in a retrospective study of 52 asthmatics (38). No pharmacogenetic effect was observed for either bronchodilator response (FEV_1, FEF25-75, PEFR) or bronchoprotection (AMP challenge), however, these data were based on only 40 wild-type homozygotes (5/5) and 12 heterozygotes [5/4 (11) and 5/6 (1)] individuals (38). In summary, therefore, ALOX5 promoter polymorphism may influence the efficacy of 5-LO inhibitors, but the role of the polymorphism in determining the efficacy of CLTR1 antagonists needs further study.

LTC4 Synthase

LTC4 synthase conjugates glutathione with LTA4 to form LTC4, the first cysteinyl-leukotriene in the 5-LO pathway (Fig. 9). The human LTC4 synthase gene (*LTC4S*) consists of five exons, ranging between 71 bp and 257 bp, spans 2.51 kb and has been mapped to chromosome 5q35. *LTC4S* is a candidate gene for aspirin-intolerant asthma (AIA), a subphenotype of the disease in which patients experience cys-LT-dependent adverse respiratory reactions to aspirin and other cyclooxygenase (COX) inhibitors. A fivefold overexpression of LTC4 synthase in bronchial biopsies of AIA patients compared with aspirin-tolerant asthma (ATA) patients was demonstrated in one study; in contrast, no significant differences were observed in other enzymes involved in the biosynthesis of Cys-LTs (39). Subsequently, a −444A/C promoter polymorphism was identified and the C variant allele was found to be more common in the AIA patients, compared with the ATA or the normal subjects (odds ratio 3.9) (40).

A small clinical study examined the role of the −444 polymorphism in severe asthmatics compared with wild-type (AA) controls. In this study, the presence of the C allele resulted in an approximate threefold increase in LTC4 production in isolated blood eosinophils stimulated with calcium ionophore A23187 in the presence of indomethacin. The response to 2-weeks treatment with zafirlukast (20 mg bd) in severe asthmatics was influenced by the −444 A/C polymorphism, with FEV_1 increasing by $9 \pm 12\%$ in individuals with the C allele and decreasing by $-12 \pm 18\%$ in the AA genotype group (41). Although based on small numbers, this suggests a possible pharmacogenetic effect due to this polymorphism at the LTC4S locus.

These data support this hypothesis that the C allele is associated with increased LTC4S levels, increased LT production, and therefore greater benefit following LTRA therapy. Subsequently, these data have been supported by a study of another LTRA, pranlukast (225 mg twice daily, four weeks) in a Japanese cohort of asthmatic subjects ($n = 50$) (42). Carriers of the C allele ($n = 17$) responded better to pranlukast compared with the individuals homozygous for the A allele ($n = 31$) ($14.3 \pm 5.3\%$ vs. $3.1 \pm 2.4\%$ improvement in FEV_1) (42). Similarly, in a study of ATA (43) and AIA (26) patients, the greatest improvements in asthma-related outcomes (morning and evening PEFR, daytime symptom scores) following montelukast treatment (10-mg tablet per day, three weeks) was observed in carriers of the −444C allele (43). These studies provide reasonable evidence that the LTC4S −444A/C promoter polymorphism, which has a frequency of around 0.3 in Caucasians (44), can influence patient responses to a range of LTRAs. The molecular mechanism of this effect remains unclear, however, with conflicting data regarding the functional effects of the −444A/C polymorphism on gene transcription (45) and the finding that other, potentially important promoter polymorphisms are present in the *LTC4S* gene (44). More recently, in a meta-analysis of eight studies examining the efficacy of LTRA to attenuate bronchial hyperresponsiveness, no correlation was observed between the LTC4S −444 polymorphism and clinical outcome (46).

FLAP and the Cys-LT Receptors

Other candidate genes that may influence patient responses to LT modifier drugs include 5-LO activating protein (FLAP) and the cognate receptors for LTD4, CYSLTR1 and -2. FLAP forms a complex with 5-LO, which facilitates the conversion of arachidonic acid to LTA4 (Fig. 9). Promoter polymorphisms within the FLAP gene (*ALOX5AP*) promoter have been identified, including a −336G/A and a CA repeat (47). The cysteinyl-LT receptor 1 (*CYSLT1R*) gene, which encodes for the receptor that is the major drug target of LTRAs, is also a strong candidate gene. The *CYSLT1R* gene is located on chromosome Xq13-q26, and a synonymous coding region polymorphism has been described at position 927C/T (48). The regulatory regions controlling the gene expression have only recently been screened for functional polymorphism (Dourodier and Hall, unpublished data), and the potential contribution of this locus to clinical response remains to be established. Because the gene is situated in the unique region of the X chromosome, it is possible that any pharmacogenetic effects resulting from variation at this locus may show sex-specific features.

GLUCOCORTICOIDS AND TREATMENT RESPONSE

Glucocorticoids remain the mainstay anti-inflammatory agents used in the management of asthma and many other inflammatory lung diseases, including most forms of interstitial lung disease, and moderate and severe COPD. In all these conditions it is clear that response is variable, with some patients responding well to inhaled or oral corticosteroids, and others having little or no response. A number of groups have therefore attempted to identify genetic markers associated with treatment response, initially concentrating on the glucocorticoid receptor itself and more recently expanding to study other potential genes that may modify the responses. In general, these studies are relatively difficult to perform mainly because it is difficult and time consuming to get a good measure of treatment response to glucocorticoids. For example, the degree of response in a condition, such as idiopathic pulmonary fibrosis, will often take weeks or months to become apparent and will also depend on the exact subtype of the disease present defined by high-resolution CT imaging or biopsy. Not all patients will have treatment with the same regimen of steroids, and follow-up may also differ between patient groups, all of which makes assessment of true treatment response more difficult. Again, the majority of studies that have been undertaken in asthma have, in particular, recognized a subgroup of "steroid-resistant" asthmatics, although again adequate phenotypic definition of these patients is difficult and time consuming.

Glucocorticoids bind to a cytoplasmic receptor, the glucocorticoid receptor, which moves to the nucleus and activates steroid-responsive genes containing the glucocorticoid response element (GRE). The receptor exists as at least two splice variants, which differ in the ninth exon. Several polymorphisms have been described in the glucocorticoid receptor (*GR*) gene, which produce functional consequences; for example, a Val641Asp polymorphism influences the binding affinity for dexamethasone (49), a Val729Ile polymorphism confers a fourfold decrease in dexamethasone activity (50), a Asn363Ser polymorphism is associated with higher sensitivity to dexamethasone (51), and 2314insA and S651F variants have suppressed GR mRNA and protein levels in a recombinant system (52). However, several of these polymorphisms are rare and their functional significance at a clinical level is unclear. Subsequently, haplotype identification across the *GR* gene identified a susceptibility haplotype associated with a lower response to dexamethasone using a suppression test in 216 U.K. Caucasians (53).

Recently, sequence variation in the corticotrophin-releasing hormone receptor 1 (*CRHR1*) gene was found to be associated with enhanced response to therapy in three asthmatic cohorts ($n = 1117$, endpoint percent change in FEV_1 following eight weeks inhaled corticosteroid treatment) (54). The CRHR1 is thought to be involved in the regulation of endogenous levels of corticosteroid and, therefore, may be predicted to influence responses to exogenously administered corticosteroid. This study is the only study to show a pharmacogenetic effect for steroid efficacy in an asthmatic cohort and involved the analysis of 131 SNPs in 14 genes prior to the identification of the positive association described previously (54).

PHARMACOGENETICS OF MUSCARINIC RECEPTOR ANTAGONISTS

Anticholinergic agents have shown efficacy in the treatment of chronic airway obstruction and have shown utility in the treatment of asthma. The M2 and M3 muscarinic receptor genes provide rational candidate genes, which might alter responses to muscarinic receptor antagonists. The M2 receptor gene (*CHRM2*) is located on chromosome 7q35-36 and several polymorphisms have been described within the *CHRM2* gene, including two degenerate SNPs (1197T/C Thr-Thr, 976A/C Arg-Arg), a 3′ UTR (1696T/A) SNP (55) and a CA repeat and C/A SNP in the promoter region (56). Functional effects have been described with different alleles of the promoter CA repeat in transfection studies, but no clinical studies have been performed to date. The M3 receptor gene (*CHRM3*) is located on chromosome 1q41-q44, and the coding region is contained within one exon. Several polymorphisms have been described including: −708A/G, −627G/C, −513C/A, 492C/T, a CTTT repeat, and a GT repeat (57). Functional data are not currently available on these polymorphisms. In summary, therefore, the significance of individual polymorphism or haplotypes in determining the efficacy of anticholinergic therapy remains to be resolved. These genes are also likely to be of interest outside the area of respiratory disease, for example, in CNS disorders including endogenous depression.

SUMMARY

It is clear from these details that pharmacogenetics has considerable potential in the management of patients with a range of airway diseases and, in particular, in diseases, such as

COPD and asthma, that are characterized by either fixed or variable airflow obstruction, and it is likely that the cost-effectiveness of these approaches will be assessed in the near future. Increasing knowledge of the extent to which genetic factors can be used to identify subgroups of patients should lead both to better use of existing medication, and potentially through pharmacogenomic approaches to novel treatments for the management of these conditions.

REFERENCES

1. Drazen JM, Silverman EK, Lee TH. Heterogeneity of therapeutic responses in asthma. Br Med Bull 2000; 56(4):1054–1070.
2. Sears MR. Role of β-agonists in asthma fatalities. In: Sheffer AL, ed. Fatal Asthma. New York: Marcel Dekker, Inc., 1998:457–481.
3. Burgess CD, Beasley R, Crane J, Pearce N. Adverse effects of beta$_2$-agonists. In: Pauwels R, O'Byrne PM, eds. Beta$_2$-Agonists in Asthma Treatment. New York: Marcel Dekker, Inc., 1997:257–282.
4. McGraw DW, Almoosa KF, Paul RJ, Kobilka BK, Liggett SB. Antithetic regulation by β-adrenergic receptors of Gq-receptor signaling via phospholipase-C underlies the airway β-agonist paradox. J Clin Invest (in press).
5. Reihsaus E, Innis M, MacIntyre N, Liggett SB. Mutations in the gene encoding for the β_2-adrenergic receptor in normal and asthmatic subjects. Am J Resp Cell Mol Biol 1993; 8:334–339.
6. Green SA, Cole G, Jacinto M, Innis M, Liggett SB. A polymorphism of the human β_2-adrenergic receptor within the fourth transmembrane domain alters ligand binding and functional properties of the receptor. J Biol Chem 1993; 268:23116–23121.
7. Green S, Turki J, Innis M, Liggett SB. Amino-terminal polymorphisms of the human β_2-adrenergic receptor impart distinct agonist-promoted regulatory properties. Biochem 1994; 33:9414–9419.
8. Green SA, Turki J, Bejarano P, Hall IP, Liggett SB. Influence of β_2-adrenergic receptor genotypes on signal transduction in human airway smooth muscle cells. Am J Resp Cell Mol Biol 1995; 13:25–33.
9. Drysdale CM, McGraw DW, Stack CB, Stephens JC, Judson RS, Nandabalan K, Arnold K, Ruano G, Liggett SB. Complex promoter and coding region β_2-adrenergic receptor haplotypes alter receptor expression and predict in vivo responsiveness. Proc Natl Acad Sci USA 2000; 97:10483–10488.
10. Green SA, Rathz DA, Schuster AJ, Liggett SB. The Ile164 β_2-adrenoceptor polymorphism alters salmeterol exosite binding and conventional agonist coupling to G_s. Eur J Pharmacol 2001; 421:141–147.
11. Scott MGH, Swan C, Wheatley AP, Hall IP. Identification of novel polymorphisms within the promoter region of the human beta2 adrenergic receptor gene. Br J Pharmacol 1999; 126(4):841–844.
12. Collins S, Bouvier M, Bolanowski MA, Caron MG, Lefkowitz RJ. cAMP stimulates transcription of the β_2-adrenergic receptor gene in response to short-term agonist exposure. Proc Natl Acad Sci USA 1989; 86(13):4853–4857.
13. Cornett LE, Hiller FC, Jacobi SE, Cao W, McGraw DW. Identification of a glucocorticoid response element in the rat β_2-adrenergic receptor gene. Mol Pharmacol 1998; 54:1016–1023.
14. McGraw DW, Forbes SL, Kramer LA, Liggett SB. Polymorphisms of the 5′ leader cistron of the human β_2-adrenergic receptor regulate receptor expression. J Clin Invest 1998; 102:1927–1932.
15. Small KM, Tanguay DA, Nandabalan K, Zhan P, Stephens JC, Liggett SB. Gene and protein domain-specific patterns of genetic variability within the G-protein coupled receptor superfamily. Am J Pharmacogenomics 2003; 3(1):65–71.

16. Stephens JC, Schneider JA, Tanguay DA, Choi J, Acharya T, Stanley SE, Jiang R, Messer CJ, Chew A, Han J-H, Duan J, Carr JL, Lee MS, Koshy B, Kumar AM, Zhang G, Newell WR, Windemuth A, Xu C, Kalbfleisch TS, Shaner SL, Arnold K, Schulz V, Drysdale CM, Nandabalan K, Judson RS, Ruano G, Vovis GF. Haplotype variation and linkage disequilibrium in 313 human genes. Science 2001; 293:489–493.
17. Johnatty SE, Abdellatif M, Shimmin L, Clark RB, Boerwinkle E. β_2 adrenergic receptor 5′ haplotypes influence promoter activity. Br J Pharmacol 2002; 137:1213–1216.
18. Lipworth B, Koppelman GH, Wheatley AP, Le Jeune I, Coutie W, Meurs H, Kauffman HF, Postma DS, Hall IP. β_2 adrenoceptor promoter polymorphisms: extended haplotypes and functional effects in peripheral blood mononuclear cells. Thorax 2002; 57:61–66.
19. Weir TD, Mallek N, Sandford AJ, Bai TR, Awadh N, FitzGerald JM, Cockcroft D, James A, Liggett SB, Pare PD. β_2 adrenergic receptor haplotypes in mild, moderate and fatal/near fatal asthma. Am J Respir Crit Care Med 1998; 158:787–791.
20. Holloway JW, Dunbar PR, Riley GA, Sawyer GM, Fitzharris PF, Pearce N, Le Gros GS, Beasley R. Association of beta2-adrenergic receptor polymorphisms with severe asthma. Clin Exp Allergy 2000; 30(8):1097–1103.
21. Ramsay CE, Hayden CM, Tiller KJ, Burton PR, Goldblatt J, LeSouef PN. Polymorphisms in the beta2-adrenoceptor gene are associated with decreased airway responsiveness. Clin Exp Allergy 1999; 29(9):1151–1154.
22. Ulbrecht M, Hergeth MT, Wjst M, Heinrich J, Bickeböller H, Wichmann H-E, Weiss EH. Association of β_2-adrenoceptor variants with bronchial hyperresponsiveness. Am J Respir Crit Care Med 2000; 161:469–474.
23. Dewar JC, Wilkinson J, Wheatley A, Thomas NS, Doull I, Morton N, Lio P, Harvey J, Liggett SB, Holgate IS, Hall IP. The glutamine 27 β_2 adrenoceptor polymorphism is associated with elevated immunoglobulin E levels in asthmatic families. J Allergy Clin Immunol 1997; 100:261–265.
24. Turki J, Pak J, Green S, Martin R, Liggett SB. Genetic polymorphisms of the β_2-adrenergic receptor in nocturnal and non-nocturnal asthma: evidence that Gly16 correlates with the nocturnal phenotype. J Clin Invest 1995; 95:1635–1641.
25. Kotani Y, Nishimura Y, Maeda H, Yokoyama M. Beta2-adrenergic receptor polymorphisms affect airway responsiveness to salbutamol in asthmatics. J Asthma 1999; 36(7):583–590.
26. Lima JJ, Thomason DB, Mohamed MHN, Eberle LV, Self TH, Johnson JA. Pharmacodynamics and drug action: impact of genetic polymorphisms of the β_2-adrenergic receptor on albuterol bronchodilator pharmacodynamics. Clin Pharmacol Ther 1999; 65:519–525.
27. Martinez FD, Graves PE, Baldini M, Solomon S, Erickson R. Association between genetic polymorphisms of the beta2-adrenoceptor and response to albuterol in children with and without a history of wheezing. J Clin Invest 1997; 100(12):3184–3188.
28. Israel E, Drazen JM, Liggett SB, Boushey HA, Cherniack RM, Chinchilli VM, Cooper DM, Fahy JV, Fish JE, Ford JG, Kraft M, Kunselman S, Lazarus SC, Lemanske RF, Martin RJ, McLean DE, Peters SP, Silverman EK, Sorkness CA, Szefler SJ, Weiss ST, Yandava CN. The effect of polymorphisms of the β_2-adrenergic receptor on the response to regular use of albuterol in asthma. Am J Respir Crit Care Med 2000; 162(1):75–80.
29. Taylor DR, Drazen JM, Herbison GP, Yandava CN, Hancox RJ, Town GI. Asthma exacerbations during long term β agonist use: influence of β_2 adrenoceptor polymorphism. Thorax 2000; 55:762–767.
30. Tan S, Hall IP, Dewar J, Dow E, Lipworth B. Association between beta 2-adrenoceptor polymorphism and susceptibility to bronchodilator desensitisation in moderately severe stable asthmatics. Lancet 1997; 350(9083):995–999.
31. Drazen JM, Israel E, Boushey HA, Chinchilli VM, Fahy JV, Fish JE, Lazarus SC, Lemanske RF, Martin RJ, Peters SP, Sorkness C, Szefler SJ. Comparison of regularly scheduled with as-needed use of albuterol in mild asthma. N Engl J Med 1996; 335(12):841–847.

32. Lipworth BJ, Hall IP, Tan S, Aziz I, Coutie W. Effects of genetic polymorphism on ex vivo and in vivo function of β_2-adrenoceptors in asthmatic patients. Chest 1999; 115:324–328.
33. Liggett SB. Polymorphisms of the β_2-adrenergic receptor. N Engl J Med 2002; 346(7): 536–538.
34. Israel E, Chinchilli VM, Ford JG, et al. Use of regularly scheduled albuterol in asthma: genotype-stratified, randomized, placebo controlled trial. Lancet 2004; 364:1505–1512.
35. In KH, Asano K, Beier D. Naturally occurring mutations in the human 5-lipoxygenase gene promoter that modify transcription factor binding and reporter gene transcription. J Clin Invest 1997; 99:1130–1137.
36. Silverman ES, Du J, De Sanctis GT. Egr-1 and Sp1 interact functionally with the 5-lipoxygenase promoter and its naturally occurring mutants. Am J Respir Cell Mol Biol 1998; 19: 316–323.
37. Drazen JM, Yandava CN, Dube L. Pharmacogenetic association between ALOX5 promoter genotype and the response to anti-asthma treatment. Nat Genet 1999; 22:168–170.
38. Fowler SJ, Hall IP, Wilson AM. 5-Lipoxygenase polymorphism and in-vivo response to leukotriene receptor antagonists. Eur J Clin Pharmacol 2002; 58:187–190.
39. Sampson AP, Cowburn AS, Sladek K. Profound overexpression of leukotriene C4 synthase in bronchial biopsies from aspirin-intolerant asthmatic patients. Int Arch Allergy Immunol 1997; 113:355–357.
40. Sanak M, Simon HU, Szczeklik A. Leukotriene C4 synthase promoter polymorphism and risk of aspirin-induced asthma [letter]. Lancet 1997; 350:1599–1600.
41. Sampson AP, Siddiqui S, Buchanan D. Variant LTC(4) synthase allele modifies cysteinyl leukotriene synthesis in eosinophils and predicts clinical response to zafirlukast. Thorax 2000; 55(suppl 2):S28–S31.
42. Asano K, Shiomi T, Hasegawa N. Leukotriene C4 synthase gene A(−444)C polymorphism and clinical response to a CYS-LT(1) antagonist, pranlukast, in Japanese patients with moderate asthma. Pharmacogenetics 2002; 12:565–570.
43. Mastalerz L, Nizankowska E, Sanak M. Clinical and genetic features underlying the response of patients with bronchial asthma to treatment with a leukotriene receptor antagonist. Eur J Clin Invest 2002; 32:949–955.
44. Sayers I, Barton S, Rorke S. Allelic association and functional studies of promoter polymorphism in the leukotriene C4 synthase gene (LTC4S) in asthma. Thorax 2003; 58:417–424.
45. Sayers I, Sampson A. Genetic regulation of leukotriene production and activity. In: Holgate ST, ed. The Hereditary Basis of Allergic Diseases. Blackwell, 2002:137–166.
46. Currie GP, Lima JJ, Sylvester JE. Leukotriene C4 synthase polymorphisms and responsiveness to leukotriene antagonists in asthma. Br J Clin Pharmacol 2003; 56:422–426.
47. Sayers I, Barton S, Rorke S. Promoter polymorphism in the 5-lipoxygenase (ALOX5) and 5-lipoxygenase-activating protein (ALOX5AP) genes and asthma susceptibility in a Caucasian population. Clin Exp Allergy 2003; 33:1103–1110.
48. Choi JH, Park HS, Oh HB. Leukotriene-related gene polymorphisms in ASA-intolerant asthma: an association with a haplotype of 5-lipoxygenase. Hum Genet 2004; 114:337–344.
49. Hurley DM, Accili D, Stratakis CA. Point mutation causing a single amino acid substitution in the hormone binding domain of the glucocorticoid receptor in familial glucocorticoid resistance. J Clin Invest 1991; 87:680–686.
50. Malchoff DM, Brufsky A, Reardon G. A mutation of the glucocorticoid receptor in primary cortisol resistance. J Clin Invest 1993; 91:1918–1925.
51. Huizenga NA, Koper JW, De Lange P. A polymorphism in the glucocorticoid receptor gene may be associated with and increased sensitivity to glucocorticoids in vivo. J Clin Endocrinol Metab 1998; 83:144–151.
52. Koyano S, Saito Y, Nagano M. Functional analysis of three genetic polymorphisms in the glucocorticoid receptor gene. J Pharmacol Exp Ther 2003; 307:110–116.
53. Stevens A, Ray DW, Zeggini E. Glucocorticoid sensitivity is determined by a specific glucocorticoid receptor haplotype. J Clin Endocrinol Metab 2004; 89:892–897.

54. Tantisira KG, Lake S, Silverman ES. Corticosteroid pharmacogenetics: association of sequence variants in CRHR1 with improved lung function in asthmatics treated with inhaled corticosteroids. Hum Mol Genet 2004; 13:1353–1359.
55. Fenech AG, Ebejer MJ, Felice AE. Mutation screening of the muscarinic M(2) and M(3) receptor genes in normal and asthmatic subjects. Br J Pharmacol 2001; 133:43–48.
56. Fenech AG, Billington CK, Swan C. Novel polymorphisms influencing transcription of the human CHRM2 gene in airway smooth muscle. Am J Respir Cell Mol Biol 2004; 30:678–686.
57. Donfack J, Kogut P, Forsythe S. Sequence variation in the promoter region of the cholinergic receptor muscarinic 3 gene and asthma and atopy. J Allergy Clin Immunol 2003; 111: 527–532.

7
Hematological Pharmacogenetics

Howard L. McLeod[a], **Charles Eby**[a], **and Brian Gage**[a]
Department of Medicine, Washington University School of Medicine, Saint Louis, Missouri, U.S.A.

INTRODUCTION

The hematopoietic system is critical for the viability of the human body. Erythrocytes play the major role in tissue oxygenation, platelets keep the vasculature intact, and white cells are a primary line of defense against infectious pathogens, among their other roles. In addition, the hematopoietic system is an important component of many common diseases, including cardiovascular, central nervous system (CNS), renal, and cancer. Major advances in the treatment of hematologic disorders have resulted from the recent revolution in medical interventions. However, significant heterogeneity in the efficacy and toxicity of drugs is consistently observed across the human population (1). Administration of the same dose of a given drug to a population of patients results in a range of toxicity, from unaffected to lethal events (2,3). Although many clinical variables have been associated with drug response (age, gender, diet, organ function, disease biology), genetic differences in drug disposition and drug targets can have a great impact on treatment outcome (1,4,5). The metabolic enzymes and cellular targets for the majority of chemotherapeutic agents contain genetic polymorphisms (6), but prospective identification of patients likely to benefit from (or be harmed by) chemotherapy is not currently possible for most treatments. This is particularly important in the current health care environment, where cost containment and evidence-based initiatives are having a significant influence on patient care.

Pharmacogenomics is the study of how genetic inheritance influences response to drugs. A greater understanding of the genetic determinants of drug response has the potential to revolutionize the use of many medications, particularly in the challenging field of oncology. By increasing our ability to prospectively identify patients at risk for severe toxicity, or those likely to benefit from a particular treatment, pharmacogenomics promises to help us move toward the ultimate goal of individualized cancer therapy. This chapter will discuss distinct clinically relevant examples of hematologic pharmacogenetics.

[a]The authors are supported in part by National Institutes of Health grants GM63340, R01HL074724, and R01HL071083.

WARFARIN PHARMACOGENETICS

Vitamin K antagonists have been used for more than 50 years to prevent the formation and extension of thrombosis. In the North America, warfarin is the most commonly prescribed vitamin K antagonist. In other continents, acenocoumarol, anisindione, dicumarol, and phenprocoumon are also prescribed. Although the half-lives and relative potency of these compounds differ, their chemical structure, mechanism of action, and need for monitoring are similar to that of warfarin.

Pharmacology of Warfarin

After oral administration, warfarin is completely absorbed, and then 99% of it is bound to albumin in the plasma. Warfarin, which is free, is taken up by the liver where it is biologically active and metabolized by the cytochrome P450 complex (CYP2C9). Commercially available warfarin (Coumadin™ and others) is a racemic mixture with each of the two enantiomers having its own route of metabolism (Fig. 1). The *S*-enantiomer is converted to 6- and 7-hydroxywarfarin by CYP2C9 and eventually excreted in the bile, whereas the *R*-enantiomer is metabolized by CYP1A1, CYP1A2, and CYP3A4 to an inactive alcohol that is excreted in the urine (7). The *S*-enantiomer more strongly blocks the regeneration of the reduced form of vitamin K, thereby interfering with the vitamin K-dependent carboxylation of glutamic acid residues on coagulation factors prothrombin II, VII, IX, and X. Although warfarin also inhibits the synthesis of the anticoagulant proteins C, S, and Z, its pharmacologic effect is inhibition of the synthesis of functional clotting factors.

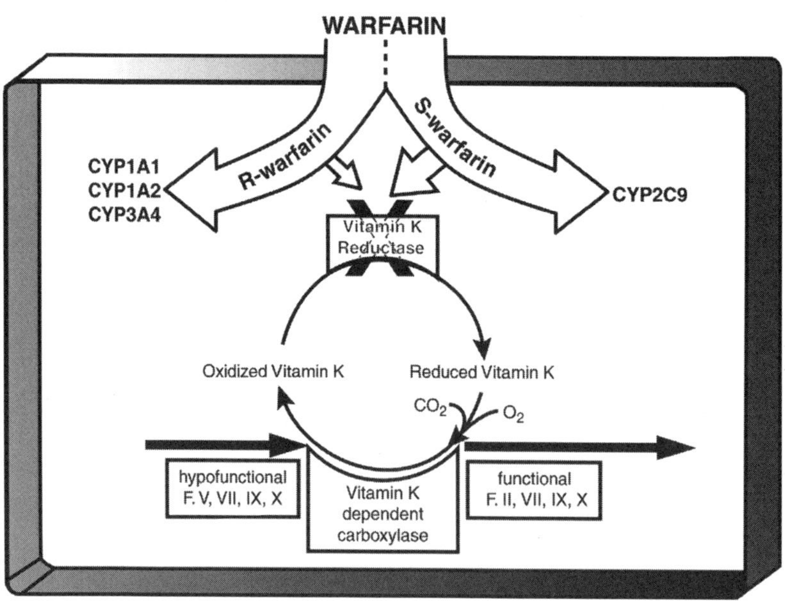

Figure 1 After oral absorption, warfarin is transported to the liver, where CYP1A1, CYP1A2, and CYP3A4 metabolize the *R*-enantiomer and CYP2C9 metabolizes the more potent *S*-enantiomer. By impairing the regeneration of the reduced form of vitamin K, *R*- and *S*-warfarin interfere with the vitamin K–dependent carboxylation of clotting factors prothrombin VII, IX, and X.

Stereo-Specific Metabolism of Warfarin

In patients who are homozygous for the wild-type allele of (CYP2C9*1), *S*-warfarin is cleared normally, resulting in a modest elevation of the international normalized ratio (INR). In contrast, patients with specific single-nucleotide polymorphisms (SNPs) in this enzyme (e.g., CYP2C9*2 or CYP2C9*3) have slow clearance of *S*-warfarin (8) and an exaggerated INR elevation during warfarin induction (9,10) (Table 1).

Pharmacogenetic Determinants of Warfarin Metabolism

In vivo, these SNPs are associated with increased responsiveness to warfarin (9,11–15). Aithal et al. (11) compared controls who required typical warfarin doses to patients whose therapeutic warfarin dose was $\leq$10.5 mg/wk. Patients requiring low doses were more likely to have a supratherapeutic INR at the time of warfarin induction and six times more likely to have the CYP2C9*2 or CYP2C9*3 SNPs (9,11). Others found that CYP2C9*3 decreased the selectivity of CYP2C9 for *S*-warfarin and that amino acid residue 359 is a component of the warfarin-binding site (16,17).

Increased Risk of Hemorrhage with CYP2C9*2 or CYP2C9*3 SNPs

Recent studies suggest that the CYP2C9*2 and CYP2C9*3 variants are associated with hemorrhage during warfarin induction but not during maintenance therapy. In their retrospective cohort of 180 patients who were given warfarin, Margaglione et al. (10) found that the odds of bleeding was increased 2.6-fold in patients with the CYP2C9*2 and/or the CYP2C9*3 SNPs than in the carriers of the wild type. They also found a statistical interaction between these variants and the presence of a local bleeding source, but the etiology and significance of that interaction are unclear. In their retrospective cohort of 185 patients who were given warfarin, Higashi et al. (9) found a 2.4-fold increased risk of hemorrhage among patients with either of the two variant alleles. In contrast to these two positive studies, Taube et al. (18) found no association between CYP2C9 genotype and bleeding in 561 patients who were taking warfarin for more than 2 months. The most likely explanation for the association between genotype and bleeding is that patients with the CYP2C9*2 and/or the CYP2C9*3 SNPs metabolize warfarin more slowly than wild-type patients and, therefore are more likely to be overdosed when beginning warfarin with a traditional dose. Indeed, Aithal et al. (11) found that patients who required tiny doses of warfarin ($\leq$1.5 mg/day) were six times more likely to have the CYP2C9*2 and/or CYP2C9*3 SNPs and four times more likely to bleed during warfarin induction.

Table 1 Cytochrome P450 2C9 SNPs that Are Known to Affect Warfarin Metabolism

Designation	Protein change	SNP	Effect on warfarin dose	Allele frequency[a]	References
CYP2C9*1	None	None	Referent	81.5–93%	
CYP2C9*2	Arg144Cys	*C430T*	−14% to −20%	5.6–12.8%	(8,10,12,18,19)
CYP2C9*3	Ile359Leu	A1061C	−21% to −49%	1.4–5.7%	(10,12,18,19)

[a]CYP2C9*2 and *3 are most common in white populations.
Abbreviations: SNP, single-nucleotide polymorphism; CYP2C9*1, wild-type allele.

Promise of Combining Genetic and Clinical Factors to Prevent Bleeding During Warfarin Induction

The associations between genotype, warfarin dose, and hemorrhage during warfarin induction suggest that tailoring the initial warfarin dose based on CYP2C9 genotype might avoid iatrogenic hemorrhages. Several investigators have combined clinical and pharmacogenetic information to estimate the maintenance warfarin dose (Table 2). Loebstein et al. (19) found that the maintenance warfarin dose was correlated with plasma warfarin levels and body surface area (BSA) and inversely correlated with CYP2C9 SNPs, age, and amiodarone use. Tabrizi et al. (14) found that warfarin dose was correlated with weight and inversely correlated with CYP2C9 SNPs and age. Gage et al. (12) found that warfarin dose was correlated with BSA, race, and target INR value and inversely correlated with age and use of amiodarone or simvastatin. Although these studies correlated the maintenance warfarin dose to genotype retrospectively, once validated they can be used to estimate the warfarin prospectively.

Newly Discovered CYP2C9 SNPs Also May Slow Warfarin Metabolism

While genotyping 32 Japanese patients who were slow metabolizers of phenytoin, Imai et al. (20) found a new polymorphism designated as CYP2C9*4: a T1076C transversion that leads to an Ile359Thr substitution. This mutation was not present in 100 unselected Japanese volunteers. The effect on warfarin metabolism is unknown, but because it alters the same amino acid (359) similar to the 2C9*3 mutation, it could decrease the metabolism of *S*-warfarin. Dickman et al. (21) found a C1080G transversion that leads to an Asp360Glu substitution. They found this mutation, CYP2C9*5, in four out of 120 African American participants and in zero of out 140 European American participants. The intrinsic clearance (V_{max}/K_m) was estimated as 8% of that of the wild type, suggesting that carriers of CYP2C9*5 will eliminate *S*-warfarin more slowly than non-carriers. Kidd et al. (22) reported a null polymorphism, 818delA, which they named CYP2C9*6. The patient presented with an overdose of phenytoin (an anticonvulsant that is metabolized by CYP2C9) and was found to have a phenytoin clearance that was only 17% of the normal. Finally, in a cohort of 89 Chinese patients who were prescribed warfarin, Leung et al. (23) found several CYP2C9 SNPs in exon 4. The Leu208Val variant was relatively common in this population and was associated with a decreased warfarin dose.

Table 2 Independent Predictors of Warfarin Dose in Three Studies

Variable	Reference 19	Reference 14	Reference 12
Model R^2	35%	26%	38%
Sample size	156	153	297
Age, yr	*	*	*
BSA, m^2	*	Not examined	*
2C9*3, per allele	*	*	*
2C9*2, per allele	*	*	*
Target INR	Not examined	Not examined	*
Amiodarone	*	Not examined	*
Dietary vitamin K	NS	Not examined	NS

*Statistically significant, $p < 0.05$.
Abbreviations: R^2, percent of variability explained by the model; BSA, body surface area; NS, not significant; INR, international normalized ratio.

Table 3 New Cytochrome P450 2C9 SNPs that May Affect Warfarin Metabolism

Designation	Protein change	SNP	Effect on warfarin dose	References
CYP2C9*4	Ile359Thr	T1076C	Not examined	(20)
CYP2C9*5	Asp360Glu	C1080G	Not examined	(21)
CYP2C9*6	Null allele	818delA	Not examined	(22)
Unnamed	Tyr358Cys	G1061A	Not examined	(30)

Abbreviation: SNP, single-nucleotide polymorphism.

However, more recent studies suggest that these apparent variants are actually results from PCR amplification of a pseudogene and are not likely to be of functional relevance. In summary, further research is needed to determine if these new CYP2C9 SNPs (Table 3) affect warfarin metabolism significantly.

Long-Term Clinical and Laboratory Outcomes with CYP2C9 SNPs

Two studies have found an association between bleeding during warfarin induction and the presence of the CYP2C9*2 and CYP2C9*3 SNPs (9,10). In contrast, Taube et al. (18) found no association between these SNPs and either INR control stability or risk of excessive anticoagulation during long-term treatment. Thus, it seems likely that CYP2C9 genotype (and clinical factors) could be used to estimate the maintenance a priori but that genotyping would not be very helpful in patients who have already found their maintenance dose empirically.

Warfarin Resistance

The widespread use of blood anticoagulants as rodenticides have selected for warfarin resistance in the mouse (24) and rat (25–27). In rodents, warfarin resistance (denoted as *Rw* in the rat) is inherited as a single autosomal gene with dominant effect. Kohn and Pelz (26) have placed Rw in relation to several positionally mapped gene-anchored microsatellite loci in the rat genome, but the gene is yet to be identified.

Case reports have identified warfarin resistance in humans with transmission that also appears to be autosomal dominant (28). The high plasma levels of warfarin observed in these patients, suggest that the resistance has a pharmacodynamic basis, rather than a pharmacokinetic one. Kohn and Pelz (26) identified homologous regions to Rw on human chromosomes 10q25.3-26, 12q23-q24.3, and 16p13.1-p11 and use positional cloning to identify the putative gene. Once the human gene for warfarin resistance is identified and validated, then it could be used to identify rare patients who have warfarin resistance and who require unusually large warfarin doses to elevate their INR value.

The Future of Oral Anticoagulants

Eventually, safer drugs with a wider therapeutic index may supplant warfarin. For example, ximelagatran is an oral thrombin inhibitor that may be a safe and effective alternative to warfarin therapy, at least for patients undergoing knee arthroplasty who have no preexisting liver disease (29). However, until the safety and effectiveness of newer anticoagulants is clear, warfarin and other vitamin K anticoagulants will be used extensively. The hypothesis that pharmacogenetic-based dosing will prevent iatrogenic hemorrhages during warfarin induction should be tested prospectively.

GENETIC POLYMORPHISMS IN HEMOSTATIC SYSTEMS

Multiple cellular and protein activation pathways are involved in formation, and subsequent remodeling, of a hemostatic plug at the site of a vascular injury (Fig. 2). Hemostasis protein levels vary widely in healthy populations, with typical reference ranges of 60% to 160% of the mean. Estimates of the genetic contribution to the observed variation for different proteins range from 22% to 55%, representing the largest identifiable determinant (31). ABO blood type is a major determinant of both von Willebrandfactor (vWF) (32), and factor VIII levels. However, even after adjusting for blood type, there is a genetic component to factor VIII levels that is not associated with polymorphisms within the factor VIII gene (33). It is likely that multiple genes are involved in the regulation of expression of most hemostatic proteins. Environmental factors and gene–environment interactions also contribute to hemostatic protein variability. Factor VIII and vWF levels rise during pregnancy and acute stress, and factor VII

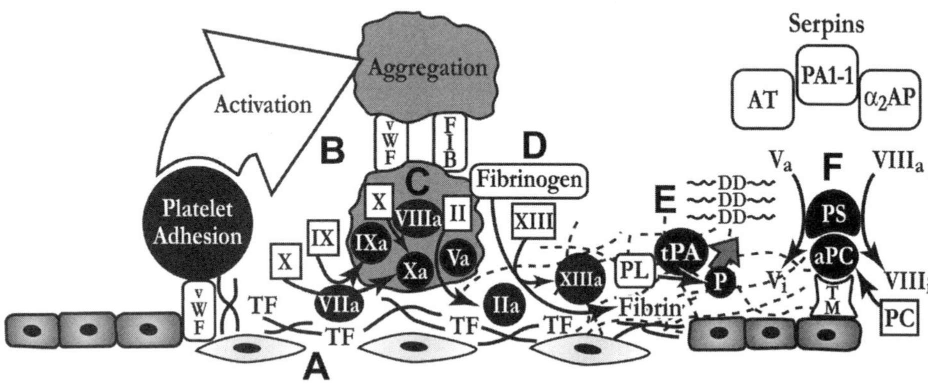

Figure 2 Formation of a hemostatic plug. (**A**) Vascular injury: Endothelial disruption exposes blood to subendothelial collagen (~), vWF, and TF. (**B**) Primary hemostasis: Circulating platelets adhere to collagen and vWF via specific surface receptor complexes and undergo activation and release of prothrombotic granule contents. Conformational changes in the platelet surface integrin glycoprotein IIbIIIa permit fibrinogen (FIB) and vWF-dependent aggregation of activated platelets. (**C**) Secondary hemostasis: TF accelerates activation of factor VII to VIIa, which converts factor X to Xa and factor IX to IXa. The phospholipid surface of activated platelets is the primary site of subsequent coagulation factor activation. Factors IXa and VIIIa activate factor X and factors Xa and Va convert Prothrombin (factor II) to thrombin (factor IIa). Sustained thrombin generation requires factor IIa activation of nonenzymatic cofactors V and VIII to accelerate activation of factors X and factor II. (**D**) Fibrin clot formation: Factor IIa converts fibrinogen to fibrin through distal amino terminal cleavages of alpha- and beta-chains. Fibrin molecules spontaneously polymerize and are covalently cross-linked by factor XIIIa, a thrombin-activated transglutaminase. (**E**) Fibrinolysis: PL binds to fibrin molecules during polymerization. tPA, released from endothelial cells, enters the fibrin clot and activates PL to P. Plasmin degrades fibrin into FDP. (**F**) Inhibitors: Thrombin generation and fibrinolysis are highly regulated processes. The major direct inhibitor of thrombin is AT, a member of the serine protease inhibitor (serpin) family. Factors Va and VIIIa are degraded by aPC and its cofactor, PS. When bound to TM, an endothelial surface protein, factor IIa activates PC to aPC. When not bound to fibrin, tPA and plasmin are rapidly inhibited by the serpin PAI-1 and α_2AP, respectively. *Abbreviations*: vWF, von Willebrand factor; TF, tissue factor; PL, plasminogen; tPA, tissue plasminogen activator; P, plasmin; FDP, fibrin degradation products; AT, antithrombin; aPC, activated protein C; TM, thrombomodulin; PS, protein S; PC, protein C; PAI-1, plasminogen activator inhibitor-1; α_2AP, alpha-2 antiplasmin.

levels decline with the lowering of plasma lipoproteins. Fibrinogen levels also rise in response to stress. However, a polymorphism in the fibrinogen beta-chain promoter is associated with a greater change in fibrinogen concentration after physical exertion compared with the wild type (34).

The most overt clinical expression of monogenetic mutations affecting hemostasis occurs in hemophilia, a congenital bleeding disorder due to deficiency of a single clotting factor. The most common types are hemophilia A and B, characterized by sex-linked inherited deficiencies of factor VIII and IX, respectively. Other types of hemophilia are rare and inherited in an autosomal recessive manner. More common than hemophilia A or B, but with a generally milder bleeding phenotype, is von Willebrand disease. Both quantitative and qualitative defects of vWF synthesis can cause autosomal dominant inherited bleeding disorders with incomplete penetrance. Mutations that cause qualitative vWF defects are clustered within exons that code for specific functional domains (35). However, mutations that would predict a quantitative deficiency of vWF are rarely identified at the *vWF* gene locus, and the range of vWF levels in obligate carriers of vWF deficiency are wide and overlap with vWF reference ranges, reflecting the combined impact of both heritable and noninheritable sources of variation on levels of hemostasis proteins (36).

Platelet activation and aggregation are complex cellular events, involving the interaction of various ligands with specific platelet surface receptors and multiple post-receptor signal transduction pathways, culminating in platelet shape change, release of granule contents, and activation of a surface heterodimer, glycoprotein IIbIIIa, which binds fibrinogen to form attachments to other activated platelets. Inherited quantitative and qualitative platelet defects are rare, produce mild to moderate bleeding symptoms, and are usually autosomal recessive heritable disorders. Drug-induced acquired platelet dysfunction is both a common complication (37) and also an effective therapeutic intervention: aspirin and clopidogrel for prevention of arterial thromboembolic complications.

Gene polymorphisms affecting platelet membrane receptors and integrins have been inconsistently associated with arterial thrombotic outcomes without convincing evidences of biological mechanisms (38).

It is now evident that most heritable risk factors for arterial and venous thromboembolic events are relatively weak, and it is the combination of multiple genetic risk factors plus environmental interactions that produce thrombotic phenotypes (39). Congenital, heterozygous deficiencies of antithrombin, protein C, and protein S (Fig. 2F), are identified in 1% to 5% of the patients with spontaneous venous thromboembolic events (VTE). However, two recently discovered gains of function coagulation factor polymorphisms have much higher prevalence in patients with VTEs (40). Factor V Leiden (FVL), a 1691 G to A mutation that substitutes glutamine for arginine at amino acid 506, slows the rate of factor Va cleavage by activated protein C. The allelic frequency of FVL is 2% to 15% in people of European ancestry, and it is identified in up to 40% of the patients with spontaneous VTE. The 20210 G to A mutation in the untranslated 3′ region of the prothrombin gene is associated with higher prothrombin levels and an increased risk for VTE. It is present in approximately 2% of the Caucasians, and it is identified in up to 20% of the patients with VTEs.

The list of coagulation, fibrinolysis, and platelet membrane protein gene polymorphisms with putative links to arterial thrombosis continues to grow (40–42). However, due to the complexity of the atherosclerotic process and the hemostatic system, it is likely that the attributable risk will be small for such polymorphisms. Changes in clinical trial designs, including much larger sample size, will be necessary to validate the significance of current and future candidate polymorphisms.

Pharmacogenetic Interactions in Hormone Replacement Therapy

Combined estrogen and progesterone therapy, whether in the form of oral contraceptive pills (OCP), in premenopausal, or hormone replacement therapy (HRT), in postmenopausal women, is associated with an increased risk for VTE. Although the absolute risk of pulmonary embolism (PE), or deep vein thrombosis (DVT), is low in healthy young women, users of OCP have a three- to sixfold increased risk of VTE compared with the nonusers (43). Traditionally, the estrogen content has been implicated as the cause for increased VTE risk. However, third generation OCP containing <50 ug of estrogen and synthetic progesterones, desogertrel or gestodone, are associated with a higher risk of VTE than second generation OCPs containing levonorgestrel and norgestrel, supporting a combined hormonal risk model (44). Based on a recent meta-analysis, the increase risk of VTE among HRT users was estimated to be 2.14, compared with the controls (45). The Women's Health Initiative study randomized 16,1809 postmenopausal women to daily conjugated equine estrogen (0.625 mg), medroxyprogesterone (2.5 mg), or placebo. The study was terminated prematurely due to an increase in breast cancer, cardiovascular endpoints, and VTEs in the treatment arm. The relative risk for VTE was 2.11 in the treatment arm (46).

Both OCP and HRT enhance procoagulant and diminish anticoagulant activities in the plasma. When estrogen/progesterone therapy is combined with inherited prothrombotic risk factors, the risk of VTE is further increased, confirming a pharmacogenetic interaction for this adverse drug reaction. Case-control studies of young women with and without a history of spontaneous DVT confirm a genetic–drug interaction (47,48). The risk of DVT was 3.8 and 6 times greater with OCP use, 7.9 and 9 times greater for carriers of FVL, and 6 times greater for carriers of PG 20210 (48). The relative risks for OCP and FVL were 20 and 34.7 and for OCP and PG20210, 16.3 (48), respectively, indicating a multiplicative interaction between drug and heritable risk factors. Both FVL and PG 20210 mutations are associated with an increased risk for cerebral vein thrombosis, and the risk is markedly increased with OCP use (49).

In a case-control study involving postmenopausal women with and without DVT or PE, HRT was associated with a 3.3-fold risk, FVL with a 3.9-fold risk, and HRT + FVL with a 15.5-fold risk for VTE, respectively, again confirming a synergistic interaction between hormone therapy and an inherited thrombophilic risk factor (50). The results from the HERS trial are similar, and predict the risk for VTE in postmenopausal women who are FVL-negative and not taking HRT to be 2/1000 patient-years compared with 5.8 and 15.2/1000 patient-years in HRT+ women who are FVL-negative and -positive, respectively (51). It is plausible to predict a similar interaction between PG 20210 and HRT, although published studies to date have not contained adequate numbers of carriers for analysis (50).

Estrogen/progesterone replacement therapy is associated with an increased risk for strokes and myocardial infarctions for premenopausal women with additional risk factors (smoking, hypertension, diabetes) (52) who use OCP, and for postmenopausal women taking HRT (46). However, there are inconsistent data regarding a pharmacogenetic interaction between FVL or PR20210 and OCP/HRT and cardiovascular ischemic events (53,54).

Heparin-Induced Thrombocytopenia

A common adverse drug reaction is heparin-induced thrombocytopenia (HIT). The pathogenesis of HIT begins with the formation of antibodies (typically IgG), against platelet factor 4 (PF4), a protein released from platelet granules that binds to and inactivates heparin (55). IgG–heparin–PF4 complexes bind to platelet immunoglobin Fc receptors (FCγ RIIa), leading to rapid uptake by splenic macrophages and thrombocytopenia. In addition, FCγ RIIa-mediated platelet activation accelerates thrombin generation, contributing to an acquired hypercoagulable state. The risk of developing HIT is dependent upon many variables, including dose and duration of heparin exposure, heparin formulation (unfractionated $\gg$ low molecular weight heparin, bovine > porcine), and clinical setting (orthopedic surgery > cardiac surgery > medical patients) (56). Thrombocytopenia rarely is severe enough to cause bleeding, but thrombotic complications occur in up to 50% of the HIT patients (57).

Although 7.5% to 50% of the patients exposed to heparin form PF4 antibodies, most do not become thrombocytopenic or develop thrombotic complications (56). In addition, when exposed to heparin and serum-containing PF4 antibodies, the degree of platelet activation varies widely among normal donors. Investigations into this variable platelet response have focused on the G507A polymorphism in the platelet FCγ RIIa receptor that substitutes histidine (H), for arginine (R), at amino acid position 131. When exposed to HIT-positive serum in vitro, platelets homozygous for 131 H/H polymorphism are more reactive than platelets homozygous for 131 R/R (58), suggesting that the G507A polymorphism could be a risk factor for HIT and thrombotic complications. Five published studies have compared the frequency of FCγ RIIa R/H 131 polymorphism in HIT patients and controls with inconsistent findings. Three reported a significant increase in H131 frequency (58–60), one no difference (61), and one an increase in A131 frequency compared with the control populations (62). PF4 polymorphisms are another potential source of genetic predisposition for developing HIT. However, no polymorphisms were found when 10 HIT patients and 10 control PF4 sequences were compared (63).

Thus, currently, there are no convincing candidate gene polymorphisms to explain the variable clinical consequences of heparin–PF4 immune complex interaction with platelets.

Warfarin-Induced Skin Necrosis

Warfarin-induced skin necrosis (WSN) is a rare thrombotic complication that occurs during initiation of oral anticoagulation therapy in patients with acute thromboembolic events. The presentation begins with intense skin pain quickly followed by erythema, hemorrhagic blisters, and, finally, full thickness skin necrosis, typically involving the breast, buttock, and thigh (64). The incidence of WSN was probably higher when it was customary to use warfarin loading doses of 15–30 mg, to rapidly obtain a therapeutic prothrombin time, compared with the current standard practice of starting with 5–10 mg and adjusting subsequent doses based on daily INR results. A plausible mechanism for this rare adverse drug reaction is a rapid fall in protein C activity paralleling the decline in factor VII activity during the first 24 to 48 hours of warfarin therapy because both proteins have half-lives of approximately 6 hours and their synthesis is vitamin K-dependent (65). Although the prothrombin time is prolonged due to the decrease in factor VII activity, an anticoagulated state is not obtained until both factor X and prothrombin activities decline, which occurs more slowly. The result is a temporary hypercoaguable state and the potential to form subdermal venous thrombi and skin necrosis. Support for a pharmacogenetic mechanism is found in sporadic case reports of WSN occurring in patients with hereditary deficiencies of the natural anticoagulants [protein C (66), protein S (67), and antithrombin (68)], and FVL (69)]. This model is supported by the spontaneous occurrence of skin necrosis in neonates born with a homozygous deficiency of protein C (70). Due to the rarity of WSN, it is not possible to accurately calculate the risk of this adverse drug reaction in patients with or without inherited hypercoaguable risk factors. Rather than screening patients with acute VTE for these risk factors before starting warfarin, following standard anticoagulation practice guidelines for parenteral anticoagulation with heparin and warfarin is recommended (71).

Aspirin Resistance

Aspirin is an effective drug for prevention of myocardial infarctions, strokes, and peripheral arterial occlusions (72). However, in vitro tests indicate only partial or no inhibition of platelet function in some patients taking aspirin (73), and aspirin resistance has been associated with arterial thrombotic complications (74). Although there may be many potential factors involved in aspirin treatment failures, a genetic resistance to the antithrombotic action of aspirin would appear plausible.

Aspirin irreversibly inhibits platelet synthesis of thromboxane A_2 (TxA_2), by acetylating cyclooxygenase-1 (*COX*-1) enzyme (75). TxA_2 activates platelets through a specific platelet membrane receptor, although the downstream steps are unknown at this time. Inactivation of *COX*-1 enzyme does diminish platelet activation by weak agonists, such as ADP and epinephrine, and low concentrations of collagen but does not prevent activation by such stronger agonists as thrombin.

Presently, there is no standard laboratory criterion for aspirin resistance. Typically, resistance has been defined as in vitro platelet aggregation in response to arachadonic acid (the substrate for *COX*-1), epinephrine, or adenosine diphosphate (ADP) that exceeds an arbitrary threshold (73,76). In most studies, documentation of aspirin ingestion in patients labeled as aspirin-resistant has been limited to patient reporting without salicylate level confirmation to assess for poor compliance. Using these laboratory criteria, reported prevalences for aspirin resistance range from 8% to 45% (77).

Possible mechanisms for platelet resistance to aspirin include alternative sources of the product of *COX*-1 metabolism, prostaglandin H2, from monocytes or endothelial cells through *COX*-2, or replenished *COX*-1 enzyme activity (76). Alternatively, *COX*-1 mutations could make the enzyme less vulnerable to acetylation. To date, no likely polymorphisms have been identified in this gene.

However, considerable attention has been focused on a common polymorphism in the beta integrin β_3 that combines with the alpha integrin α_{IIb} to form the platelet fibrinogen receptor glycoprotein IIbIIIa. The nucleotide substitution T1565C encodes for amino acid change leucine to proline at position 33 (78). This is one of the eight SNPs in the GPIIIa protein that can cause platelet alloimmunization during pregnancy or following platelet transfusion. In platelet serology nomenclature, the wild-type allele is Pl^{A1} or HPA-1a, and the polymorphic one is PL^{A2} or HPA-1b. The allelic frequency of HPA-1b is approximately 15% among the Caucasians, and 1–2% are homozygous. In 1996, Weiss et al. (79) reported that HPA-1b was a risk factor for myocardial infarction based on a retrospective case-control study involving 71 subjects. Subsequent studies reported conflicting findings (80,81), including the Physicians Health study (81), which showed no increased risk for myocardial infarction (MI), stroke, or DVT associated with the HPA-1b phenotype. HPA-1b has been associated with an increased risk for reocclusions following percutaneous coronary artery stenting in some (82,83), but not all, studies (84). At present, the evidence for a link between glycoprotein IIIa HPA-1b polymorphism and atherosclerotic complications is inconclusive.

Meanwhile, the search for a biological mechanism whereby HPA-1b could affect a prothrombotic phenotype has lead to divergent findings. Feng et al. (85) reported increased platelet aggregability in response to epinephrine in HPL-1b compared with HPA-1a subjects among 1336 participants in the Framingham Offspring Study. However, Bray et al. (86,87), reported similar in vitro platelet aggregation responses to epinephrine and ADP for HPA-1a homozygous, HPA-1b heterozygous, and HPA-1b homozygous subjects. When exposed to aspirin, HPA-1b heterozygous platelets were significantly more sensitive to inhibition of epinephrine-induced platelet aggregation than HPA-1a or HPA-1b homozygous platelets, which do not support clinical aspirin resistance due to HPA-lb polymorphism (87). Undas (88) indirectly monitored aspirin inhibition of platelet activation by measuring thrombin generation in blood shed from a bleeding time wound. Baseline thrombin generation rates were similar for HPA-1a homozygotes (wild-type), and HPA-1b heterozygotes. After aspirin ingestion, thrombin generation was reduced in both groups but significantly less so in HPA-1b carriers. The results of a subsequent study by these investigators, measuring additional markers of thrombin activity in shed blood, showed that prior to aspirin ingestion, HPA-1b carriers had enhanced prothrombin activation compared with the HPA-1a subjects and that suppression of thrombin generation by aspirin was impaired in the HPA-1b group (89).

Given the complexities of the molecular mechanisms involved in platelet function, it is possible that the HPA-1b polymorphism could both increase platelet aggregation and decrease aspirin suppression of activated platelet generation of thrombin. However, no conclusions can be drawn from these in vitro data regarding the physiologic consequences of the PLA-1b polymorphism in terms of atherosclerotic disease progression and choice of antithrombotic therapy.

THIOPURINE PHARMACOGENETICS

Thiopurines are a family of drugs that include mercaptopurine (MP) [a daily component of maintenance therapy for childhood acute lymphoblastic leukemia (ALL) treatment (89) and commonly used in the treatment of inflammatory bowel disease], thioguanine (used to treat acute myeloblastic lukemias), and azathioprine (a commonly prescribed immunosuppressant used in solid organ transplants, rheumatic disease, and dermatologic disorders). The principal cytotoxic mechanism of these agents is the incorporation of thioguanine nucleotides (TGN) into DNA (Fig. 3). Thus, thiopurines are inactive prodrugs

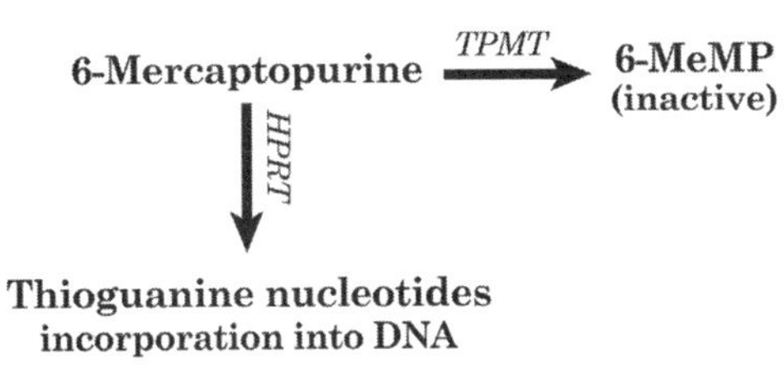

Figure 3 6-MP is converted by HPRT to TGN, its active metabolites. Thioguanine nucleotides exert anticancer effects and myelotoxicity via incorporation into DNA. 6-MP is inactivated via methylation by TPMT to the active metabolite 6-MeMP. Inactivation can also occur through oxidation by xanthine oxidase (XO, not shown). *Abbreviations*: 6-MP, 6-mercapropurine; HPRT, hypoxanthine phosphoribosyl transferase; TGN, thioguanine nucleotides; TPMT, thiopurine methyltransferase; 6-MeMP, 6-methylmercaptopurine.

that require metabolism to TGN to exert cytotoxicity. This activation is catalyzed by multiple enzymes, of which the first one is hypoxanthine phosphoribosyl transferase (HPRT). Alternatively, these agents can be inactivated via oxidation by xanthine oxidase (XO) or via methylation by thiopurine methyltransferase (TPMT). TPMT catalyzes the *S*-methylation of the thiopurine agents, such as azathioprine, MP, and thioguanine (89,90), thereby shunting the drug away from TGN formation.

TPMT polymorphisms have been associated with the therapeutic efficacy and toxicity of MPs. TPMT activity is highly variable and polymorphic in all large populations studied to date; approximately 90% of the individuals have high activity, 10% have intermediate activity, and 0.3% have low or no detectable enzyme activity (91,92). Although eight *TPMT* alleles have been identified, three alleles (*TPMT*2, TPMT*3A, TPMT*3C*) account for about 95% of the intermediate or low enzyme activity cases (89,93–96). All three alleles are associated with lower enzyme activity due to enhanced rates of proteolysis of the mutant proteins (97). The presence of *TPMT*2*, *TPMT*3A*, or *TPMT*3C* is predictive of *TPMT* activity; patients heterozygous for these alleles all have intermediate activity, and subjects homozygous for these alleles are TPMT-deficient (96,98). In addition, compound heterozygotes (*TPMT*2/3A, TPMT*2/TPMT*3C, TPMT*3A/3C*) are also TPMT-deficient, as would be expected (96). Numerous studies have shown that *TPMT*-deficient patients are at very high risk of developing severe hematopoietic toxicity if treated with conventional doses of thiopurines (99,100). Studies have also shown that patients who are heterozygous at the *TPMT* locus are at intermediate risk of dose-limiting toxicity (101,102). In a study of 67 patients treated with azathioprine for rheumatic disease, six patients (9%) were heterozygous for mutant *TPMT* alleles, and therapy was discontinued in five of the six patients because of low leukocyte count within 1 month of starting the treatment (101). The sixth patient had documented noncompliance with azathioprine therapy. Patients with wild-type *TPMT* received therapy for a median of 39 weeks without complications, compared with a median of two weeks in patients heterozygous for mutant *TPMT* alleles. Futhermore, Relling et al. (102) showed that *TPMT*-deficient patients tolerated full doses of MP for only 7% of the scheduled weeks, whereas heterozygous and homozygous wild-type patients tolerated full doses for 65% and 84% of the scheduled weeks of therapy over the 2.5 years of treatment, respectively (102). However, another study using lower doses of 6-MP found no significant difference between heterozygous and homozygous wild-type *TPMT* patients in the median number of weeks in which 6-MP treatment could not be given at full dose due to hematological toxicity (103).

These studies demonstrate that the influence of *TPMT* genotype on hematopoietic toxicity is most dramatic for homozygous mutant patients but is also of clinical relevance for heterozygous individuals, which represent about 10% of the patients treated with these medications. The remaining 90% of the population carry two wild-type *TPMT* alleles; these individuals have full TPMT activity and do not require dose reduction. By using polymerase chain reaction (PCR)-based assays to detect the three signature mutations in these alleles, a rapid and relatively inexpensive assay is available to identify >90% of all mutant alleles (96,104). These results can then be used prospectively to determine safe starting doses for thiopurine therapy. Prospective analysis of *TPMT* genotype and/or phenotype are now integrating into standard practice for many areas of medicine, in particular the treatment of inflammatory bowel disease, rheumatologic disease, and dermatological disorders. However, the use of *TPMT* testing would benefit from additional prospective studies of *TPMT*-guided dosing or some other method for objectively evaluating the utility of testing the patient's outcome.

THE FUTURE

The aforementioned examples are only the beginning. There are many areas of hematology where unexplained variability in drug effect is the norm, including response to hematopoietic growth factors and efficacy of new clotting agents. In addition, hematologic toxicity is a common side effect of HIV therapy, new antipsychotics, and other drugs used to treat chronic disorders. Therefore, a greater degree of investigation is needed to clarify the role of genetics (vs. environmental influences) in these adverse events. There is also a greater need for definitive clinical trials. Interesting associations do not change patient care. We need data that mandates a particular therapy or dose of therapy in order to allow pharmacogenetics to reach its potential as a revolution in medical practice.

REFERENCES

1. Weinshilboum R. Inheritance and drug response. N Engl J Med 2003; 348:529–537.
2. Phillips KA, Veenstra DL, Oren E, Lee JK, Sadee W. Potential role of pharmacogenomics in reducing adverse drug reactions: a systematic review. J Am Med Assoc 2001; 286:2270–2279.
3. Pirmohamed M, Park BK. Adverse drug reactions: back to the future. Br J Clin Pharmacol 2003; 55:486–492.
4. McLeod HL, Evans WE. Pharmacogenomics: unlocking the human genome for better drug therapy. Annu Rev Pharmacol Toxicol 2001; 41:101–121.
5. Watters JW, McLeod HL. Cancer pharmacogenomics: current and future applications. Biochim Biophys Acta 2003; 1603:99–111.
6. Evans WE, McLeod HL. Pharmacogenomics—drug disposition, drug targets, and side effects. N Engl J Med 2003; 348:538–549.
7. Redman AR. Implications of cytochrome P450 2C9 polymorphism on warfarin metabolism and dosing. Pharmacotherapy 2001; 21:235–242.
8. Scordo MG, Pengo V, Spina E, Dahl ML, Gusella M, Padrini R. Influence of CYP2C9 and CYP2C19 genetic polymorphisms on warfarin maintenance dose and metabolic clearance. Clin Pharmacol Ther 2002; 72:702–710.
9. Higashi MK, Veenstra DL, Kondo LM, Wittkowsky AK, Srinouanprachanh SL, Farin FM, Rettie AE. Association between CYP2C9 genetic variants and anticoagulation-related outcomes during warfarin therapy. J Am Med Assoc 2002; 287:1690–1698.
10. Margaglione M, Colaizzo D, D'Andrea G, Brancaccio V, Ciampa A, Grandone E, Di Minno G. Genetic modulation of oral anticoagulation with warfarin. Thromb Haemost 2000; 84:775–778.
11. Aithal GP, Day CP, Kesteven PJL, Daly AK. Association of polymorphisms in the cytochrome P450 CYP2C9 with warfarin dose requirement and risk of bleeding complications. Lancet 1999; 353:717–719.
12. Gage BF, Eby C, Banet G, Milligan P, McLeod H. Use of pharmacogenetics and clinical factors to predict the maintenance dose of warfarin (abstract). J Gen Intern Med 2002; 17:111.
13. Steward DJ, Haining RL, Henne KR, et al. Genetic association between sensitivity to warfarin and expression of CYP2C9*3. Pharmacogenetics 1997; 7:361–367.
14. Tabrizi AR, Zehnbauer BA, Borecki IB, McGrath SD, Buchman TG, Freeman BD. The frequency and effects of cytochrome P450 (CYP) 2C9 polymorphisms in patients receiving warfarin. J Am Coll Surg 2002; 194:267–273.
15. Takahashi H, Kashima T, Nomoto S, et al. Comparisons between in-vitro and in-vivo metabolism of (S)-warfarin: catalytic activities of cDNA-expressed CYP2C9, its Leu359 variant and their mixture versus unbound clearance in patients with the corresponding CYP2C9 genotypes. Pharmacogenetics 1998; 8:356–373.

16. Gotoh O. Substrate recognition sites in cytochrome P450 family 2 (CYP2) proteins inferred from comparative analyses of amino acid and coding nucleotide sequences. J Biol Chem 1992; 267:83–90.
17. Kaminsky LS, de Morais SM, Faletto MB, Dunbar DA, Goldstein JA. Correlation of human cytochrome P4502C substrate specificities with primary structure: warfarin as a probe. Mol Pharmacol 1993; 43:234–239.
18. Taube J, Halsall D, Baglin T. Influence of cytochrome P-450 CYP2C9 polymorphisms on warfarin sensitivity and risk of over-anticoagulation in patients on long-term treatment. Blood 2000; 96:1816–1819.
19. Loebstein R, Yonath H, Peleg D, et al. Interindividual variability in sensitivity to warfarin—Nature or nurture? Clin Pharmacol Ther 2001; 70:159–164.
20. Imai J, Ieiri I, Mamiya K, et al. Polymorphism of the cytochrome P450 (CYP) 2C9 gene in Japanese epileptic patients: genetic analysis of the CYP2C9 locus. Pharmacogenetics 2000; 10:85–89.
21. Dickmann LJ, Rettie AE, Kneller MB, et al. Identification and functional characterization of a new CYP2C9 variant (CYP2C9*5) expressed among African Americans. Mol Pharmacol 2001; 60:382–387.
22. Kidd RS, Curry TB, Gallagher S, Edeki T, Blaisdell T, Goldstein JA. Identification of a null allele of CYP2C9 in an African-American exhibiting toxicity to phenytoin. Pharmacogenetics 2001; 11:803–808.
23. Leung AY, Chow HC, Kwong YL, et al. Genetic polymorphism in exon 4 of cytochrome P450 CYP2C9 may be associated with warfarin sensitivity in Chinese patients. Blood 2001; 98:2584–2587.
24. Wallace WE, MacSwiney FJ. A major gene controlling warfarin-resistance in the house mouse. J Hyg (Lond) 1976; 76:173–181.
25. Greaves JH, Ayres P. Linkages between genes for coat colour and resistance to warfarin in *Rattus norvegicus*. Nature 1969; 224:284–285.
26. Kohn MH, Pelz HJ. A gene-anchored map position of the rat warfarin-resistance locus, Rw, and its orthologs in mice and humans. Blood 2000; 96:1996–1998.
27. Kohn MH, Pelz HJ, Wayne RK. Natural selection mapping of the warfarin-resistance gene. Proc Natl Acad Sci USA 2000; 97:7911–7915.
28. Hulse ML. Warfarin resistance: diagnosis and therapeutic alternatives. Pharmacotherapy 1996; 16:1009–1017.
29. Francis CW, Davidson BL, Berkowitz SD, et al. Ximelagatran versus warfarin for the prevention of venous thromboembolism after total knee arthroplasty. A randomized, double-blind trial. Ann Intern Med 2002; 137:648–655.
30. Wang SL, Huang J, Lai MD, Tsai JJ. Detection of CYP2C9 polymorphism based on the polymerase chain reaction in Chinese. Pharmacogenetics 1995; 5:37–42.
31. Souto JC, Almasy L, Borrell M, Gari M, Martinez E, et al. Genetic determinants of hemostasis phenotypes in Spanish families. Circulation 2000; 101:1546–1551.
32. Gill JC, Endres-Brooks J, Bauer PJ, Marks WJ, Montgomery RR. The effect of ABO blood group on the diagnosis of von Willebrand Disease. Blood 1987; 69:1691–1695.
33. Kamphuisen PW, Eikenboom JCJ, Rosendaal FR, Koster T, Blann AD, et al. High factor VIII antigen levels increase the risk of venour thrombosis but are not associated with polymorphisms in the von Willebrand factor and factor VIII gene. Br J Haematology 2001; 115:156–158.
34. Humphries SE, Thomas A, Montgomery HE, Green F, Winder A, Miller G. Gene-environmental interaction in the determination of plasma levels of fibrinogen. Fibrinol Proteol 1997; 11(suppl):3–7.
35. Sadler JE. Biochemisty and genetics of von Willebrand factor. Annu Rev Biochem 1998; 67:395–424.
36. Sadler JE. von Willebrand Disease type I—a diagnosis in search of a disease. Blood; George JN, Shattil SJ. The clinical importance of acquired abnormalities of platelet function. NEJM 1991; 324: 27–39. In Press.

37. Eby CS. Prothrombotic states in ischemic stroke. Sem Cerebrovasc dz stroke 2002; 2:90–101.
38. Lane DA, Grant PJ. Role of hemostatis gene polymorphismx in venous and arterial thrombotic disease. Blood 2000; 95:1517–1532.
39. Kottke-Marchant K. Genetic polymorphisms associated with venous and arterial thrombosis. Arch Pathol Lab Med 2002; 126:295–304.
40. Franco RF. Gene polymorphisms of the haemostatic system and the risk of arterial thrombotic disease. Br J Haematology 2001; 115:491–506.
41. Ferrer-Antunes C. Polymorphisms of coagulation factor genes—a review. Clin Chem Lab Med 1998; 36:897–906.
42. Hannaford PC, Owen-Smith V. Using epidemiological data to guide clinical practice: review of studies on cardiovascular disease and the use of combined oral contraceptives Brit Med J 1998; 316:984–987.
43. Vandenbroucke JP, Rosing J, Bloemenkamp KWM, et al. Oral contraceptives and the risk of venous thrombosis. N Engl J Med 2001; 344:1527–1535.
44. Miller J, Chan BKS, Nelson HD. Postmenopausal estrogen replacement and risk for venous thromboembolism: a systematic review and meta-analysis for the U.S. preventive services task force. Ann Intern Med 2002; 136:680–690.
45. Writing Group for the Women's Health Initiative Investigators. Risks and benefits of estrogen plus progestin in healthy postmenopausal women. J Am Med Assoc 2002; 288:321–333.
46. Vandenbroucke JP, Koster T, Briet E, et al. Increased risk of venous thrombosis in oral-contraceptive users who are carriers of factor V Leiden mutation. The Lancet 1994; 344:1453–1457.
47. Martinelli I, Emanuela T, Bucciarelli P, et al. Interaction between the G20210A mutation of the prothrombin gene and oral contraceptive use in deep vein thrombosis. Arterioscler Thromb Vasc Biol 1999; 19:700–703.
48. Martinelli I, Sacchi E, Landi G, Taioli E, Duca F, Mannucci PM. High risk of cerebral vein thrombosis in carriers of a porthrombin gene mutation and in users of oral contraceptives. NEJM 1998; 338:1793–1797.
49. Rosendaal FR, Vessey M, Ruumley A, et al. Hormonal replacement therapy, prothrombic mutations and the risk of venous thrombosis. Br J Haematol 2002; 116:851–854.
50. Herrington DM, Vittinghoff D, Major DA, Owen J, Reboussin DM, et al. Factor V Leiden, hormone replacement therapy, and the risk for venous thromboembolic events in women with coronary disease. Arterioscler Thromb Vasc Biol 2002; 22:1012–1017.
51. Tanis BC, van den Bosch MA, Kemmeren JM, et al. Oral contraceptives and the risk of myocardial infarction. N Engl J Med 2001; 345:1841–1842.
52. Psaty BM, Smith NL, Lemaitre RN, Vos HL, Heckbert SR, et al. Hormone replacement therapy, prothombotic mutations, and the risk of incident nonfatal myocardial infarction in postmenopausal women. J Am Med Assoc 2001; 285: 906–913.
53. Glueck CJ, Wang P, Fontaine RN, Sieve-Smith L, Lang JE. Estrogen replacement therapy, thrombophilia, and atherothrombosis. Metabolism: Clin & Exp 2002; 51:724–732.
54. Fabris F, Ahmad S, Cella G, Jeske WP, Walenga JM, et al. Pathophysiology of heparin-induced thrombocytopenia. Arch Patholo Lab Med 2000; 124:1657–1665.
55. Alving BM. How I treat heparin-induced thrombocytopenia and thrombosis. Blood 2003; 101:31–37.
56. Warkentin TE, Kelton JG. A 14-year study of heparin-induced thrombocytopenia. Am J Med 1996; 101:502–507.
57. Denomme GA, Warkentin TE, Horsewood P, et al. Activation of platelets by sera containing IgG1 heparin-dependent antibodies: an explanation for the predominance of the Fc gammaR-IIa "low responder" (his131) gene in patients with heparin-induced thrombocytopenia. J Lab & Clin Med 1997; 130:242–244.
58. Burgess JK, Lindeman R, Chesterman CN, Chong BH. Single amino acid mutation of fcY receptor is associated with the development of heparin-induced thrombocytopenia. Br J Haematol 1995; 91:761.

59. Brandt JT, Isenhart CE, Osborne JM, et al. On the role of platelet FcYRIIa phenotype in heparin-induced thrombocytopenia. Thromb Haemost 1995; 74:1564.
60. Arepally G, McKenzie ST, Jiang XM, et al. FcYRIIA H/R[131] Polymorphism, subclass-specific IgG anti-heparin/platelet factor 4 antibodies and clinical course in patients with heparin-induced thrombocytopenia and thrombosis. Blood 1997; 89:370–375.
61. Carlsson LE, Santoso S, Baurichter G, et al. Heparin-induced thrombocytopenia: new insights into the impact of the FcYRIIA H/R[131] -R-H131 polymorphism. Blood 1998; 92:1526–1531.
62. Horsewood P, Kelton JG. Investigation of a platelet factor 4 polymorphism on the immune response in patients with heparin-induced thrombocytopenia. Platelets 2000; 11:23–27.
63. Eby CS. Warfarin-induced skin necrosis. Hematology/Oncology Clinics of North America 1993; 7:1291–1300.
64. D'Angelo SV, Comp PC, Esmon CT, D'Angelo A. Relationship between protein C antigen and anticoagulant activity during oral anticoagulation and in selected disease states. J Clin Invest 1986; 77:416–425.
65. Brockmans AW, Bertina RM, Loeliger EA, et al. Protein C and the development of skin necrosis during anticoagulant therapy. Thromb Haemost 1983; 49:251.
66. Gailani D, Reese EP Jr. Anticoagulant-induced skin necrosis in a patient with hereditary deficiency of protein S. Am J Hematol 1999; 60:231–236.
67. Kiehl R, Hellstern P, Wenzel E. Hereditary antithrombin III (at III) deficiency and atypical localization of a coumarin necrosis. Thromb Res 1987; 45:191–193.
68. Ng T, Tillyer ML. Warfarin-induced skin necrosis associated with Factor V Leiden and protein S. deficiency. Clinical & Laboratory Haematology 2001; 23:261–264.
69. Seligsohn U, Berger A, Abend M, et al. Homozygous protein C deficiency manifested by massive venous thrombosis in the newborn. New Engl J Med 1984; 310:559–562.
70. Ansell J, Hirsh J, Dalen J, Bussey H, Anderson D, et al. Managing oral anticoagulation therapy. Circulation 2001; 119(suppl 11):22S-38S.
71. Antiplatelet trialists' collaboration. Collaborative overview of the randomized trials of antiplatelet therapy I: prevention of death, myocardial infarction, and stroke by prolonged antiplatelet therapy in various categories of patients. Br Med J 1994; 308:81–106.
72. Helgason CM, Bolin KM, Hoff JA, Winikler SR, Mangat A, et al. Development of aspirin resistance in persons with previous ischemic stroke. Stroke 1994; 225:2331–2336.
73. Mueller MR, Salat A, Stangl P, Muratibo M, Pulaki S, et al. Variable platelet response to low-dose ASA and the risk of limb deterioration in patients submitted to peripheral arterial angioplasty. Thromb Haemsot 1997; 78:1003–1007.
74. Roth GJ, Stanford N, Majerus PW. Acetlyation of prostaglandin synthase by aspirin. Proc Natl Acad Sci USA 1975; 72:3073–3076.
75. Gum PA, Kottke-Marchant K, Poggio ED, Gurn H, Welsh PA, et al. Profile and prevalence of aspirin resistance in patients with cardiovascular disease. Am J Cardiol 2001; 88:2230–2235.
76. Newman PJ, Derbes RS, Aster RH. The human platelet alloantigens, P1A1 and P1A2, are associated with a leucine33/proline33 amino acid polymorphism in membrane glycoprotein IIIa, and are distinguishable by DNA typing. J Clin Invest 1989; 83:1778–1781.
77. Eikelboom JW, Hirst J, Weitz JI, Johnston M, Y Q, et al. Aspirin-resistant thromboxane biosynthesis and the risk of myocardial infarction, stroke, or cardiovascular death in patients at high risk for cardiovascular events. Circulation 2002; 105:1650–1655.
78. Weiss EJ, Bray PF, Tayback M, Schulman SP, Kickler TS, et al. A polymorphism of a platelet glycoprotein receptor as an inherited risk factor for coronary thrombosis. N Engl J Med 1996; 334:1090–1094.
79. Zotz RB, Klein M, Dauben HP, Moser C, Gams E, et al. Prospective analysis after coronary-artery bypass grafting: platelet GP IIIa polymorphism (HPA-1b/PI^{A2}) is a risk factor by bypass occlusion, myocardial infarction, and death. Thromb Haemost 2000; 83:404–407.
80. Ridker PM, Hennekens CH, Schmitz C, Stampfer MJ, Lindpaintner K. $PI^{A1}/^{A2}$ polymorphism of platelet glycoprotein IIIa and risks of myocardial infarction, stroke, and venous thrombosis. Lancet 1997; 349:385–388.

81. Walter DH, Schachinger V, Elsner M, Dimmeler S, Zeiher AM. Platelet glycoprotein IIIa polymorphisms and risk of restenosis after coronary stent thrombosis. Lancet 1997; 350:1217–1219.
82. Kastrati A, Schomig A, Seyfarth M, Koch W, Elezi S, et al. PI^{A} polymorphism of platelet glycoprotein IIIa and risk of restenosis after coronary stent placement. Circulation 1999; 99:1005–1010.
83. Mamotte CDS, van Bockxmeer FM, Taylor RR. $PI^{a1/a2}$ polymorphism of glycoprotein IIIa and risk of coronary artery disease and restenosis following coronary angioplasty. Am J Cardiol 1998; 82:13–16.
84. Feng D, Lindpaintner K, Larson MG, Rao VS, O'Donnell CJ, Lipinska I, Schmitz C, Sutherland PA, Silbershatz H, D'Agostino RB, Muller JE, Myers RH, Levy D, Tofler GH. Increased platelet aggregability associated with platelet GPIIIa PL^{A2} polymorphism. Arterioscler Thromb Vasc Biol 1999; 1142–1147.
85. Cooke GE, Bray PF, Hamlington JD, Pham DM, Goldschmidt-Clermont PJ. PI^{A2} polymorphism and efficacy of aspirin. Lancet 1998; 351:1253.
86. Michelson AD, Furman MI, Goldschmidt-Clermont P, Mascelli M, Hendrix C, et al. Platelet GP IIIa PI^{A} polymorphisms display different sensitivities to agonists. Circulation 2000; 101:1013–1018.
87. Undas A, Sanak M, Musial J, Szczeklik. Platelet glycoprotein IIIa polymorphism, aspirin, and thrombin generation. The Lancet 1999; 353:982–983.
88. Undas A, Brummel K, Musial J, Mann KG, Szczeklik A. PI^{A2} polymorphism of β_3 integrins is associated with enhanced thrombin generation and impaired antithrombotic action of aspirin at the site of microvascular injury. Circulation 2001; 104:2666–2672.
89. McLeod HL, Krynetski EY, Relling MV, Evans WE. Genetic polymorphism of thiopurine methyltransferase and its clinical relevance for childhood acute lymphoblastic leukemia. Leukemia 2000; 14:567–572.
90. Krynetski EY, Evans WE. Pharmacogenetics of cancer therapy: getting personal. Am J Hum Genet 1998; 63:11–16.
91. Weinshilboum RM, Sladek SL. Mercaptopurine pharmacogenetics: monogenic inheritance of erythrocyte thiopurine methyltransferase activity. Am J Human Genet 1980; 32:651–662.
92. McLeod HL, Relling MV, Liu Q, Pui CH, Evans WE. Polymorphic thiopurine methyltransferase in erythrocytes is indicative of activity in leukemic blasts from children with acute lymphoblastic leukemia. Blood 1995; 85:1897–1902.
93. Krynetski EY, Schuetz JD, Galpin AJ, Pui CH, Relling MV, Evans WE. A single point mutation leading to loss of catalytic activity in human thiopurine S-methyltransferase. Proc Natl Acad Sci USA 1995; 92:949–953.
94. Tai HL, Krynetski EY, Yates CR, Loennechen T, Fessing MY, Krynetskaia NF, Evans WE. Thiopurine S-methyltransferase deficiency: two nucleotide transitions define the most prevalent mutant allele associated with loss of catalytic activity in Caucasians. Am J Hum Genet 1996; 58:694–702.
95. Otterness D, Szumlanski C, Lennard L, Klemetsdal B, Aarbakke J, Park-Hah JO, Iven H, Schmiegelow K, Branum E, O'Brien J, Weinshilboum R. Human thiopurine methyltransferase pharmacogenetics: gene sequence polymorphisms. Clin Pharmacol Ther 1997; 62:60–73.
96. Yates CR, Krynetski EY, Loennechen T, Fessing MY, Tai HL, Pui CH, Relling MV, Evans WE. Molecular diagnosis of thiopurine S-methyltransferase deficiency: genetic basis for azathioprine and mercaptopurine intolerance. Ann Intern Med 1997; 126:608–614.
97. Tai HL, Krynetski EY, Schuetz EG, Yanishevski Y, Evans WE. Enhanced proteolysis of thiopurine S-methyltransferase (TPMT) encoded by mutant alleles in humans (TPMT*3A, TPMT*2): mechanisms for the genetic polymorphism of TPMT activity. Proc Natl Acad Sci USA 1997; 94:6444–6449.
98. Hon YY, Fessing MY, Pui CH, Relling MV, Krynetski EY, Evans WE. Polymorphism of the thiopurine S-methyltransferase gene in African-Americans. Hum Mol Genet 1999; 8:371–376.

99. Lennard L, Van Loon JA, Weinshilboum RM. Pharmacogenetics of acute azathioprine toxicity: relationship to thiopurine methyltransferase genetic polymorphism. Clin Pharmacol Ther 1989; 46:149–154.
100. Evans WE, Horner M, Chu YQ, Kalwinsky D, Roberts WM. Altered mercaptopurine metabolism, toxic effects, and dosage requirement in a thiopurine methyltransferase-deficient child with acute lymphocytic leukemia. J Pediatr 1991; 119:985–989.
101. Black AJ, McLeod HL, Capell HA, Powrie RH, Matowe LK, Pritchard SC, Collie-Duguid ES, Reid DM. Thiopurine methyltransferase genotype predicts therapy-limiting severe toxicity from azathioprine. Ann Intern Med 1998; 129:716–718.
102. Relling MV, Hancock ML, Rivera GK, Sandlund JT, Ribeiro RC, Krynetski EY, Pui CH, Evans WE. Mercaptopurine therapy intolerance and heterozygosity at the thiopurine S-methyltransferase gene locus. J Natl Cancer Inst 1999; 91:2001–2008.
103. McLeod HL, Coulthard S, Thomas AE, Pritchard SC, King DJ, Richards SM, Eden OB, Hall AG, Gibson BE. Analysis of thiopurine methyltransferase variant alleles in childhood acute lymphoblastic leukaemia. Br J Haematol 1999; 105:696–700.
104. McLeod HL, Siva C. The thiopurine S-methyltransferase gene locus—implications for clinical pharmacogenomics. Pharmacogenomics 1999; 3:89–98.

8
Pharmacogenetics in Oncology

Romano Danesi, Antonello Di Paolo, and Mario Del Tacca
Division of Pharmacology and Chemotherapy, Department of Oncology, University of Pisa, Pisa, Italy

Filippo De Braud
Clinical Pharmacology and New Drug Development Unit, European Institute of Oncology, Milano, Italy

INTRODUCTION

The therapeutic index of most cytotoxic agents is still a matter of concern because drug activity against malignant cells is associated with toxicity to normal tissues. In addition to this, new drugs designed to inhibit specific molecular pathways critical to tumor cell survival, such as imatinib and gefitinib (1), are susceptible to therapeutic failure due to target mutation or downregulation with activation of alternative signal transduction pathways. Recent progress in analytical techniques and the sequencing of the human genome has allowed the discovery of gene variants involved in pharmacokinetic and pharmacodynamic pathways (Fig. 1), which define cancer chemosensitivity and/or drug tolerability (2).

Two branches of pharmacology have benefited from the completion of the human genome project: pharmacogenetics, the study of the genetic basis of drug response, and pharmacogenomics, the genome-wide analysis of cell and tissues to identify complex genetic alterations underlying drug responses not explained by the classical pharmacogenetic approach or to discover novel targets for drug development. A simple classification of genetic variability includes:

1. Genetic alterations occurring at low frequency, whose effects suddenly arise and negatively affect cell function (i.e., inactivating mutations affecting genes, which encode for drug-metabolizing enzymes).
2. Sequence variants situated at well-defined positions along the gene (i.e., single-nucleotide polymorphisms, SNPs), appearing at higher frequency in the case population than that of casually occurring mutations. SNPs may affect exons (i.e., the effect may be the change in the amino acid sequence), introns (likely causing the insertion of alternative splicing sites), or the regulatory region of the gene (with alteration of gene expression) (Fig. 2).

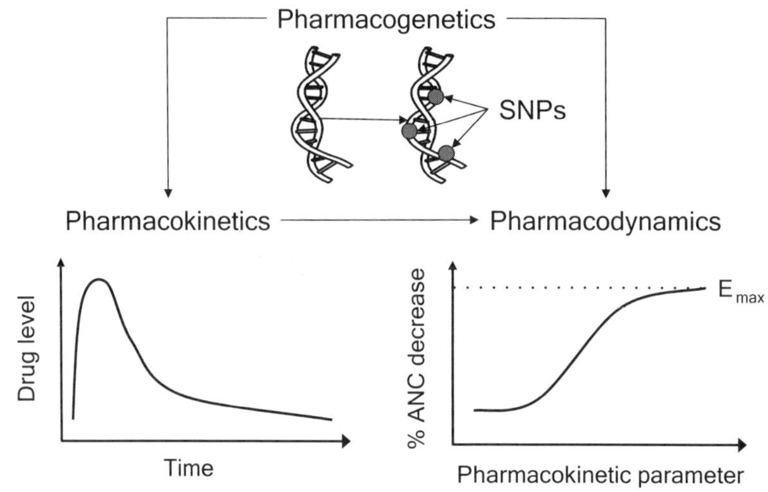

Figure 1 Influence of genetic factors on the pharmacokinetics and pharmacodynamics of anticancer agents. *Abbreviations*: SNPs, single-nucleotide polymorphisms; E_{max}, maximum effect (sigmoid effect model); ANC, absolute neutrophil count.

Genetic analysis is based on a wide variety of techniques suitable to decipher the alterations of genetic material (SNP, deletion or duplication of a few genes up to chromosomal rearrangements); and the recent development of DNA microarray technology will enable genome-wide screening for diagnostic purposes (3,4).

The identification of candidate genes for pharmacogenetic analysis is a complex process because the activity of anticancer drugs is influenced by (1) metabolic activation and inactivation (i.e., CYP450 and UGT), (2) expression of drug targets [i.e., thymidylate synthase and epidermal growth factor receptor (EGFR)], (3) integrity of pathways that recognize the cellular damage and promote or inhibit apoptosis (i.e., p53 and Bcl-2), (4) DNA repair systems (i.e., *ERCC1*, *XPD*), and (5) active drug transport outside the cell (i.e., ABC transporters) (5,6).

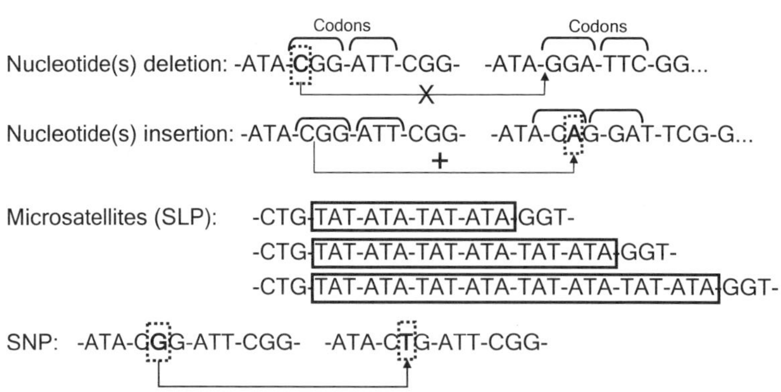

Figure 2 Major causes of genetic variability; nucleotide deletions or insertions are responsible for frame shifts, whereas microsatellites, affecting the regulatory regions of the gene, are associated with variability in translation efficiency. SNP may be silent or associated with amino acid change in the encoded protein. *Abbreviations*: SNP, single-nucleotide polymorphism; SLP, sequence length polymorphism.

PHARMACOGENETICS OF DRUG TARGETS: THEORETICAL BACKGROUND

From a theoretical point of view, the chemosensitivity of a tumor may be influenced by the genetic background of a disease in three different ways. First, if the drug target plays an important role in the process of tumor progression (i.e., *HER2/neu*) and its expression in tumor tissue is low at the time of drug treatment, despite efficient target saturation by the drug, the therapeutic effect is likely to be unsatisfactory. On the contrary, high expression may indicate a critical dependence of the cancer cell on the specific function of the target, and thus drug treatment is likely to result in effective cell killing (Fig. 3).

Second, if the drug target is not involved in neoplastic transformation and/or progression, being an enzyme of nucleotide synthesis, and its expression is low at the time of drug treatment, it will be saturated, and a high cytotoxic effect will be obtained. On the contrary, high expression will result in the residual drug target being available for cell survival with the treatment producing low cell killing. Typical examples of such targets are thymidylate synthase [TS (7)] and ribonucleotide reductase (RR) (Fig. 4).

Third, mutations may reduce the affinity of the drug for the target, thus resulting in unbound target and drug resistance (i.e., mutations affecting the kinase domain of *c-kit*). Less frequently, mutations affecting the coding sequence may increase the drug affinity of the target resulting in effective target saturation, high cytotoxicity, and optimal tumor sensitivity (Fig. 5).

Finally, genetic variation in the drug-metabolizing enzymes may be associated with a poor- or extensive-metabolizer phenotype. Examples of well-characterized polymorphic

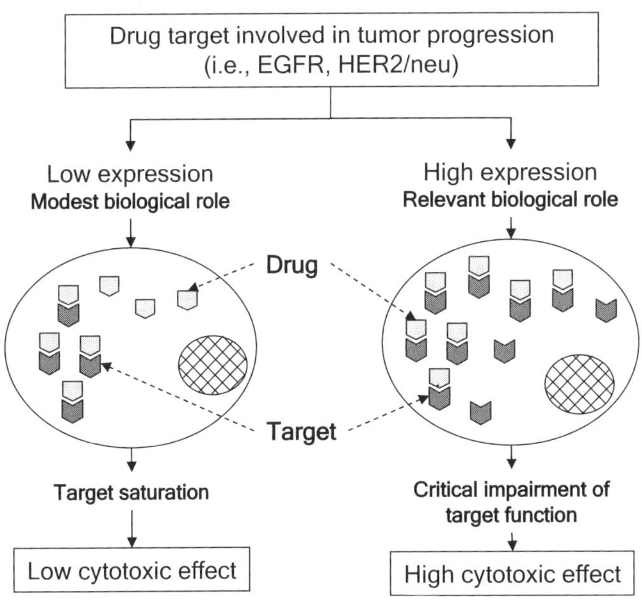

Figure 3 Relationship between chemosensitivity and the expression of drug targets involved in neoplastic transformation and/or progression. If the expression is low at the time of drug treatment, this reflects a secondary role played by the drug target, and, despite efficient saturation, the therapeutic effect is likely to be low. In contrast, high expression indicates critical dependence of the cancer cell on the specific function of the target, and drug treatment is likely to result in effective cytotoxicity. A typical example of such a target in solid tumors is *HER2/neu*. *Abbreviations*: EGFR, epidermal growth factor receptor; *HER2/neu*, human epidermal receptor 2/neu.

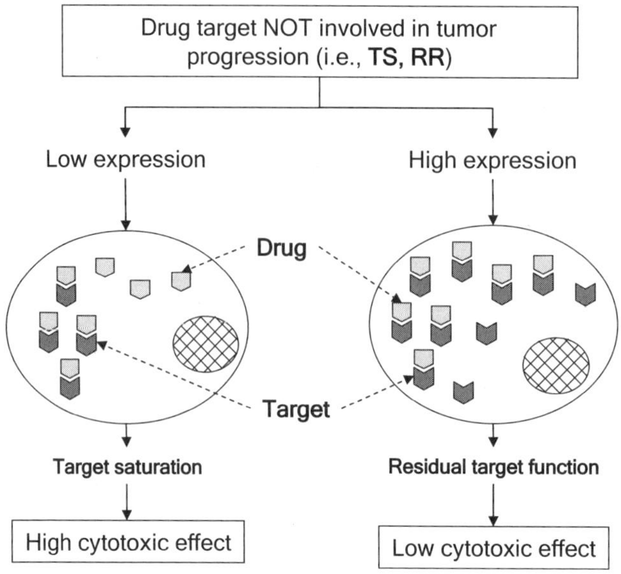

Figure 4 The relationship between chemosensitivity and expression of the drug target not involved in neoplastic transformation and/or progression. If the expression is low at the time of drug treatment, the drug target will be saturated, and a high cytotoxic effect will be obtained. In contrast, high expression will result in the residual drug target being available for the cell to survive and treatment will produce low cytotoxicity. Typical examples of such targets are: TS and RR. *Abbreviations*: TS, thymidylate synthase; RR, ribonucleotide reductase.

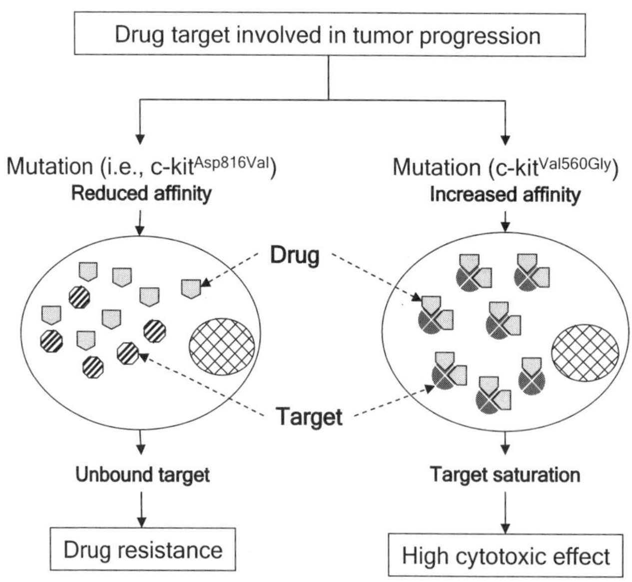

Figure 5 Relationship between chemosensitivity and the genotype of the drug target. Mutations may reduce drug affinity with the target (i.e., $c\text{-}kit^{\mathrm{Asp816Val}}$), thus resulting in unbound target and drug resistance. Conversely, drug-target affinity may be increased (i.e., $c\text{-}kit^{\mathrm{Val560Gly}}$) with effective target saturation, high cytotoxic effect, and optimal tumor sensitivity.

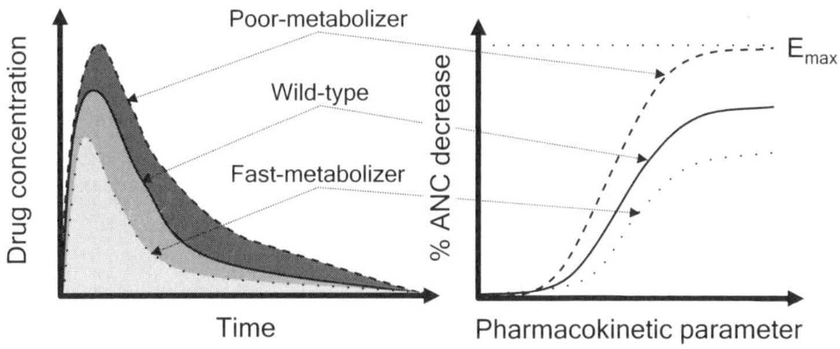

Figure 6 Poor-metabolizer, wild-type, and fast-metabolizer phenotypes and drug pharmacodynamics. Progressive increment in drug area under the concentration-time curve (area under the curve, *shaded areas on the left graph*) results in the increase in both drug exposure of peripheral tissues and drug effect (i.e., ANC decrease, *right graph*). *Abbreviation*: ANC, absolute neutrophil count.

variants are cytochrome P-450 enzymes (CYP450), folyl-polyglutamate synthase, thiopurine *S*-methyltransferase, UDP-glucuronosyl-transferase, dihydropyrimidine dehydrogenase, and glutathione *S*-transferase. The drugs affected are epipodophyllotoxins, antifolates, thiopurines, camptothecins and anthracyclines, fluoropyrimidines, and cisplatin analogs, respectively. The extensive-metabolizer phenotype, with respect to enzymes of drug inactivation, is associated with reduced drug exposure of cancer cells and normal tissues, high tolerability, but impaired activity, whereas high activity of the enzymes involved in prodrug activation (i.e., CYP450 and cyclophosphamide) is likely to result in poor tolerability but high anticancer activity (Fig. 6).

PHARMACOGENETICS OF DRUG TARGETS AND ENZYMES OF DRUG METABOLISM

5-Fluorouracil

5-Fluorouracil (5-FU) is still one of the most widely used antineoplastic agents; its effect is mainly dependent on the inhibition of TS, an enzyme involved in the de novo biosynthesis of pyrimidines, by the active metabolite 2′-deoxy-5-fluorouridine monophosphate (2′-dFUMP), whereas the triphosphate metabolites interfere with nucleic acid synthesis (Fig. 7). It was evident from the time it went into use that some tumor responses to 5-FU were lower than would have been expected, although some patients suffered from severe toxicity, suggesting that genetic factors may have been responsible for the differences. High expression of TS in tumor cells is associated with an unsatisfactory response to chemotherapy (8), and the analysis of the regulatory region of the *TS* gene led to the discovery that variability in gene expression depends, at least in part, on the presence of a polymorphism in the 5′-untranslated region of the promoter (*TSER*). This consists of a sequence of 28 bp, which is repeated from two to nine times, with the number of repetitions being related to the level of gene expression (9) (Fig. 8). Clinical studies have demonstrated that the *TSER*2/2* homozygous genotype is associated with lower levels of TS protein expression compared with individuals homozygous for the allele with three repeats (*TSER*3/3*). Higher translation efficiency is thought to be responsible for the genotype–phenotype relationship (10). Therefore, genotyping the tumor for *TSER* status, in combination with the other factors that follow, is potentially useful to predict cancer sensitivity to fluoropyrimidines.

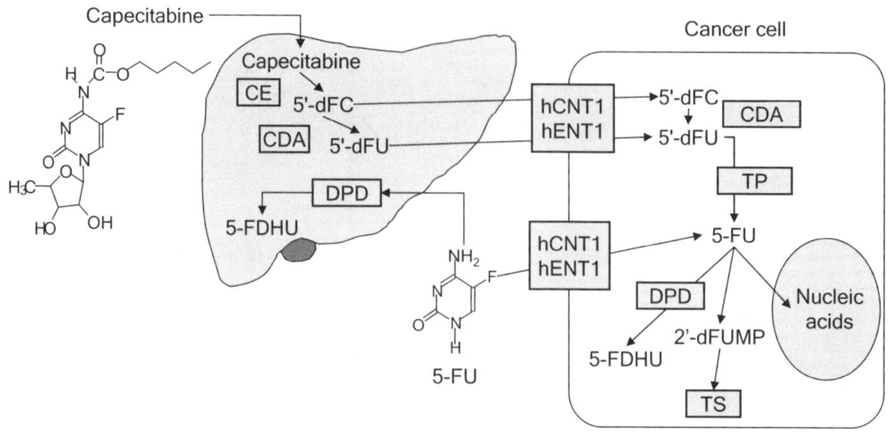

Figure 7 Overview of selected genetic determinants of activity and tolerability of fluoropyrimidines, including CE, CDA, DPD, hCNT1/hENT1, TP, and TS. *Abbreviations*: CE, carboxylesterase; CDA, cytidine deaminase; DPD, dihydropyrimidine dehydrogenase; hCNT1/hENT1, nucleotide concentrative and equilibrative transport systems; TP, thymidine phosphorylase; TS, thymidylate synthase; 5′-dFC, 5′-deoxy-5-fluorocytidine; 5′-dFU, 5′-deoxy-5-fluorouridine; 5-FU, 5-fluorouracil; 5-FDHU, 5-fluoro-5,6-dihydrouracil; 2′-dFUMP, 2′-deoxy-5-fluorouridine monophosphate.

Dihydropyrimidine dehydrogenase (DPD) is the rate-limiting step in 5-FU catabolism with 85% of the dose of 5-FU being inactivated by the enzyme; therefore, a genetically determined deficiency of the enzyme is associated with a profound alteration in metabolism and severe toxicity (Fig. 9) (11). The most common alteration associated with severe toxicity is the A → G transition at position 1986 (*DPYD*2A* allele) leading

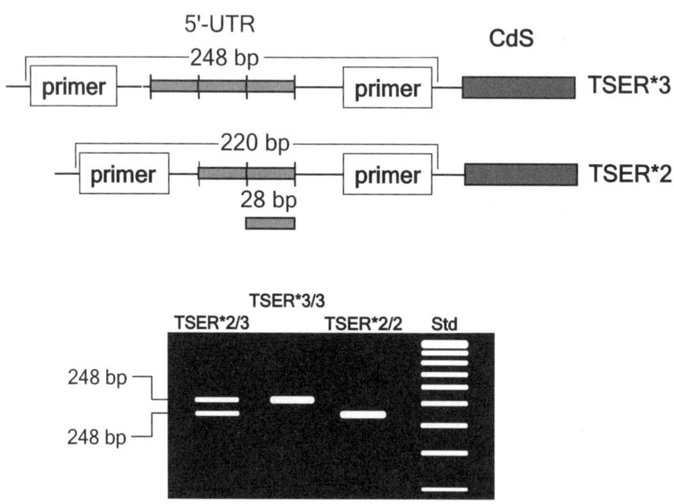

Figure 8 Characterization of SLP variants of the TSER. In this example, PCR amplification with specific primers (*top*) yields fragments of different lengths; separation on an agarose gel (*bottom*) shows three genotypes corresponding to heterozygotes for 2/3 repeats (*TSER*2/3*) and homozygotes for two (*TSER*2/2*) and three repeats (*TSER*3/3*). *Abbreviations*: SLP, sequence length polymorphic; TSER, enhancer region of the promoter of thymidylate synthase; 5′-UTR, 5′-untranslated region of the gene; CdS, coding sequence; bp, base pair.

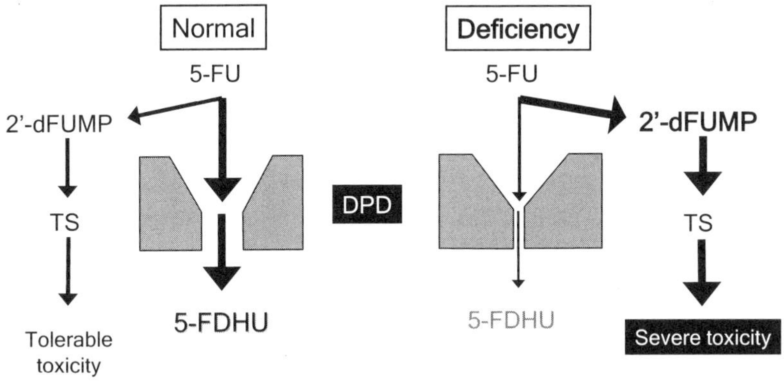

Figure 9 Mechanism of 5-FU toxicity depending on the deficiency of DPD. In the normal phenotype (*left*), a substantial proportion of the 5-FU dose is metabolized to the inactive metabolite 5-FDHU, while a minor proportion is anabolized to the active metabolite 2′-dFUMP, which inhibits TS. If metabolism through DPD is impaired, an excessive amount of 5-FU is converted into 2′-dFUMP, thus resulting in marked TS inhibition and severe damage to normal tissues (*right*). *Abbreviations*: DPD, dihydropyrimidine dehydrogenase; 5-FDHU, 5-dihydro-FU; 2′-dFUMP, 2′-deoxy-5-fluorouridine monophosphate; TS, thymidylate synthase.

to the skipping of exon 14 and production of an inactive enzyme (12). This variant is present in up to 3% of the individuals (13). Other mutations have also been discovered (14,15), and DPD genotyping may be a useful pharmacogenetic test for identifying patients at risk of life-threatening toxicities. Moreover, low levels of DPD expression in tumors are associated with poor 5-FU inactivation and higher efficacy rates in patients with colorectal cancer (16).

Oral bioavailability of 5-FU is poor because of high DPD activity in the gut and liver; therefore, administration of 5-FU and a DPD inhibitor (i.e., ethynyluracil) or a 5-FU prodrug, such as capecitabine, has proved to be an effective strategy. Capecitabine is a promising tumor-specific agent because it releases 5-FU in the cancer cells expressing high levels of thymidine phosphorylase (TP), an enzyme of drug anabolism (Fig. 7). TP, also known as platelet-derived-endothelial cell growth factor, is associated with high proliferation rate, angiogenesis, and inhibition of apoptosis (17). It has been demonstrated that higher expression of TP in tumors, with respect to healthy tissues, is associated with extensive metabolism of 5′-deoxy-5-fluorouridine (5′-dFU) to 5-FU (18). Therefore, genetic stratification of patients to be given capecitabine may include the analysis of TP gene expression, together with *TS* and *DPD*, to assess their likelihood of response to the treatment (Fig. 7) (16). Indeed, the probability of survival is higher in patients with metastatic colorectal cancers that have a low expression of TS, DPD, and TP genes (16). Furthermore, the TP/DPD gene expression ratio was significantly different between sensitive and resistant tumors (19).

Retrospective studies have correlated microsatellite instability (MSI) and survival with the benefit of adjuvant 5-FU chemotherapy in patients with stages II and III colon cancer. Patients not given adjuvant chemotherapy, whose tumors displayed high-frequency MSI (H-MSI), had a better five-year survival with respect to patients with low-frequency MSI (L-MSI) or microsatellite stability (MSS). On the contrary, adjuvant chemotherapy with 5-FU improved overall survival among patients with MSS or L-MSI tumors, whereas no benefit was obtained with adjuvant chemotherapy in the group with H-MSI (20). However, the predictive value of these genetic markers, including *TP53*, has not been fully validated, and cDNA microarray-generated gene expression profiles of tumors may allow a much more accurate analysis of 5-FU sensitivity (21).

Methotrexate

Methotrexate (MTX) is a wide-spectrum antimetabolite active against solid and hematologic malignancies. MTX penetrates the cells through the reduced folate carrier (RFC) and is activated by folylpoly-gamma-glutamate synthase (FPGS); in cancer cells resistant to MTX, defective polyglutamation due to the loss of FPGS activity (22), reduced expression of RFC (23), and increased levels of DHFR due to the C829C SNP in the 3′-untranslated region of the gene (24) have been described. In contrast, DHFR mutations occur rarely, and it seems unlikely that they play a major role in the acquired resistance to MTX (25). The 5,10-methylentetrahydrofolate reductase (MTHFR) enzyme is targeted by MTX; two of the best characterized variants in the genes are the *C677T* and *A1298C* SNPs. The common MTHFR C677T polymorphism decreases enzyme activity; in TT homozygous patients activity is decreased by 70% with respect to CC subjects, while TT subjects have significantly lower plasma folate concentrations than the CT and CC subjects (26). The TT genotype is associated with severe MTX-induced oral mucositis and delayed hematological recovery (27), suggesting that MTHFR genotyping could have a role in MTX dosing strategies in patients. Finally, screening of the RFC gene revealed at least seven SNPs, with one resulting in an amino acid substitution (Arg → His) at position 27 of the carrier, although it was considered not to be relevant for folate and antifolate uptake (28). In contrast, a CATG frameshift causes the synthesis of a nonfunctional carrier, resulting in low MTX transport rates in cancer cells, and is a mechanism for drug resistance (28).

Gemcitabine

Gemcitabine (difluorodeoxycitidine, dFdC) is an antimetabolite pyrimidine analog clinically used in the treatment of pancreas, lung, breast, and bladder cancers. The drug inhibits RR by the diphosphate metabolite dFdCDP and DNA synthesis by incorporation of the triphosphate metabolite (dFdCTP) during the *S*-phase of the cell cycle. Biochemical studies have demonstrated that the prodrug gemcitabine is converted into dFdCMP by deoxycytidine kinase (dCK), the rate-limiting enzyme of the *salvage* pathway of nucleotide synthesis, while cytidine deaminase (CdA) and 5′-nucleotidase (5′-NT) play an important role in drug catabolism (29,30). Preclinical studies have demonstrated that the sensitivity of tumor cells to dFdC depends, at least in part, on the expression of activating and inactivating enzymes, on the intracellular amount of dFdCTP, and also on the cellular target enzyme RR (29,31). These findings underscore the potential role of RR, an essential enzyme of DNA synthesis and repair, because it maintains a large deoxyribonucleotide pool by reduction of ribonucleotides (32). Indeed, chemosensitive tumors have low expression of RR, while dCK is upregulated; thus gemcitabine is converted into active metabolites, inhibits RR, lowers the deoxynucleotide pool, and thereby facilitates the incorporation of dFdCTP into the DNA (33) (Fig. 10). Conversely, in tumors resistant to gemcitabine, the expression of RR is high and dCK is low (34). Experimental studies have demonstrated that downregulation of the catalytic subunit of RR (RRM2) enhances chemosensitivity to gemcitabine (35) and clinical studies are underway to test the clinical advantage achieved by individually tailored chemotherapy on the basis of gene profiling of the tumor, which includes the regulatory subunit of RR (RRM1) (36). Finally, alternatively spliced dCK transcripts have been detected at high frequency in

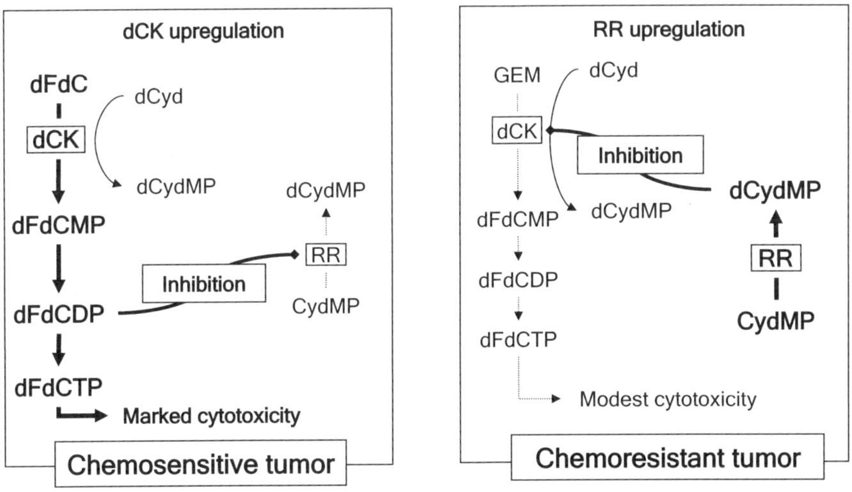

Figure 10 Overview of molecular determinants of gemcitabine (dFdC) activity and opposite regulation of dCK and RR activity. A chemosensitive tumor (*left*) is characterized by elevated expression of dCK and low expression of RR; the opposite genetic signature is associated with the resistant tumor (*right*). *Abbreviations*: MP, DP, TP, mono-, di-, and tri-phosphate metabolites; dCK, deoxycytidine kinase; RR, ribonucleotide reductase; dCyd, deoxycytidine.

cytarabine-resistant leukemic cell lines and preliminary data indicate that this also occurs in solid tumors; since this genetic abnormality does not have a dominant-negative inhibitory effect on normal dCK activity, cells must have lost wild-type dCK expression (37).

Irinotecan

Irinotecan is a wide spectrum anticancer agent with a preeminent role in the therapy of colorectal cancer. Cleavage of the bispiperidine moiety of irinotecan by carboxylesterases releases the active metabolite SN-38 (Fig. 11), which is up to 1000 times more potent than the parent compound in inhibiting nuclear topoisomerase I through the formation of the SN-38–topoisomerase I–DNA ternary complex. This results in DNA fragmentation during replication (38). Gene sequencing has revealed the presence of several non-synonymous mutations, potentially associated with drug resistance and mainly involving exons 12, 13, 15, and 20. Most of them occur in the DNA-binding domain, resulting in amino acid changes (Gly717Val, Ile721Arg, Asn722Ser, Asn722Ala, Thr729Ile, and Thr729Ala); others affect exons 12 and 13 (Phe361Ser, Arg362Leu, Gly363Cys, Arg364Gly, Met370Thr, and Glu418Lys), whereas the Ala653Pro mutation in the linker domain of topoisomerase I results in a marked increase in the re-ligation rate relative to the wild-type enzyme (39–41). Therefore, it is conceivable that mutational analysis of topoisomerase I might be considered to exclude patients from receiving irinotecan chemotherapy if their genotype suggests drug resistance. Likewise, selection of patients on the basis of their risk of toxicity is an important goal of clinical pharmacogenetics. Uridine diphosphate-glucuronosyl transferase, and in particular the *UGT1A1* isoform, plays a pivotal role in SN-38 detoxification, leading to the formation of the inactive metabolite SN-38 glucuronate (SN-38G) (42) (Figs. 11, 12). The rate of SN-38 glucuronidation is genetically determined and variants of uridine glucuronyl transferase (UGT) with low activity have been described, thus providing a potential reason for the severe neutropenia

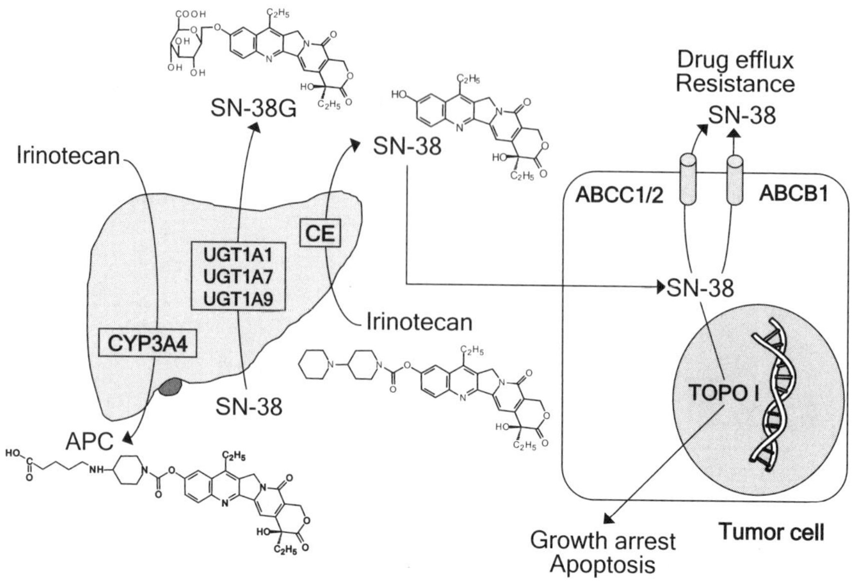

Figure 11 Overview of selected molecular determinants of irinotecan activity and tolerability. *Abbreviations*: APC, 7-ethyl-10-[4-N-(5-aminopentanoic acid)-1-piperidino]-carbonyloxy-camptothecin; SN-38G, glucuronide metabolite of SN-38; *CYP3A4*, cytochrome P450 3A4 isoform; *UGT1A1/7/9*, *UGT1A 1*, *-7*, and *-9* isoforms; CE, carboxylesterase; *ABCB1-C1/2*, ATP-binding cassette drug transporters B1-C1/2; TOPO I, topoisomerase I.

and dose-limiting diarrhea suffered by some patients. However, the clinical relevance and utility of UGT variants in irinotecan toxicity remains to be firmly established. The most common cause of reduced glucuronidation is a polymorphism in the promoter region of *UGT1A1*, which consists of a variable number of TA tandem sequences (43). Individuals who have a high number of TA repeats, that is, TA_7 (*UGT1A1*28*) versus wild-type TA_6 (*UGT1A1*1*), have reduced gene expression and diminished *UGT1A1* production (44). Additional nucleotide changes in the *UGT1A1* gene generate a number of variants with reduced activity (*UGT1A1*6*, *UGT1A1*7*, *UGT1A1*27*, *UGT1A1*29*, Fig. 12) (45). Other UGT isoforms involved in irinotecan metabolism also show missense mutations with moderate to profound reduction in UGT activity, including Met33Thr Asp256Asn in *UGT1A9* (46,47) and Trp208Arg, Asn129Lys, and Arg131Lys in *UGT1A7* (46). Finally, the influence of irinotecan oxidation to 7-ethyl-10-[4-*N*-(5-aminopentanoic acid)-1-piperidino]-carbonyloxy-camptothecin (APC) and to 7-ethyl-10-(4-amino-1-piperidino)-carbonyloxy-camptothecin (NPC) by *CYP3A4* and its genetic variants is an attractive field of research that awaits further investigation (48).

Taxanes

In mammalian cells, tubulin is a structurally heterogeneous 100-kDa $\alpha\beta$ heterodimer with six α- and seven ß-tubulin isotypes. The antimitotics used in chemotherapy, including taxanes and vinca alkaloids, primarily target ß-I tubulin. Paclitaxel is the prototype of the taxane family of antitumor drugs, which also includes docetaxel. It was the first natural product shown to induce the formation of microtubule bundles in cells, followed by impairment of depolymerization and apoptosis by aberrant mitosis or a multinucleated

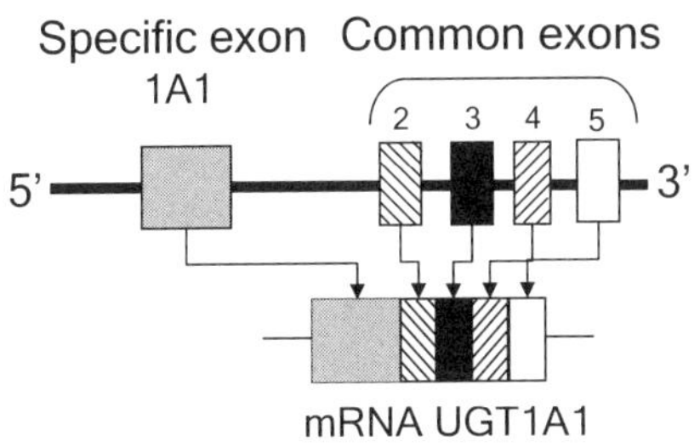

Alleles	Polymorphism	Exons	UGT activity
UGT1A1*1	Normal		Normal
UGT1A1*6	211G>A	1	Reduced
UGT1A1*7	1456T>G	1	Reduced
UGT1A1*27	686C>A	5	Reduced
UGT1A1*28	$(TA)_7TAA$	Promoter	Reduced expression
UGT1A1*29	1099C>G	4	Reduced

Figure 12 *UGT1A1* gene structure and a partial list of genetic variants affecting promoter sequences and gene expression (*UGT1A1*28*) and coding sequences (*UGT1A1*6*, *UGT1A1*7*, *UGT1A1*27*, and *UGT1A1*29*), thus resulting in reduced UGT activity.

G1-like state. Disruption of microtubules also results in the induction of *TP53* and inhibition of cyclin-dependent kinases. As a consequence, cells are arrested in the G2-M phase of the cell cycle, after which they may either undergo cell death by apoptosis or overcome the G2-M stop and continue in the division cycle depending on the tumor cell type. However, the mechanisms by which taxanes induce caspase activation and apoptosis are not yet defined. A possibility is that taxanes are able to induce the phosphorylation of $Bcl\text{-}_{XL}$/Bcl-2 members and thereby inactivate their antiapoptotic activity and also upregulate p53 and p21/WAF-1 (49).

A major mechanism of resistance to taxanes involves the overexpression or mutation of specific tubulin isotypes. Upregulation of the ß-III isotype is an important marker of resistance (50), and high concentrations of α-tubulin are associated with a decrease in paclitaxel sensitivity in MCF-7 breast cancer cells (51). More recently, the overexpression of *HER2/neu* oncoprotein in NIH3T3 cells was shown to be associated with a threefold increase in the expression of the ß-IVa isotype in comparison with the parental line, leading to paclitaxel resistance in transformed cells (52).

Tubulin mutations are important determinants of paclitaxel sensitivity. The amino acid residues 1–31 and 217–233 have a relevant role in paclitaxel binding to the protein and mutations near these sites, such as Thr274Ile and Arg282Gln, may be associated with a drug-resistant phenotype (53). Therefore, mutational and gene expression analysis of tubulin isotypes might be of critical importance in assessing the degree of sensitivity of cancer cells towards taxanes.

Metabolism of paclitaxel in tissues is primarily dependent on inactivating biotransformation through hydroxylation at the C6′ or C3′ position of the C-13 side chain by cytochrome P450 (CYP) 2C8 and 3A4 isoforms, respectively. Several polymorphisms have been described in the encoding genes, such as *CYP2C8*2*, *CYP2C8*3*, *CYP3A4*17*, and *CYP3A4*18* (54,55), thereby providing a partial explanation for interpatient variability in drug pharmacokinetics (56,57).

Alkylating Agents

The oxazaphosphorine alkylating agents cyclophosphamide (CTX) and ifosfamide (IFX) are prodrugs that undergo extensive P450-catalyzed metabolism to yield both active (4-hydroxylated, i.e., 4-hydroxy-CTX/IFX and ifo/phosphoramide mustard) and therapeutically inactive but neurotoxic *N*-dechloroethylated metabolites (i.e., dechloroethyl-CTX/IFX and chloroacetaldehyde). Metabolism studies using cDNA-expressed CYP isoforms have shown that the production of active cytotoxic metabolites mainly depends on the activity of, in decreasing order of importance, *CYP2B6* $\gg$ 3A4 for CTX and *CYP3A4* $\gg$ 2B6 for IFX, whereas the production of neurotoxic metabolites almost exclusively occurs through the *CYP3A4* isozyme for CTX and CYP3A4 $>$ 2B6 for IFX (58). Overexpression of the type 1 (cytosolic) isoform of aldehyde dehydrogenase (ALDH1), which irreversibly oxidizes aldophosphamide, the major circulating metabolite of CTX, to the inactive metabolite carboxyphosphamide may be associated with drug resistance. Indeed, a retrospective analysis has shown that cellular levels of ALDH1A1 were significantly higher in metastatic tumor cells that (*i*) had survived exposure to CTX and (*ii*) did not respond to subsequent treatment with CTX-based chemotherapeutic regimens than in those that did respond to such regimens. The therapeutic outcome of CTX-based chemotherapy corresponded to cellular ALDH1A1 levels in 77% of the cases, and partial or complete responses to CTX-based chemotherapy occurred 2.3 times more often when the ALDH1A1 level was low than when it was high (59). Finally, variability in CYP2B6 activity (60) could be responsible for severe neurological toxicities induced by IFX, because of the overproduction of dechloroethyl-IFX and chloroacetaldehyde, although this is yet to be shown.

The glutathione-*S*-transferase (*GST*) gene locus is located on chromosome 11q13 and encodes the A, M, P, and T isozymes. The GST enzymes conjugate electrophilic groups of toxic compounds, including chemotherapeutic agents, with glutathione. Amplification of the *GSTP* gene locus is a common event in head and neck squamous cell cancer; indeed, tumors with a normal *GSTP* copy number responded completely to cisplatin-based neoadjuvant chemotherapy, whereas patients showing *GSTP* gene amplification did not respond and died within nine months of the diagnosis (61). The *GSTP1* gene product shows a Ile104Val polymorphism; survival of patients with advanced colorectal cancer when given 5-FU/oxaliplatin therapy varied according to the *GSTP1* genotype and was 24.9 months (homozygous 105Val/105Val), 13.3 months (heterozygous 105Ile/105Val), and 7.9 months (homozygous 105Ile/105Ile) (62). A second *GSTP1* variant (Ala113Val) displays higher activity (from 2.5- to 15-fold) with chlorambucil than other variants of GSTP1 (Ile104/Val113, Val104/Ala113, and Val104/Val113) (63). Finally, a promoter region polymorphism in the *GSTA1*B* gene is associated with reduced expression of the enzyme with respect to the wild-type allele. Breast cancer patients given cyclophosphamide-containing chemotherapy showed a 5-year survival rate of 66% (0 or 1 *GSTA1*B*) or 86% (*GSTA1*B/*B*), the risk of death during the first five years after diagnosis being significantly reduced in *GSTA1*B/*B* subjects (64).

Inhibitors of Growth Factor Receptor Tyrosine Kinases

The rationale to target growth factor receptors is compelling; they are frequently upregulated in human cancers and confer either more aggressive clinical behavior or are responsible for malignant transformation (1). The well-characterized drug targets in solid tumors are erbB1 (*EGFR* or *HER1*) and erbB2 (*HER2/neu*), two proteins belonging to the erbB family, and also the *c-kit*/stem cell factor receptor (SCFR). ErbB1 is a 170-kD transmembrane glycoprotein that forms homo- (erbB1/erbB1) or heterodimers (erbB1/erbB2, erbB1/erbB3) with other members of the family upon binding with EGF or other ligands, including transforming growth factor-α (TGF-α) (65). The erbB2 is a 185-kD tyrosine kinase anchored to the cell membrane; although a ligand for erbB2 has not been identified, this protein is the preferred heterodimerization partner within the family (65). Gene amplification, mutation, and increased expression of the erbB members have been reported in glioblastomas, breast, lung, colon, bladder, and head and neck malignancies (65). The receptor tyrosine kinase (RTK) inhibitors, gefitinib and erlotinib, block the activation of the signal transduction pathway initiated by the RTK of erbB1, whereas the monoclonal antibodies, cetuximab and trastuzumab, target erbB1 and erbB2, respectively (65). Treatment with these drugs results in clinically significant responses in patients with non-small cell lung cancer (NSCLC) [gefitinb, erlotinib (66)], colorectal cancer (cetuximab), and breast cancer (trastuzumab) (65). The activity of trastuzumab is dependent on gene amplification and overexpression of erbB2, whereas the role of target expression and/or activation of signal transduction pathway of erbB1 is less clear (67). Resistance to EGF-RTK inhibitors and anti-erbB1 monoclonal antibodies is likely to occur in tumors bearing the most common EGFR mutation, namely *EGFRvIII* (ΔEGFR or del2-7EGFR), which is characterized by the deletion of exons 2–7 in EGFR mRNA as a result of alternative splicing or gene rearrangements, and encodes for a truncated extracellular EGF-binding domain with ligand-independent constitutive activation (68).

Imatinib is an effective inhibitor of the *c-kit*/SCFR and platelet-derived growth factor receptor A (PDGFRA); this receptor is mutated and overfunctioning in a selected group of malignancies, particularly gastrointestinal stromal tumors (GIST). Activating mutations of *c-kit* gene, mostly involving exons 9 and 11, are present in up to 92% of the GISTs and are likely to play a critical role in the development of these tumors (69). In patients with GIST-harboring exon 11 *c-kit* mutations, the partial response rate was 83.5%, whereas patients with tumors containing an exon 9 mutation or no detectable mutations of *c-kit* or PDGFRA had partial response rates significantly lower (47.8% and 0.0%, respectively) (69). Finally, cells bearing the Asp816Phe, Asp816Tyr, and Asp816Val mutations in the kinase domain of *c-kit* are resistant to imatinib, whereas the Val560Gly mutant displays increased affinity for the drug (Fig. 5) (70).

PHARMACOGENETICS OF DNA REPAIR SYSTEMS AND APOPTOSIS

Antimetabolites

Damage to DNA induced by antimetabolites is recognized by the cell and generates a signal that blocks proliferation in order to repair the alteration and allows the proliferation to either resume or depending on the extent of the damage, triggers cell death by apoptosis. The regulation of this machinery is finely regulated by proapoptotic factors, such as p53, Bax, and related proteins, and antiapoptotic factors, which are mainly members of the Bcl-2 superfamily (71).

Defects in the ability of tumor cells to undergo apoptosis may result in drug resistance and poor clinical outcome. The *TP53* gene product is characterized by a 3′–5′ exonuclease activity (72) and controls the transactivation of proapoptotic factors (i.e., Bax, Bak) and the repression of antiapoptotic pathways (i.e., Bcl-2, Bcl-X_L), hence favoring the death of cells with irrepairable DNA damage (Fig. 13). Given that *TP53* is a tumor suppressor gene, a defective *TP53* pathway will allow cell proliferation to proceed in the presence of damaged DNA, thereby causing accumulation of DNA mutations (73). Reduced sensitivity of tumor cells to antimetabolites, such as 5-FU, may thus be due to *TP53* gene mutations (74), which is unable to upregulate Bax and downregulate Bcl-2.

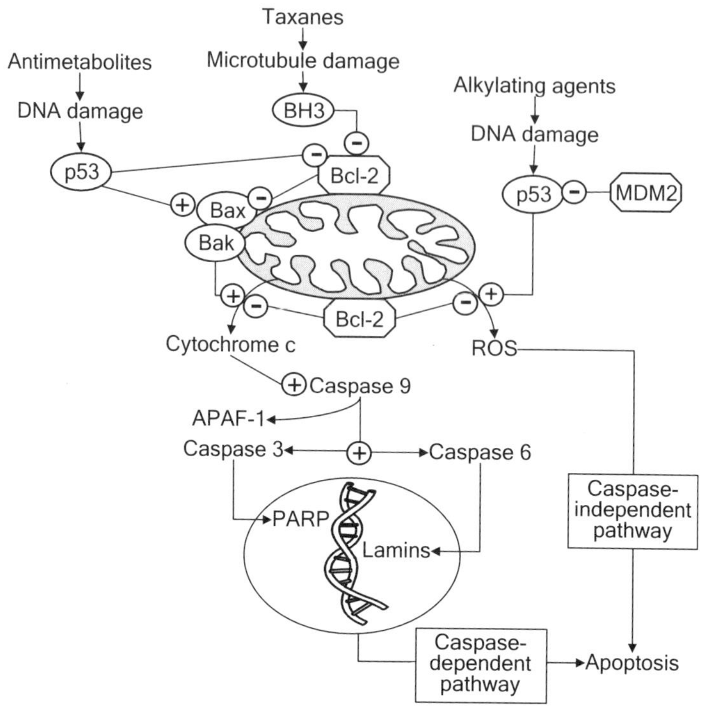

Figure 13 Schematic representation of apoptosis pathways triggered by antimetabolites, alkylating, and antimicrotubule agents. Proapototic factors (Bax and Bak) are activated by p53, which is in turn suppressed by MDM2; Bcl-2 inhibits caspase-dependent and -independent apoptosis initiated by the release of cytochrome c and ROS, respectively. *Abbreviations*: PARP, poly (ADP-ribose) polymerase; BH3, Bcl-2 homology 3 domain; APAF-1, apoptosis protease activating factor 1; −, inhibition; +, induction; ROS, reactive oxygen species.

Similar findings have been obtained in ovarian cancer, where p53 overexpression or missense mutations were associated with resistance to platinum compounds, early relapse, and shortened overall survival (75). Indeed, the ratio between Bcl-x_L and Bax is significantly associated with 5-FU chemosensitivity in colorectal carcinoma cell lines (76), whereas Bax overexpression in gliomas is sufficient to render the cells more sensitive to apoptosis even in the presence of a deficient *TP53* pathway (77). Finally, the mismatch repair (MMR) system is the crucial mutation avoidance machinery that recognizes and repairs mismatched and unpaired bases that arise from replication errors and DNA-damaging agents. In MMR-proficient cells, inability to repair sublethal damage to the DNA results in cell cycle arrest and apoptosis; conversely, MMR-deficient cells are not deleted and accumulate mutations that may result in aberrant biological behavior and potentially cancerogenesis. The expression of two important MMR members, hMLH1 and hMSH2, is significantly correlated with response to the chemotherapy regimen comprising cyclophosphamide, methotrexate, and 5-FU (CMF) in patients with advanced ductal breast cancer and lymph node metastasis. Patients with low hMLH1 immunoreactivity have a significantly higher failure rate with the CMF regimen than those with high hMLH1 expression (78). MMR-deficient tumor cells are resistant to the cytotoxic effects of 5-FU, and demethylation of the hMLH1 promoter in hypermethylated colorectal cancer cells restores MMR proficiency and drug sensitivity to 5-FU (79). Finally, loss of chemosensitivity to gemcitabine may arise as a consequence of cisplatin-mediated selection of

MMR-deficient cells, and the presence of such cells in a tumor may predispose to drug resistance and treatment failure (80).

Alkylating Agents

Cisplatin and related drugs, including carboplatin and oxaliplatin, inhibit cell proliferation by irreversibly damaging DNA through the formation of intra- and interstrand cross-links. Drug resistance occurs because of poor cisplatin accumulation, detoxification, or efficient repair of damaged DNA by the nucleotide excision repair (NER) system. The NER superfamily is composed of numerous members, including *ERCC1*, *XPA*, *XPB*, *XPC*, *XPD*, and *XPF*, which display different functions (helicases, 3′- and 5′-endonucleases, and ligases) (81). Among those factors, the *ERCC1* (excision repair cross complementing 1) gene product forms a heterodimer with *XPF*, and the complex is responsible for the endonuclease activity required to repair the DNA damage (Fig. 14). In vitro studies have demonstrated that upregulation of *ERCC1-XPF* is associated with cisplatin resistance (82). However, in another study, DNA repair activity was not correlated with cytotoxicity of cisplatin and melphalan in ovary and colon cancer cells (83).

ERCC1 gene expression affects the clinical outcome of patients with NSCLC and colorectal cancer treated with cisplatin and oxaliplatin, with response and survival being improved in the presence of low *ERCC1* expression (84,85). The survival of patients with relapsed colorectal cancer treated with oxaliplatin/5-FU was 17.4 months in subjects with the wild-type 751Lys/Lys XPD, whereas survival of patients with 751Lys/Gln and 751Gln/Gln polymorphism was reduced to 12.8 and 3.3 months, respectively (86). The O6-alkyl(methyl)guanine-DNA alkyl(methyl)transferase (AGAT/MGMT) is capable of protecting cells from the mutagenic effect of DNA alkylation and, therefore, from the cytotoxicity induced by chemotherapeutic drugs, such as BCNU (87,88). Correlation between pretreatment expression of AGAT/MGMT and response to treatment has so far been established in primary brain tumors only. Patients with malignant astrocytoma treated with BCNU had a better objective response when the AGAT/MGMT expression levels were low (89). Furthermore, low AGAT/MGMT activity, due to promoter methylation, was associated with statistically significant prolongation of survival and improved

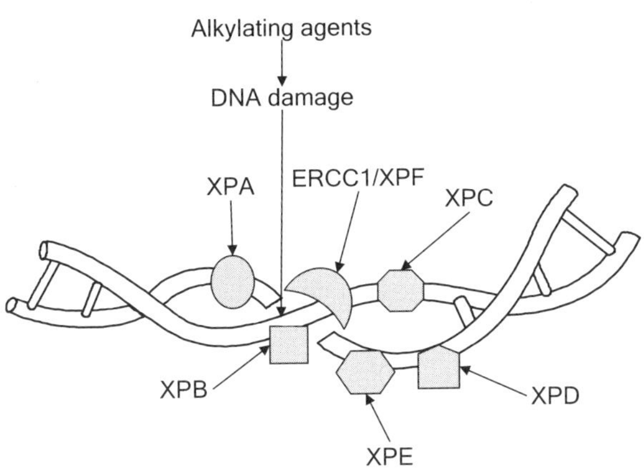

Figure 14 Members of the NER system. XPA, XPC, and XPE are involved in DNA damage recognition by alkylating agents; *ERCC1*/XPF have 5′-endonuclease activity, XPG has 3′-endonuclease activity, while XPB and XPD have helicase activity (109). *Abbreviation*: NER, nucleotide excision repair.

disease-free survival in patients with gliomas treated with the combination of BCNU and cisplatin (90). Similar results were observed in patients with astrocytomas and glioblastomas; a 60% response rate to temozolomide was obtained if tumor expression of AGAT/MGMT was low, but the response rate was only 9% in those with high enzyme activity; tumor MMR status was less predictive of response than AGAT/MGMT (91).

THE ATP-BINDING CASSETTE SUPERFAMILY OF DRUG TRANSPORTERS

The ATP-binding cassette (ABC) superfamily includes P-glycoprotein (MDR1, *ABCB1*), multidrug resistance-associated protein 1 (MRP1, *ABCC1*), canalicular multiorganic anion transporter (cMOAT, *ABCC2*), and breast cancer resistance protein/mitoxantrone resistance protein (BCRP/MXR, *ABCG2*). These transporters play an important role in drug distribution and elimination, being expressed in the lower intestinal tract, liver, kidney, and blood-brain. The transporters also play an important role in resistance to structurally unrelated anticancer drugs, including mitoxantrone, anthracyclines, paclitaxel, SN-38, vinca alkaloids, and epipodophyllotoxins (92,93). Many tumors overexpress more than one ABC transporter; however, *ABCB1* is the most important member of the family, and drug resistance characterized by its overexpression is associated with altered distribution and reduced drug levels intracellularly (94). The *ABCB1* gene is polymorphic, and several SNPs have been identified, including *A61G*, *G1199A*, *C1236T*, and *G2677T*; the *C3435T* variant is associated with a lower expression of MDR1 (*ABCB1*) in homozygous TT patients with respect to the CC genotype (95,96). Clinical studies on the effect of the *C3435T* SNP on MDR1 function have produced discrepant results and led to the suggestion that haplotype analysis of the gene should be considered instead of simple SNP detection (97). Expression levels of BCRP, LRP, MRP1, MRP2, and MDR1 in breast cancers responding to anthracycline-based chemotherapy were markedly lower when compared with nonresponding tumors. Furthermore, high expression of MDR1 was found to be significantly associated with a poor progression-free survival (98). In addition to this, MDR1 expression correlated with shorter progression-free survival in locally advanced bladder cancer. MRP1 expression significantly predicted for higher likelihood of response and bladder preservation following neoadjuvant chemotherapy and high lung resistance–related protein/major vault protein (LRP/MVP) expression was associated with worse response to neoadjuvant chemotherapy and a decrease in the probability of bladder preservation (99). Moreover, patients with LRP-positive metastatic testicular germ-cell tumors had significantly shorter progression-free and overall survival than LRP-negative patients, suggesting that LRP upregulation at the time of diagnosis is associated with an adverse clinical outcome (100). Finally, LRP expression correlated inversely with response to platinum-based chemotherapy in NSCLC (response rates, 33% and 100% for patients with LRP-positive and LRP-negative tumors, respectively) (101).

CLINICAL PHARMACOGENETICS

The determination of the clinical utility of pharmacogenetics is currently a high research priority in oncology. A large number of important genetic determinants have been identified thus far in tumors, but the clinical relevance of most of them currently remains unconfirmed because the data correlating specific tumor markers with survival or therapeutic response have been limited by the (*i*) small number of patients screened due to the difficulties in obtaining suitable tissue samples, (*ii*) lack of studies primarily designed to detect specific correlations between gene abnormalities and drug response or disease prognosis, and (*iii*) marked variability in analytical methodology and lack of quality controls among different studies. TP53 and ErbB2 represent a sound example of the problematic link between the choice of reference methodology and the determination of clinical utility. These genes may be analyzed by different methods, including sequencing, fluorescence in situ hybridization, and immunohistochemistry, but even for a single type of analysis, the specific methodological procedure and the interpretation criteria may be subjected to considerable variability.

TP53 is the most widely studied gene in gastrointestinal cancer; however, it has not been validated as a prognostic marker, despite the large number of articles published in the scientific literature and the continuous interest in methodologic improvement with the aim of making genetic analysis feasible for routine use. Indeed, there is no single guideline in gastrointestinal oncology that currently recommends the routine analysis of *TP53* status for the assessment of prognosis or drug response. This is despite the evidence that a high proportion of mutations are present in colorectal tumors (upto 73.4% cases). Furthermore, using multivariate Cox proportional-hazards analysis, *TP53* gene mutations were found to be a significant and independent predictor of poor prognosis in colorectal cancer (102). To facilitate the transition of molecular markers from the laboratory to the clinic, rigorous standardization of analytical methods and tissue banking (i.e., neoplastic tissue sampling, lymphocytes, tumor protein, and DNA recovered from peripheral blood) (Fig. 15), and the incorporation of these into large clinical studies, is required. Therefore, accurate genetic profiling of tumors and optimally designed human trials are the most important points for future application of pharmacogenetics to the management of patients with cancer. With respect to the genetic profiling of tumors, it will be crucial to identify (*i*) the genetic abnormalities involved in tumorigenesis and disease prognosis, (*ii*) the genes affecting drug response, and (*iii*) the degree of overlap between the two groups. With respect to clinical trial design, the relevant genetic markers associated with disease progression and prognosis could be characterized in

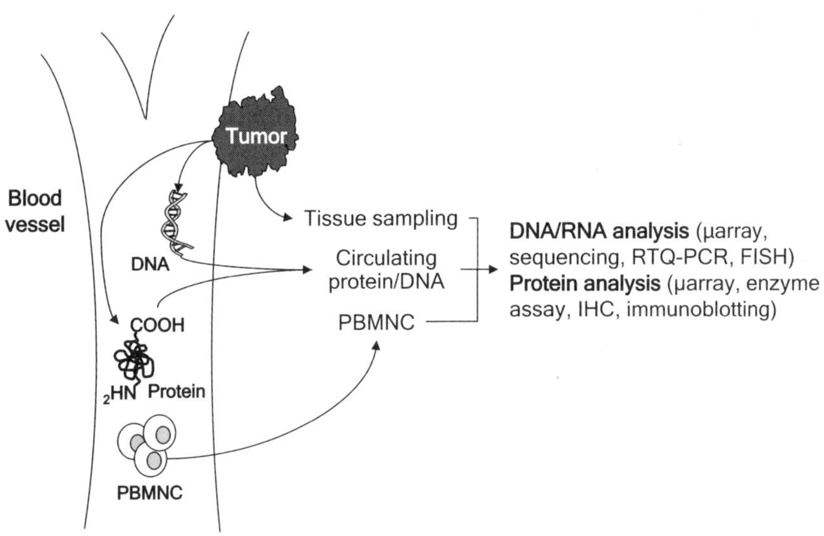

Figure 15 Sources of nucleic acids and proteins for genomic and proteomic profiling of tumors and patients. *Abbreviations*: RTQ-PCR, real-time, quantitative polymerase chain reaction; FISH, fluorescence, in situ hybridization; IHC, immunohistochemistry; PBMNC, peripheral blood mononucleated cells. *Source*: From Ref. 92.

case-control studies, while retrospective analysis may be used to identify genetic alterations associated with drug efficacy (predictivity) (Fig. 16). For example, a recent population-based case-control study demonstrated the presence of a common A870G polymorphism in the cyclin D1 (*CCND1*) gene, the *CCND1* 870A genetic variant being associated with clinically aggressive colorectal cancer (103). The complexity of the problem is evidenced by the observation in another case-control study of *CCND1* A870G genotype, which showed no correlation between the presence of the A allele and tumor pathology or patient survival (104). Retrospective studies revealed important correlations between MSI, survival, and the benefit of adjuvant 5-FU chemotherapy in stages II and III colon cancer. Patients not given adjuvant chemotherapy, whose tumors displayed high-frequency MSI (H-MSI), had a better 5-year survival than patients with low-frequency MSI (L-MSI) or MSS. In contrast, adjuvant chemotherapy with 5-FU improved overall survival among patients with MSS or L-MSI tumors, but no benefit was obtained with adjuvant chemotherapy in the group with H-MSI (105).

Therefore, a critical reappraisal of the role and clinical burden of the many genetic abnormalities detected in solid tumors is needed. Despite the tremendous advances in the comprehension of the molecular and genetic pathways leading to solid tumors, such progress has not yet been translated into better management of patients with cancer (106). Hopefully, translation of novel knowledge into clinical practice may be overcome by the results of well-designed prospective clinical trials in which direct comparison is performed between patient treatment selected on the basis of conventional criteria versus treatment selection based on tumor genotype (Fig. 16).

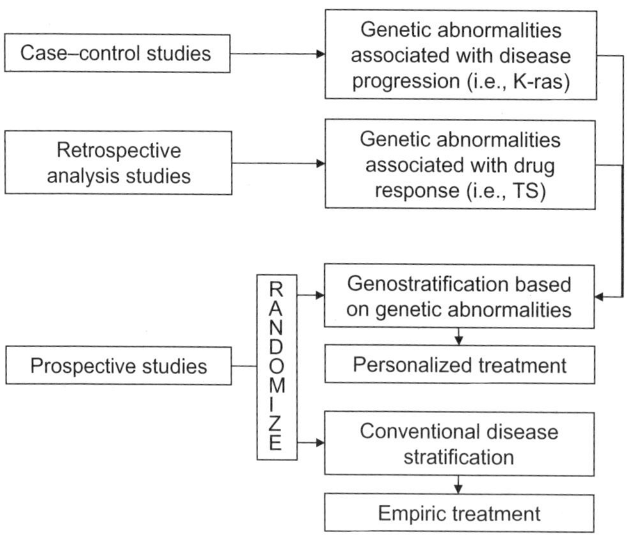

Figure 16 Identification of genetic abnormalities associated with disease progression in case–control studies and those associated with drug response in retrospective studies. The validation of the predictive power of genetic profiling within the clinical setting requires the design of ad hoc randomized clinical trials in which patients are stratified according to their disease genotype and managed specifically or treated empirically with conventional stratification based on clinicopathologic factors known to influence disease outcome. *Abbreviation*: TS, thymidylate synthase.

CONCLUSIONS AND FUTURE PROSPECTS

Despite the pessimism, interest in pharmacogenetics is unlikely to vanish in the future. However, before being stably integrated into the clinical practice, pharmacogenetics needs to be shown to significantly improve the outcome of drug treatment in order to outweigh the extra costs associated with the widespread application of genetic techniques to patient management. The identification of genes implicated in the response to anticancer agents has created the scientific basis for novel approaches, for example, using proteomics, to evaluate the role of gene products in the response of cells to drugs (107). The rationale behind this approach may be summarized as follows: (*i*) several mutations are silent and do not interfere with the function of gene products, (*ii*) the SNPs affecting a gene may be so numerous and their different combinations (haplotypes) so complex that the evaluation of protein function turns out to be simple and more informative, (*iii*) some genes are characterized by posttranscriptional regulation, such as TS (108), therefore gene expression may not be directly related to the synthesis of the protein product, and (*iv*) many additional factors may contribute to the function of proteins, making it difficult to predict the final effect of all factors considered as a whole.

The time delay between drug introduction into clinical practice and the search for genetic factors affecting outcome and tolerability may be significantly reduced by the introduction of pharmacogenetics and pharmacogenomics in clinical studies, and it should be of value in identifying patients at risk of major toxicity or therapeutic failure.

In conclusion, advances in molecular techniques have led to the discovery of genetic factors related to drug sensitivity or resistance within cancer cells, including those in metabolic pathways and cellular targets. The ultimate aim of pharmacogenetics will thus be the segmentation of patients into discrete categories according to their likelihood of response to drugs and the identification, on an individual basis, of subjects with "rare" unfavorable genotypes at risk of major toxicities following treatment administration.

REFERENCES

1. Rowinsky EK. Signal events: cell signal transduction and its inhibition in cancer. Oncologist 2003; 8(suppl 3):5–17.
2. Danesi R, De Braud F, Fogli S, Di Paolo A, Del Tacca M. Pharmacogenetic determinants of anti-cancer drug activity and toxicity. Trends Pharmacol Sci 2001; 22:420–426.
3. Kwok P-Y. Methods for genotyping single nucleotide polymorphisms. Annu Rev Genomics Hum Genet 2001; 2:235–258.
4. Zhang W, Labordé PM, Coombes KR, Berry DA, Hamilton SR. Cancer genomics: promises and complexities. Clin Cancer Res 2001; 7:2159–2167.
5. Krishna R, Mayer LD. Multidrug resistance (MDR) in cancer. Mechanisms, reversal using modulators of MDR and the role of MDR modulators in influencing the pharmacokinetics of anticancer drugs. Eur J Pharm Sci 2000; 11:265–283.
6. Danesi R, De Braud F, Fogli S, De Pas TM, Di Paolo A, Curigliano G, Del Tacca M. Pharmacogenetics of anticancer drug sensitivity in non-small cell lung cancer. Pharmacol Rev 2003; 55:57–103.
7. Peters GJ, Backus HH, Freemantle S, van Triest B, Codacci-Pisanelli G, van der Wilt CL, Smid K, Lunec J, Calvert AH, Marsh S, et al. Induction of thymidylate synthase as a 5-fluorouracil resistance mechanism. Biochim Biophys Acta 2002; 1587:194–205.
8. Aschele C, Debernardis D, Bandelloni R, Cascinu S, Catalano V, Giordani P, Barni S, Turci D, Drudi G, Lonardi S, Gallo L, Maley F, Monfardini S. Thymidylate synthase protein expression in colorectal cancer metastases predicts for clinical outcome to leucovorin-modulated bolus

or infusional 5-fluorouracil but not methotrexate-modulated bolus 5-fluorouracil. Ann Oncol 2002; 13:1882–1892.

9. Pullarkat ST, Stoehlmacher J, Ghaderi V, Xiong YP, Ingles SA, Sherrod A, Warren R, Tsao-Wei D, Groshen S, Lenz HJ. Thymidylate synthase gene polymorphism determines response and toxicity of 5-FU chemotherapy. Pharmacogenomics J 2001; 1:65–70.
10. Kawakami K, Salonga D, Park JM, Danenberg KD, Uetake H, Brabender J, Omura K, Watanabe G, Danenberg PV. Different lengths of a polymorphic repeat sequence in the thymidylate synthase gene affect translational efficiency but not its gene expression. Clin Cancer Res 2001; 7:4096–4101.
11. Di Paolo A, Danesi R, Vannozzi F, Falcone A, Mini E, Cionini L, Ibrahim T, Amadori D, Del Tacca M. Limited sampling model for the analysis of 5-fluorouracil pharmacokinetics in adjuvant chemotherapy for colorectal cancer. Clin Pharmacol Ther 2002; 72:627–637.
12. van Kuilenburg AB, De Abreu RA, van Gennip AH. Pharmacogenetic and clinical aspects of dihydropyrimidine dehydrogenase deficiency. Ann Clin Biochem 2003; 40:41–52.
13. van Kuilenburg AB, Muller EW, Haasjes J, Meinsma R, Zoetekouw L, Waterham HR, Baas F, Richel DJ, van Gennip AH. Lethal outcome of a patient with a complete dihydropyrimidine dehydrogenase (DPD) deficiency after administration of 5-fluorouracil: frequency of the common IVS14 + 1G>A mutation causing DPD deficiency. Clin Cancer Res 2001; 7:1149–1153.
14. Johnson MR, Wang K, Diasio RB. Profound dihydropyrimidine dehydrogenase deficiency resulting from a novel compound heterozygote genotype. Clin Cancer Res 2002; 8:768–774.
15. van Kuilenburg ABP, Haasjes J, Richel DJ, Zoetekouw L, Van Lenthe H, De Abreu RA, Maring JG, Vreken P, van Gennip AH. Clinical implications of dihydropyrimidine dehydrogenase (DPD) deficiency in patients with severe 5-fluorouracil-associated toxicity: identification of new mutations in the DPD gene. Clin Cancer Res 2000; 6:4705–4712.
16. Salonga D, Danenberg KD, Johnson M, Metzger R, Groshen S, Tsao-Wei DD, Lenz HJ, Leichman CG, Leichman L, Diasio RB, Danenberg PV. Colorectal tumors responding to 5-fluorouracil have low gene expression levels of dihydropyrimidine dehydrogenase, thymidylate synthase, and thymidine phosphorylase. Clin Cancer Res 2000; 6:1322–1327.
17. Matsuura T, Kuratate I, Teramachi K, Osaki M, Fukuda Y, Ito H. Thymidine phosphorylase expression is associated with both increase of intratumoral microvessels and decrease of apoptosis in human colorectal carcinomas. Cancer Res 1999; 59:5037–5040.
18. Schuller J, Cassidy J, Dumont E, Roos B, Durston S, Banken L, Utoh M, Mori K, Weidekamm E, Reigner B. Preferential activation of capecitabine in tumor following oral administration to colorectal cancer patients. Cancer Chemother Pharmacol 2000; 45:291–297.
19. Ishikawa T, Sekiguchi F, Fukase Y, Sawada N, Ishitsuka H. Positive correlation between the efficacy of capecitabine and doxifluridine and the ratio of thymidine phosphorylase to dihydropyrimidine dehydrogenase activities in tumors in human cancer xenografts. Cancer Res 1998; 58:685–690.
20. Ribic CM, Sargent DJ, Moore MJ, Thibodeau SN, French AJ, Goldberg RM, Hamilton SR, Laurent-Puig P, Gryfe R, Shepherd LE, Tu D, Redston M, Gallinger S. Tumor microsatellite-instability status as a predictor of benefit from fluorouracil-based adjuvant chemotherapy for colon cancer. N Engl J Med 2003; 349:247–257.
21. Mariadason JM, Arango D, Shi Q, Wilson AJ, Corner GA, Nicholas C, Aranes MJ, Lesser M, Schwartz EL, Augenlicht LH. Gene expression profiling-based prediction of response of colon carcinoma cells to 5-fluorouracil and camptothecin. Cancer Res 2003; 63:8791–8812.
22. Takemura Y, Kobayashi H, Miyachi H. Antifolate resistance and its circumvention by new analogues. Hum Cell 2001; 14:185–202.
23. Serra M, Reverter-Branchat G, Maurici D, Benini S, Shen JN, Chano T, Hattinger CM, Manara MC, Pasello M, Scotlandi K, Picci P. Analysis of dihydrofolate reductase and reduced folate carrier gene status in relation to methotrexate resistance in osteosarcoma cells. Ann Oncol 2004; 15:151–160.

24. Goto Y, Yue L, Yokoi A, Nishimura R, Uehara T, Koizumi S, Saikawa Y. A novel single-nucleotide polymorphism in the 3′-untranslated region of the human dihydrofolate reductase gene with enhanced expression. Clin Cancer Res 2001; 7:1952–1956.
25. Banerjee D, Mayer-Kuckuk P, Capiaux G, Budak-Alpdogan T, Gorlick R, Bertino JR. Novel aspects of resistance to drugs targeted to dihydrofolate reductase and thymidylate synthase. Biochim Biophys Acta 2002; 1587:164–173.
26. de Bree A, Verschuren WM, Bjorke-Monsen AL, van der Put NM, Heil SG, Trijbels FJ, Blom HJ. Effect of the methylene-tetrahydrofolate reductase 677C>T mutation on the relations among folate intake and plasma folate and homocysteine concentrations in a general population sample. Am J Clin Nutr 2003; 77:687–693.
27. Ulrich CM, Yasui Y, Storb R, Schubert MM, Wagner JL, Bigler J, Ariail KS, Keener CL, Li S, Liu H, Farin FM, Potter JD. Pharmacogenetics of methotrexate: toxicity among marrow transplantation patients varies with the methylenetetrahydrofolate reductase C677T polymorphism. Blood 2001; 98:231–234.
28. Whetstine JR, Gifford AJ, Witt T, Liu XY, Flatley RM, Norris M, Haber M, Taub JW, Ravindranath Y, Matherly LH. Single nucleotide polymorphisms in the human reduced folate carrier: characterization of a high-frequency G/A variant at position 80 and transport properties of the His^{27} and Arg^{27} carriers. Clin Cancer Res 2001; 7:3416–3422.
29. Giovannetti E, Mey V, Danesi R, Mosca I, Del Tacca M. Synergistic cytotoxicity and pharmacogenetics of gemcitabine and pemetrexed combination in pancreatic cancer cell lines. Clin Cancer Res 2004; 10:2936–2943.
30. Bergman AM, Pinedo HM, Peters GJ. Determinants of resistance to 2′,2′-difluorodeoxycytidine (gemcitabine). Drug Resist Updat 2002; 5:19–33.
31. Kroep JR, Loves WJ, van der Wilt CL, Alvarez E, Talianidis L, Boven E, Braakhuis BJ, van Groeningen CJ, Pinedo HM, Peters GJ. Pretreatment deoxycytidine kinase levels predict in vivo gemcitabine sensitivity. Mol Cancer Ther 2002; 1:371–376.
32. Burton TR, Kashour T, Wright JA, Amara FM. Cellular signaling pathways affect the function of ribonucleotide reductase mRNA binding proteins: mRNA stabilization, drug resistance, and malignancy. Int J Oncol 2003; 22:21–31.
33. Obata T, Endo Y, Murata D, Sakamoto K, Sasaki T. The molecular targets of antitumor 2′-deoxycytidine analogues. Curr Drug Targets 2003; 4:305–313.
34. Goan Y-G, Zhou B, Hu E, Mi S, Yen Y. Overexpression of ribonucleotide reductase as a mechanism of resistance to 2,2-difluorodeoxycytidine in the human KB cancer cell line. Cancer Res 1999; 59:4204–4207.
35. Duxbury MS, Ito H, Zinner MJ, Ashley SW, Whang EE. RNA interference targeting the M2 subunit of ribonucleotide reductase enhances pancreatic adenocarcinoma chemosensitivity to gemcitabine. Oncogene 2004; 23:1539–1548.
36. Rosell R, Crino L, Danenberg K, Scagliotti G, Bepler G, Taron M, Alberola V, Provencio M, Camps C, De Marinis F, Sanchez JJ, Penas R. Targeted therapy in combination with gemcitabine in non-small cell lung cancer. Semin Oncol 2003; 30(4 suppl 10):19–25.
37. Veuger MJ, Heemskerk MH, Honders MW, Willemze R, Barge RM. Functional role of alternatively spliced deoxycytidine kinase in sensitivity to cytarabine of acute myeloid leukemic cells. Blood 2002; 99:1373–1380.
38. Pommier Y, Pourquier P, Fan Y, Strumberg D. Mechanism of action of eukaryotic DNA topoisomerase I and drugs targeted to the enzyme. Biochim Biophys Acta 1998; 1400:83–106.
39. Chang JY, Liu JF, Juang SH, Liu TW, Chen LT. Novel mutation of topoisomerase I in rendering cells resistant to camptothecin. Cancer Res 2002; 62:3716–3721.
40. Wang LF, Ting CY, Lo CK, Su JS, Mickley LA, Fojo AT, Whang-Peng J, Hwang J. Identification of mutations at DNA topoisomerase I responsible for camptothecin resistance. Cancer Res 1997; 57:1516–1522.
41. Fiorani P, Bruselles A, Falconi M, Chillemi G, Desideri A, Benedetti P. Single mutation in the linker domain confers protein flexibility and camptothecin resistance to human topoisomerase I. J Biol Chem 2003; 278:43268–43275.

42. Cummings J, Boyd G, Ethell BT, Macpherson JS, Burchell B, Smyth JF, Jodrell DI. Enhanced clearance of topoisomerase I inhibitors from human colon cancer cells by glucuronidation. Biochem Pharmacol 2002; 63:607–613.
43. Iyer L, Das S, Janisch L, Wen M, Ramirez J, Karrison T, Fleming GF, Vokes EE, Schilsky RL, Ratain MJ. UGT1A1*28 polymorphism as a determinant of irinotecan disposition and toxicity. Pharmacogenomics J 2002; 2:43–47.
44. Burchell B, Soars M, Monaghan G, Cassidy A, Smith D, Ethell B. Drug-mediated toxicity caused by genetic deficiency of UDP-glucuronosyltransferases. Toxicol Letters 2000; 112–113:333–340.
45. Ando Y, Saka H, Ando M, Sawa T, Muro K, Ueoka H, Yokoyama A, Saitoh S, Shimokata K, Hasegawa Y. Polymorphisms of UDP-glucuronosyltransferase gene and irinotecan toxicity: a pharmacogenetic analysis. Cancer Res 2000; 60:6921–6926.
46. Villeneuve L, Girard H, Fortier LC, Gagne JF, Guillemette C. Novel functional polymorphisms in the UGT1A7 and UGT1A9 glucuronidating enzymes in Caucasian and African-American subjects and their impact on the metabolism of 7-ethyl-10-hydroxycamptothecin and flavopiridol anticancer drugs. J Pharmacol Exp Ther 2003; 307:117–128.
47. Jinno H, Saeki M, Saito Y, Tanaka-Kagawa T, Hanioka N, Sai K, Kaniwa N, Ando M, Shirao K, Minami H, Ohtsu A, Yoshida T, Saijo N, Ozawa S, Sawada J. Functional characterization of human UDP-glucuronosyltransferase 1A9 variant, D256 N, found in Japanese cancer patients. J Pharmacol Exp Ther 2003; 306:688–693.
48. Toffoli G, Cecchin E, Corona G, Boiocchi M. Pharmacogenetics of irinotecan. Curr Med Chem Anti-Canc Agents 2003; 3:225–237.
49. Ganansia-Leymarie V, Bischoff P, Bergerat JP, Holl V. Signal transduction pathways of taxanes-induced apoptosis. Curr Med Chem Anti-Canc Agents 2003; 3:291–306.
50. Verdier-Pinard P, Wang F, Martello L, Burd B, Orr GA, Horwitz SB. Analysis of tubulin isotypes and mutations from taxol-resistant cells by combined isoelectrofocusing and mass spectrometry. Biochemistry 2003; 42:5349–5357.
51. Kyu-Ho Han E, Gehrke L, Tahir SK, Credo RB, Cherian SP, Sham H, Rosenberg SH, Ng S. Modulation of drug resistance by α-tubulin in paclitaxel-resistant human lung cancer cell lines. Eur J Cancer 2000; 36:1565–1571.
52. Montgomery RB, Guzman J, O'Rourke DM, Stahl WL. Expression of oncogenic epidermal growth factor receptor family kinases induces paclitaxel resistance and alters β-tubulin isotype expression. J Biol Chem 2000; 275:17358–17363.
53. Giannakakou P, Gussio R, Nogales E, Downing KH, Zaharevitz D, Bollbuck B, Poy G, Sackett D, Nicolaou KC, Fojo T. A common pharmacophore for epothilone and taxanes: molecular basis for drug resistance conferred by tubulin mutations in human cancer cells. Proc Natl Acad Sci USA 2000; 97:2904–2909.
54. Dai D, Zeldin DC, Blaisdell JA, Chanas B, Coulter SJ, Ghanayem BI, Goldstein JA. Polymorphisms in human CYP2C8 decrease metabolism of the anticancer drug paclitaxel and arachidonic acid. Pharmacogenetics 2001; 11:597–607.
55. Dai D, Tang J, Rose R, Hodgson E, Bienstock RJ, Mohrenweiser HW, Goldstein JA. Identification of variants of CYP3A4 and characterization of their abilities to metabolize testosterone and chlorpyrifos. J Pharmacol Exp Ther 2001; 299:825–831.
56. Soyama A, Saito Y, Hanioka N, Murayama N, Nakajima O, Katori N, Ishida S, Sai K, Ozawa S, Sawada JI. Non-synonymous single nucleotide alterations found in the CYP2C8 gene result in reduced in vitro paclitaxel metabolism. Biol Pharm Bull 2001; 24:1427–1430.
57. Goh BC, Lee SC, Wang LZ, Fan L, Guo JY, Lamba J, Schuetz E, Lim R, Lim HL, Ong AB, Lee HS. Explaining interindividual variability of docetaxel pharmacokinetics and pharmacodynamics in Asians through phenotyping and genotyping strategies. J Clin Oncol 2002; 20:3683–3690.
58. Huang Z, Roy P, Waxman DJ. Role of human liver microsomal CYP3A4 and CYP2B6 in catalyzing N-dechloroethylation of cyclophosphamide and ifosfamide. Biochem Pharmacol 2000; 59:961–972.

59. Sladek NE, Kollander R, Sreerama L, Kiang DT. Cellular levels of aldehyde dehydrogenases (ALDH1A1 and ALDH3A1) as predictors of therapeutic responses to cyclophosphamide-based chemotherapy of breast cancer: a retrospective study. Cancer Chemother Pharmacol 2002; 49:309–321.
60. Jinno H, Tanaka-Kagawa T, Ohno A, Makino Y, Matsushima E, Hanioka N, Ando M. Functional characterization of cytochrome P450 2B6 allelic variants. Drug Metab Dispos 2003; 31:398–403.
61. Cullen KJ, Newkirk KA, Schumaker LM, Aldosari N, Rone JD, Haddad BR. Glutathione S-transferase pi amplification is associated with cisplatin resistance in head and neck squamous cell carcinoma cell lines and primary tumors. Cancer Res 2003; 63:8097–8102.
62. Stoehlmacher J, Park DJ, Zhang W, Groshen S, Tsao-Wei DD, Yu MC, Lenz HJ. Association between glutathione S-transferase P1, T1, and M1 genetic polymorphism and survival of patients with metastatic colorectal cancer. J Natl Cancer Inst 2002; 94: 936–942.
63. Pandya U, Srivastava SK, Singhal SS, Pal A, Awasthi S, Zimniak P, Awasthi YC, Singh SV. Activity of allelic variants of Pi class human glutathione S-transferase toward chlorambucil. Biochem Biophys Res Commun 2000; 278:258–262.
64. Sweeney C, Ambrosone CB, Joseph L, Stone A, Hutchins LF, Kadlubar FF, Coles BF. Association between a glutathione S-transferase A1 promoter polymorphism and survival after breast cancer treatment. Int J Cancer 2003; 103:810–814.
65. Mendelsohn J, Baselga J. Status of epidermal growth factor receptor antagonists in the biology and treatment of cancer. J Clin Oncol 2003; 21:2787–2799.
66. Herbst RS, Bunn PA Jr. Targeting the epidermal growth factor receptor in non-small cell lung cancer. Clin Cancer Res 2003; 9(16 Pt 1):5813–5824.
67. Ciardiello F, Tortora G. Epidermal growth factor receptor (EGFR) as a target in cancer therapy: understanding the role of receptor expression and other molecular determinants that could influence the response to anti-EGFR drugs. Eur J Cancer 2003; 39: 1348–1354.
68. Heimberger AB, Learn CA, Archer GE, McLendon RE, Chewning TA, Tuck FL, Pracyk JB, Friedman AH, Friedman HS, Bigner DD, Sampson JH. Brain tumors in mice are susceptible to blockade of epidermal growth factor receptor (EGFR) with the oral, specific, EGFR-tyrosine kinase inhibitor ZD1839 (Iressa). Clin Cancer Res 2003; 8:3496–3502.
69. Heinrich MC, Corless CL, Demetri GD, Blanke CD, von Mehren M, Joensuu H, McGreevey LS, Chen CJ, Van den Abbeele AD, Druker BJ, et al. Kinase mutations and imatinib response in patients with metastatic gastrointestinal stromal tumor. J Clin Oncol 2003; 21:4342–4349.
70. Frost MJ, Ferrao PT, Hughes TP, Ashman LK. Juxtamembrane mutant V560G-Kit is more sensitive to imatinib (STI571) compared with wild-type c-kit whereas the kinase domain mutant D816V-Kit is resistant. Mol Cancer Ther 2002; 1:1115–1124.
71. Loni L, Del Tacca M, Danesi R. Pharmacogenetics of anticancer drugs in non-Hodgkin lymphomas. Br J Cancer 2001; 85:1425–1431.
72. Lilling G, Elena N, Sidi Y, Bakhanashvili M. p53-associated $3'\rightarrow5'$ exonuclease activity in nuclear and cytoplasmic compartments of cells. Oncogene 2003; 22:233–245.
73. Wang Y-C, Chen C-Y, Chen S-K, Chang Y-Y, Lin P. p53 codon 72 polymorphism in Taiwanese lung cancer patients: association with lung cancer susceptibility and prognosis. Clin Cancer Res 1999; 5:129–134.
74. Bunz F, Hwang PM, Torrance C, Waldman T, Zhang Y, Dillehay L, Williams J, Lengauer C, Kinzler KW, Vogelstein B. Disruption of p53 in human cancer cells alters the responses to therapeutic agents. J Clin Invest 1999; 104:263–269.
75. Reles A, Wen WH, Schmider A, Gee C, Runnebaum IB, Kilian U, Jones LA, El-Naggar A, Minguillon C, Schönborn I, Reich O, Kreienberg R, Lichtenegger W, Press MF. Correlation of p53 mutations with resistance to platinum-based chemotherapy and shortened survival in ovarian cancer. Clin Cancer Res 2001; 7:2984–2997.

76. Nita ME, Nagawa H, Tominaga O, Tsuno N, Fujii S, Sasaki S, Fu CG, Takenoue T, Tsuruo T, Muto T. 5-Fluorouracil induces apoptosis in human colon cancer cell lines with modulation of Bcl-2 family proteins. Br J Cancer 1998; 78:986–992.
77. Vogelbaum MA, Tong JX, Perugu R, Gutmann DH, Rich KM. Overexpression of bax in human glioma cell lines. J Neurosurg 1999; 91:483–489.
78. Son BH, Ahn SH, Ko CD, Ka IW, Gong GY, Kim JC. Significance of mismatch repair protein expression in the chemotherapeutic response of sporadic invasive ductal carcinoma of the breast. Breast J 2004; 10:20–26.
79. Arnold CN, Goel A, Boland CR. Role of hMLH1 promoter hypermethylation in drug resistance to 5-fluorouracil in colorectal cancer cell lines. Int J Cancer 2003; 106:66–73.
80. Lin X, Howell SB. Effect of loss of DNA mismatch repair on development of topotecan-, gemcitabine-, and paclitaxel-resistant variants after exposure to cisplatin. Mol Pharmacol 1999; 56:390–395.
81. McHugh PJ, Spanswick VJ, Hartley JA. Repair of DNA interstrand crosslinks: molecular mechanisms and clinical relevance. Lancet Oncol 2001; 2:483–490.
82. Ferry KV, Hamilton TC, Johnson SW. Increased nucleotide excision repair in cisplatin-resistant ovarian cancer cells role of ERCC1–XPF. Biochem Pharmacol 2000; 60:1305–1313.
83. Damia G, Guidi G, D'Incalci M. Expression of genes involved in nucleotide excision repair and sensitivity to cisplatin and melphalan in human cancer cell lines. Eur J Cancer 1998; 34:1783–1788.
84. Lord RV, Brabender J, Gandara D, Alberola V, Camps C, Domine M, Cardenal F, Sanchez JM, Gumerlock PH, Taron M, Sanchez JJ, Danenberg KD, Danenberg PV, Rosell R. Low ERCC1 expression correlates with prolonged survival after cisplatin plus gemcitabine chemotherapy in non-small cell lung cancer. Clin Cancer Res 2002; 8:2286–2291.
85. Shirota Y, Stoehlmacher J, Brabender J, Xiong YP, Uetake H, Danenberg KD, Groshen S, Tsao-Wei DD, Danenberg PV, Lenz HJ. ERCC1 and thymidylate synthase mRNA levels predict survival for colorectal cancer patients receiving combination oxaliplatin and fluorouracil chemotherapy. J Clin Oncol 2001; 19:4298–4304.
86. Park DJ, Stoehlmacher J, Zhang W, Tsao-Wei DD, Groshen S, Lenz HJ. A xeroderma pigmentosum group D gene polymorphism predicts clinical outcome to platinum-based chemotherapy in patients with advanced colorectal cancer. Cancer Res 2001; 61:8654–8658.
87. Gerson SL. Clinical relevance of MGMT in the treatment of cancer. J Clin Oncol 2002; 20:2388–2399.
88. Middleton MR, Margison GP. Improvement of chemotherapy efficacy by inactivation of a DNA-repair pathway. Lancet Oncol 2003; 4:37–44.
89. Jaeckle KA, Eyre HJ, Townsend JJ, Schulman S, Knudson HM, Belanich M, Yarosh DB, Bearman SI, Giroux DJ, Schold SC. Correlation of tumor O6-methylguanine-DNA methyltransferase levels with survival of malignant astrocytoma patients treated with bischloroethylnitrosourea: a Southwest Oncology Group Study. J Clin Oncol 1998; 16:3310–3315.
90. Esteller M, Garcia-Foncillas J, Andion E, Goodman SN, Hidalgo OF, Vanaclocha V, Baylin SB, Herman JG. Inactivation of the DNA-repair gene *MGMT* and the clinical response of gliomas to alkylating agents. N Engl J Med 2000; 343:1350–1354.
91. Friedman HS, McLendon RE, Kerby T, Dugan M, Bigner SH, Henry AJ, Ashley DM, Krischer J, Lovell S, Rasheed K, et al. DNA mismatch repair and O6-alkylguanine-DNA alkyltransferase analysis and response to temodal in newly diagnosed malignant glioma. J Clin Oncol 1998; 16:3851–3857.
92. Sparreboom A, Danesi R, Ando Y, Chan J, Figg WD. Pharmacogenomics of ABC transporters and its role in cancer chemotherapy. Drug Resist Updat 2003; 6:71–84.
93. Lage H, Dietel M. Effect of the breast-cancer resistance protein on atypical multidrug resistance. Lancet Oncol 2000; 1:169–175.
94. Larsen AK, Escargueil AE, Skladanowski A. Resistance mechanisms associated with altered intracellular distribution of anticancer agents. Pharmacol Ther 2000; 85:217–229.

95. Brinkmann U, Roots I, Eichelbaum M. Pharmacogenetics of the human drug transporter gene MDR1: impact of polymorphisms on pharmacotherapy. Drug Disease Treat 2001; 6:835–839.
96. Johne A, Kopke K, Gerloff T, Mai I, Rietbrock S, Meisel C, Hoffmeyer S, Kerb R, Fromm MF, Brinkmann U, Eichelbaum M, Brockmoller J, Cascorbi I, Roots I. Modulation of steady-state kinetics of digoxin by haplotypes of the P-glycoprotein MDR1 gene. Clin Pharmacol Ther 2002; 72:584–594.
97. Sakaeda T, Nakamura T, Okumura K. Pharmacogenetics of MDR1 and its impact on the pharmacokinetics and pharmacodynamics of drugs. Pharmacogenomics 2003; 4:397–410.
98. Burger H, Foekens JA, Look MP, Meijer-van Gelder ME, Klijn JG, Wiemer EA, Stoter G, Nooter K. RNA expression of breast cancer resistance protein, lung resistance-related protein, multidrug resistance-associated proteins 1 and 2, and multidrug resistance gene 1 in breast cancer: correlation with chemotherapeutic response. Clin Cancer Res 2003; 9:827–836.
99. Diestra JE, Condom E, Del Muro XG, Scheffer GL, Perez J, Zurita AJ, Munoz-Segui J, Vigues F, Scheper RJ, Capella G, Germa-Lluch JR, Izquierdo MA. Expression of multidrug resistance proteins P-glycoprotein, multidrug resistance protein 1, breast cancer resistance protein and lung resistance related protein in locally advanced bladder cancer treated with neoadjuvant chemotherapy: biological and clinical implications. J Urol 2003; 170:1383–1387.
100. Zurita AJ, Diestra JE, Condom E, Garcia Del Muro X, Scheffer GL, Scheper RJ, Perez J, Germa-Lluch JR, Izquierdo MA. Lung resistance-related protein as a predictor of clinical outcome in advanced testicular germ-cell tumours. Br J Cancer 2003; 88:879–886.
101. Harada T, Ogura S, Yamazaki K, Kinoshita I, Itoh T, Isobe H, Yamashiro K, Dosaka-Akita H, Nishimura M. Predictive value of expression of P53, Bcl-2 and lung resistance-related protein for response to chemotherapy in non-small cell lung cancers. Cancer Sci 2003; 94:394–399.
102. Haseba M, Hidaka S, Tsuji T, Yano H, Komatsu H, Sawai T, Yasutake T, Nakagoe T, Tagawa Y, Ayabe H. Detection of p53 gene mutations by nonisotopic RNase cleavage assay as a predictor of poor prognosis in colorectal cancers. Dig Dis Sci 2003; 48:1984–1989.
103. Le Marchand L, Seifried A, Lum-Jones A, Donlon T, Wilkens LR. Association of the cyclin D1 A870G polymorphism with advanced colorectal cancer. J Am Med Assoc 2003; 290:2843–2848.
104. Grieu F, Malaney S, Ward R, Joseph D, Iacopetta B. Lack of association between CCND1 G870A polymorphism and the risk of breast and colorectal cancers. Anticancer Res 2003; 23:4257–4259.
105. Ribic CM, Sargent DJ, Moore MJ, Thibodeau SN, French AJ, Goldberg RM, Hamilton SR, Laurent-Puig P, Gryfe R, Shepherd LE, Tu D, Redston M, Gallinger S. Tumor microsatellite-instability status as a predictor of benefit from fluorouracil-based adjuvant chemotherapy for colon cancer. N Engl J Med 2003; 349:247–257.
106. Nebert DW, Jorge-Nebert L, Vesell ES. Pharmacogenomics and "individualized drug therapy": high expectations and disappointing achievements. Am J Pharmacogenomics 2003; 3:361–370.
107. Loni L, De Braud F, Zinzani PL, Danesi R. Pharmacogenetics and proteomics of anticancer drugs in non-Hodgkin's lymphoma. Leuk Lympoma 2003; 44:S115-S122.
108. Lin X, Parsels LA, Voeller DM, Allegra CJ, Maley GF, Maley F, Chu E. Characterization of a cis-acting regulatory element in the protein coding region of thymidylate synthase mRNA. Nucleic Acids Res 2000; 28:1381–1389.
109. de Laat WL, Jaspers NG, Hoeijmakers JH. Molecular mechanism of nucleotide excision repair. Genes Dev 1999; 13:768–875.

9
Pharmacogenetics in Infectious Diseases

Belle L. Lee
University of California, San Francisco, California, U.S.A., and Division of Infectious Diseases, Department of Clinical Research, University Hospital, Berne, Switzerland

Laurent A. Decosterd
Division of Clinical Pharmacology, University of Lausanne, Lausanne, Switzerland

Reinhold Kerb
Experimental Medicine, Astra Zeneca, Mölndal, Sweden

Amalio Telenti
Institute of Microbiology, University Hospital, University of Lausanne, Lausanne, Switzerland

INTRODUCTION

Genetics is challenging the traditional approach to infectious diseases. Until recently, research was mostly directed to the analysis of the pathogen and of its virulence factors. However, we are now in a position to investigate the pathogen in the context of the host genetic make-up. Concepts, such as colonization versus infection and life-threatening infection versus contained disease, will be revisited to better define pathogen-specific virulence versus host-specific susceptibility. Thus, genetic susceptibility (Table 1) will be the initial step in defining the need for treatment, to be completed by analysis of pharmacogenetic determinants in order to choose the most effective and least toxic therapy for the individual patient (Fig. 1).

Both genetics of disease susceptibility and pharmacogenetics are of major interest in the field of infectious diseases: (*i*) tuberculosis (TB), HIV, malaria, pneumonia, diarrheal diseases, and sepsis, are among the great medical problems in the world, (*ii*) all can be treated but not always effectively or without toxicity, (*iii*) standard guidelines are drafted based on drug development and trials in Caucasian populations, although different ethnic groups may present significant differences in the frequency of the alleles modifying the drug metabolism (1,2), and (*iv*) many infectious diseases are treated by complex multidrug regimens. Here the issue of pharmacokinetics and drug interactions becomes critical. Genetic prediction would be of interest in preventing toxicity and also for identifying the most likely component of a multidrug regimen leading to toxicity or lack of efficacy.

The fields of genetics of disease susceptibility and of pharmacogenetics overlap with the field of immunogenetics (the genetic factors contributing to differences in immune

Table 1 Association of Genetic Polymorphisms with Disease Severity

Gene/protein	Role	Polymorphism/ allele	Associated disease
Mannose-binding lectin	Pathogen sensing	Codons 52, 54, 57	Meningococcemia, respiratory infections
Toll-like receptor 4	Pathogen sensing	D299G	Gram-negative shock
Fc gamma receptor IIA	Pathogen sensing	H131R	Meningococcemia, pneumococcemia
CD14	Pathogen sensing	C160T	Septic shock
Tumor necrosis factor A	Inflammation	TNF2	Meningococcemia, septic shock, cerebral malaria
Tumor necrosis factor B	Inflammation	TNFB2	Severe sepsis
Interleukin-1B	Inflammation	IL-1B (511)	Meningococcal disease
Interleukin-1-ra	Inflammation	IL-1 RN2	Severe sepsis
C reactive protein	Inflammation	134 bp dinucleotide repeat polymorphism	Invasive pneumococcal disease
Interferon-γ receptor 1	Inflammation	*IFNGR1* nonfunctional alleles	Susceptibility to mycobacteria
Interleukin-10	Inflammation	Promoter polymorphism	Persistence of hepatitis B and altered response to INF-α therapy in hepatitis C treatment. Accelerated progression of HIV infection
Interleukin-12	Inflammation	Deficiency	Susceptibility to mycobacteria
Interleukin-12 receptor	Inflammation	Mutation	Susceptibility to mycobacteria
CC chemokine receptor 5	Inflammation	CCR5 Δ32	Protection from HIV
		CCR5 p1/p1	Accelerated progression of HIV infection
CC chemokine receptor 2	Inflammation	CCR2-I64	Accelerated progression of HIV infection
Macrophage inflammatory prot-1α	Inflammation	*MIP-1α459T*	Accelerated progression of HIV infection
Rantes	Inflammation	*Rantes In1.1C*	Accelerated progression of HIV infection
HLA class I	Immunity	B8	Susceptibility to tuberculosis

(*Continued*)

Table 1 Association of Genetic Polymorphisms with Disease Severity (*Continued*)

Gene/protein	Role	Polymorphism/ allele	Associated disease
		B35	Susceptibility to AIDS
		B53	Protection from severe malaria
		B5701	Protection from AIDS
		*Cw*04*	Susceptibility to AIDS
HLA class II	Immunity	*DRB1*1302*	Clearance of hepatitis B
		*DRB1*1352*	Protection from severe malaria
		*DRB1*1101*	Clearance of hepatitis C
		*DRB1*04*	Protection from typhoid fever
		DR2	Susceptibility to tuberculosis and leprosy
		DR7	Susceptibility to hepatitis B
Plasminogen activator inibitor-1	Coagulation	4G/4G	Meningococcemia, severe sepsis
Solute carrier family 11 (*NRAMP1*, *SLC11A1*)	Transporter	—	Susceptibility to tuberculosis
Vitamin D receptor	Metabolism	*Taq*I restriction polymorphism	Protection from tuberculosis and leprosy

Source: From Refs. 3, 68, 185, 186.

response among individuals). The study of immunogenetic determinants may become central for those investigating allergic and hypersensitivity reaction and also disease susceptibility (3,4). The present chapter will focus on current knowledge of inherited differences in the metabolism, transport, and disposition of anti-infective drugs, and drugs' targets (pharmacogenetics sensu stricto). However, attention will also be given to other genetic determinants of disease progression, as they will help define the need for treatment or the likelihood of response.

PHARMACOGENETICS OF SPECIFIC INFECTIOUS DISEASES

Inherited differences in response to anti-infective drugs were observed several decades ago. Indeed, it is in the field of anti-infective therapy that the importance of polymorphisms in drug disposition was first encountered: the *N*-acetyltransferase 2 (NAT2) acetylation polymorphism discovered during isoniazid treatment of TB patients (5) was one of the first examples of a pharmacogenetic defect influencing drug biotransformation in human populations. A number of antibiotics and chemotherapeutic agents are substrates of polymorphic phases I and II metabolic pathways and transport genes (Table 2). However, there are currently limited data on the clinical relevance of such genetic variations. In the following, we discuss the current pharmacogenetic knowledge relevant to the treatment of four major diseases and infectious syndromes: HIV, TB, malaria, and sepsis.

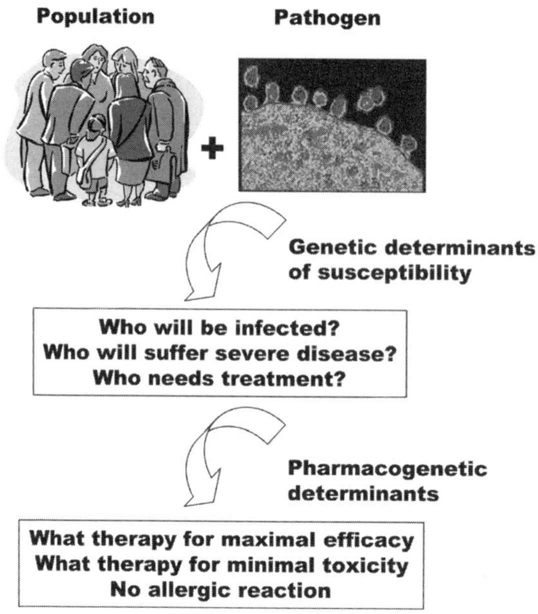

Figure 1 Genetic markers in the treatment of infection. Genetic determinants of susceptibility define who should be treated, and pharmacogenetic markers help in the choice of therapy.

HIV

The availability of effective combination antiretroviral therapy since 1995 has changed the prognosis of HIV disease dramatically. Five drug classes are currently in use: nucleoside analogs (NRTI), nucleotide analogs (NtRTI), non-nucleoside inhibitors of the HIV reverse transcriptase (NNRTI), inhibitors of the HIV protease (PI), and peptidic inhibitors of the viral-cell fusion process. PIs are moderate to strong inhibitors of various cytochrome P450 (CYP450) isoenzymes (Table 2), whereas NNRTIs are inducers of several CYP450 isoenzymes. In addition, PIs are substrates of the multidrug transporter P-glycoprotein (P-gp). There is marked interindividual variation in plasma drug levels, in efficacy, and in susceptibility to adverse reactions (6–8). Antiretroviral agents, in particular NNRTIs and PIs, are subject to significant drug–drug interactions within combination antiretroviral therapy and with medications used to treat opportunistic diseases associated with AIDS (e.g., antimycobacterial drugs). In addition, the disease itself can affect enzymatic activity. For example, patients with AIDS and acute infections have altered patterns of enzymatic drug metabolism (9). Using caffeine as a probe for NAT2 enzymatic activity, we identified an increased number of slow acetylators in AIDS patients with an acute infection, compared with the control healthy volunteers and HIV-asymptomatic patients. The patterns of oxidative metabolism (decreased demethylation, increased 8-hydroxylation) were also altered. This type of phenomenon might contribute to the increased incidence of adverse reactions observed in these patients, a phenomenon similar to that described in the treatment of TB (10–12).

Irrespective of these considerations, polymorphisms in genes encoding for metabolizing enzymes, carrier proteins, and drug transporters are expected to influence antiretroviral plasma drug levels, bound and free, and also intracompartmental and intracellular effective levels (Fig. 2). These three components and their relevance in the treatment of HIV diseases are discussed in the following sections.

(Text continues on page 162.)

Table 2 Inherited Differences in the Metabolism, Transport and Disposition, and Toxicity of Anti-infective Drugs

Gene/protein	Anti-infective drug	Polymorphism/mutation	Consequence
Phase I enzymes[a]			
CYP3A	Rifampicin, ceftriaxone, erythromycin, clarithromycin, HIV protease inhibitors	Role of polymorphisms in *CYP3A4* unclear. *CYP3A5*1* express high amounts of CYP3A5	Interindividual variation in 20% of the bioavailability of substrates
CYP2C19	Amoxicillin, clarithromycin, (plus proton pump inhibitors: omeprazole/lansoprazole/rabeprazole), ketoconazole, HIV protease inhibitors, rifampicin, isoniazid	*CYP2C19* PM, heterozygous/extensive metabolizer	*CYP2C19* PM better cure rates; EM less eradication of *H. pylori*; PM implicated in adverse drug reactions
Other *CYP*: *CYP2D6*, *CYP2C9*, *CYP2E1*, *CYP1A2*, *CYP2B6*	HIV protease inhibitors and non-nucleoside reverse transcriptase inhibitors, erythromycin, isoniazid, rifampin	All enzymes have variant alleles associated with PM	Interindividual variation in drug levels and increased adverse drug reactions
Phase II enzymes			
N-acetyltransferase (*NAT*) II	Isoniazid, sulfonamides, dapsone	Slow acetylators	Neuropathy, hematologic toxicities
Glucose 6-phosphate dehydrogenase (*G6PD*)	Primaquine, dapsone, sulfonamides	G6PD deficiency	Hemolysis
Thiopurine *S*-methyltransferase (*TPMT*)	Moxalactam, cephalosporins	TPMT deficiency	Hematopoietic toxicity—bleeding

(*Continued*)

Table 2 Inherited Differences in the Metabolism, Transport and Disposition, and Toxicity of Anti-infective Drugs (*Continued*)

Gene/protein	Anti-infective drug	Polymorphism/mutation	Consequence
Transporters			
P-glycoprotein (*MDR1*)	HIV protease inhibitors, rifampicin, ceftriaxone, erythromycin, clarithromycin, antifungals (ketoconazole, Itraconazole, amphotericin B), chloroquine, quinine	Exon 21 and exon 26 polymorphism	Drug levels of protease inhibitors, intracellular drug concentration, immune recovery in HIV-infected individuals
Multidrug resistance-related protein 1 (*MRP1, ABCC1*)	Fluoroquinolones, tetracyclines, macrolides, LTC4 inhibitors (penicillin, probenecid, rifampicin, clotrimazole)	Arg433Ser	Reduced intracellular drug concentration, reduced body clearance?
MRP2 (*ABCC2*)	Substrates: fluoroquinolones, tetracyclines, macrolides, HIV protease inhibitors, penicillin sulfinpyrazone, LTC4 inhibitors: HIV protease inhibitors, cefodizime rifampicin	Dubin-Johnson syndrome–related nonsynonymous mutations	Reduced bilirubin efflux
MRP4 (*ABCC4*)	Adefovir, azidothymidine, lamivudine, ddC, stavudine	Multiple	Unknown
MRP5 (*ABCC5*)	Adefovir, azidothymidine, lamivudine, ddC, stavudine	Multiple	Unknown
OAT1 (*SLC22A6*)	Cephalosporins, adefovir, cidofovir	n.i.	
OAT2 (*SLC22A7*)	Azidothymidine	n.i.	

OCT1 (*SLC22A1*)	Azidothymidine Inhibitors: indinavir, saquinavir, ritonavir, nefinavir	Arg61Cys Cys88Arg Gly401Ser	Reduced in vitro uptake, reduced hepatic clearance/intestinal absorption, increased susceptibility to drug–drug interaction
OCT2	Organic cations	P54S, M165I, R400C, K432Q, insertion	Reduced in vitro uptake, non-functional protein
OATP-C (*SLC21A6*)	Benzylpenicillin, rifampicin Inhibitor: rifamycin, LTC4	Phe73Ala (*2 allele) Val82Ala and Glu156Gly (*3 allele) Ile353Thr (*6), Val174Ala (*5), Gly488Ala (*9)	Reduced in vitro uptake, reduced hepatic drug clearance?
OATP8 (*SLC21A8*)	Rifampicin Inhibitor: rifamycin	n.i.	
OATP-B (*SLC21A9*)	Amphiphilic organic anions	S486F (*3)	Reduced in vitro uptake
Other			
Mitochondrial ribosomal 12S rRNA gene	Aminoglycoside antibiotics (streptomycin)	A1555G and T961C mutation of 12SrRNA gene	Irreversible deafness in maternally inherited mitochondrial mutations
HLA haplotypes	Hepatitis B vaccine abacavir	Many haplotypes are involved: haplotype *HLA-B*5701*, *HLA-DR7*, *HLA-DQ3*	Poor and nonresponse to hepatitis B vaccine Hypersensitivity reaction to abacavir

[a]See www.imm.ki.se/CYPalleles/for detailed description of *CYP* alleles and SNPs.

Abbreviations: n.i., none identified; PM, poor metabolizer; EM, extensive metabolizer; LTC4, leukotriene C4; TPMT, thiopurine *S*-methyltransferase.

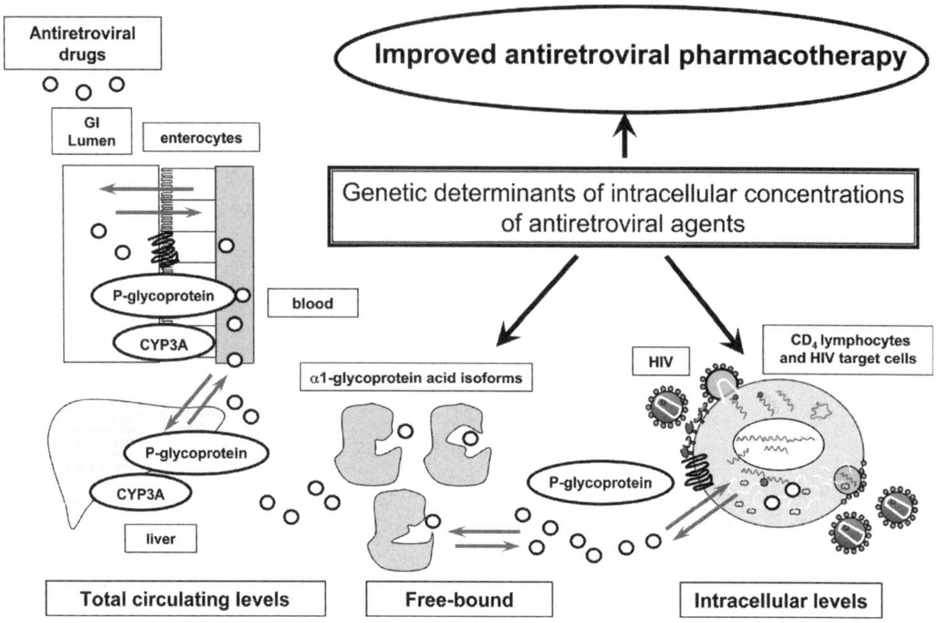

Figure 2 Schematic representation of known determinants of intracellular drug concentration of antiretroviral agents.

CYP450 Metabolism

PIs and NNRTIs, unlike NRTIs, are extensively metabolized by CYPP450 isozymes present in the liver and in the gut wall, with CYP3A being the most important isozyme: other isozymes, such as CYP2C9, CYP2C19, CYP2D6, and CYP2B6, also contribute (13–16). Most PIs are inhibitors of CYP3A, with ritonavir being the most potent and saquinavir the least (17,18). Because some PIs simultaneously inhibit and/or induce these enzymatic systems, whereas NNRTIs act as inducers, regimens combining PIs with each other or with NNRTIs are complicated by influences from both classes of drugs. In addition, and as described previously, the disease status may also modulate the enzymatic activity of CYP450. In a study addressing this question, the genotype and phenotype of CYP2D6 were investigated in 61 HIV-infected and AIDS patients. The authors found an apparent shift towards the poor metabolizer (PM) phenotype from the extensive metabolizer (EM) genotype. The authors concluded that a change might occur in HIV-positive patients such that their CYP2D6 activity approaches that of the PMs, despite having an EM genotype (19).

Fellay et al. (20) conducted a pilot study on 123 HIV-infected patients to analyze the association of CYP polymorphims and plasma drug levels and response. Investigation included *CYP3A4*1B* and **2* (21), *CYP3A5*1, CYP2D6 *3*, **4*, and **6*, and gene duplication (22–24) and *CYP2C19* exons 4 and 9 polymorphisms and also the functional analysis of CYP3A (midazolam to 1′-hydroxymidazolam oxidation). Patients who were either homozygous or heterozygous at one *CYP2D6* allele associated with a PM phenotype had higher median plasma nelfinavir levels than patients with a *CYP2D6* EM genotype. In contrast, there was no significant contribution of *CYP2C19* genotype to nelfinavir plasma drug levels, despite the fact that in vitro data identify CYP2C19 as the main P450 isoform involved in the metabolism of nelfinavir (25,26). Functional and genetic analysis of *CYP3A* alleles did not identify an association with drug levels in vivo. Virological and immunological responses to treatment did not vary among patients with the various *CYP* alleles (20). A detailed description of *CYP* alleles and single nucleotide polymorphisms is beyond the scope of this chapter; please refer to (27) for precise nomenclature and functional consequences.

P-gp

The *MDR1*gene codes for P-gp, which is an ABC transporter. PIs are substrates (as well as inhibitors and/or inducers) of this transporter. The intracellular accumulation and active transport of PIs have been studied by Jones et al. (28,29). The recent identification of polymorphisms in the *MDR1* gene associated with changes in transporter function spurred a significant amount of research, including in the field of HIV. The current state of knowledge has been reviewed recently by Kim (30), and there appears to be considerable confusion and controversy (Table 3). Hoffmeyer et al. (31) characterized the *MDR1* gene in a group of Caucasian subjects. They reported that individuals homozygous for the *MDR1* exon 26 3435T allele had significantly decreased intestinal P-gp expression and increased digoxin plasma concentrations after oral administration. In contrast, Sakaeda et al. (32) showed that digoxin plasma levels were lower in Japanese subjects carrying the 3435T allele. Nakanuma also found lower digoxin plasma levels for TT subjects, albeit with a higher MDR1 expression (33). Kim et al. (34) reported that the 3435T/T genotype was associated with high expression in vitro and low plasma concentrations of fexofenadine, a model substrate drug for the P-gp transporter. In a study investigating *MDR1* tissue expression, Goto et al. (35) reported that the 3435C/T polymorphism in exon 26 did not significantly alter the *MDR1* level expressed in intestinal enterocytes or correlate with the tacrolimus concentration/dose ratio. In our study, with a cohort of HIV-infected patients, the 3435TT genotype was associated with lower expression of P-gp (both *MDR1* mRNA and P-gp levels) in peripheral-blood mononuclear cells, and lower plasma concentrations of nelfinavir and efavirenz, as compared with the 3435CC genotype (20). This synonymous 3435T polymorphism is linked to the nonsynonymous exon 21 2677G/T (Ala893Ser) polymorphism. Therefore, the possibility exists that some of the observed differences in P-gp activity attributed to the 3435C/T polymorphism may reflect the exon 21 polymorphism and its effects on transporter activity. Several studies have compared the effects of 2677G/T SNP on P-gp activity. However, the results obtained so far have been variable and conflicting (Table 3), and thus recent activity has shifted towards determining the role of *MDR1* haplotypes on the functional activity of the protein product.

Many of the drugs that are transported by P-gp are also metabolized by the cytochrome P450 enzymes, especially CYP3A. It is likely that because P-gp can influence the intracellular concentration of many CYP3A substrates it can also affect the availability of those substrates to CYP3A and therefore the extent of their metabolism. P-gp thus plays an important role in modulating the expression of CYP3A and is likely to complicate the predictability of drug interactions among drugs that are substrates for both P-gp and CYP3A systems (33). It has been reported that carriers of the 3435T allele have reduced expression of intestinal CYP3A4 mRNA (35). It is not clear, however, how a synonymous SNP in *MDR1* can alter CYP3A4 expression. The role of other transporters is discussed in a dedicated section that follows.

Alpha1-Acid Glycoprotein

The binding of drugs to plasma proteins can influence the pharmacokinetics of that drug. A large number of drugs, including PIs, bind extensively to alpha1-acid glycoprotein (AAG). Binding is about 95% for the PIs, saquinavir, and ritonavir and 60% for indinavir (36). It has

Table 3 Functional Consequences of *MDR1* Polymorphism at Exons 26 and 21

Polymorphism	Study	Ethnicity	Tissue or cell lines	*MDR1* expression or activity in vitro	Drug tested	Effect
Exon 26						
C3435T	Hoffmeyer (31)	Caucasians	Duodenum	TT < CC	Digoxin	Plasma level higher for TT subjects
	Sakaeda (32)	Japanese			Digoxin	Plasma level lower for TT subjects
	Nakamura (187)	Japanese	Duodenum	CC < TT	Digoxin	Plasma level lower for TT subjects
	Kim (188)	European American and African American			Fexofenadine	Plasma level lower for TT subjects
	Drescher (189)	Caucasians	$CD56^+$ cells	TT < CC	Fexofenadine	No difference
	von Ahsen (190)	Caucasians			Ciclosporine	No difference
	Min (191)				Ciclosporine	No difference
	Fellay (20)	Caucasians	PBMC	TT < CC	Nelfinavir	Plasma level lower for TT subjects
	Hitzl (86)	Caucasians	$CD56^+$ cells	TT < CC	Rhodamine 123	Rhodamine 123 accumulation higher in CD56+ cells from TT subjects
	Tanabe (192)	Japanese	Placenta	TT = CC		
	Goto (35)	Japanese	Upper jejunum	TT = CC	Tacrolimus	No difference

	Roberts (193)	Caucasians			Nortriptyline	TT associated with nortriptline-associated hypotension, with no statistical difference in blood levels
Exon 21						
G2677T/A (Ala893Ser/Thr)	Kim (188)	European American and Africanm American	NIH-3T3 cells	GG < TT	Fexofenadine	Plasma level lower for TT subjects
	Tanabe (192)	Japanese	Placenta	TT < GG[a] AA < GG[a]		
	Kimchi-Sarfety (194)		HeLa cells	TT = GG		Multiple drugs tested in vitro. No difference in expression or activity
Exons 21 and 26						
Haplotype 2677/3435	Johne (195)	Caucasians		ND	Digoxin	Highest plasma levels for Haplotype 12 (*2677G/3435T*)
	Kurata (196)	Japanese		ND	Digoxin	Highest plasma levels for Haplotype *2677T/3435T*

[a]Not statistically significant.
Abbreviations: ND, not done; PBMC, peripheral blood mononuclear cells.
Source: From Ref. 30.

been shown in AAG overexpressing transgenic mice that elevated AAG levels reduce the volume of distribution and systemic clearance of saquinavir (37). Unbound drug represents not only the drug available for exerting the pharmacological effect, but it also influences the tissue and cellular penetration of drugs into cells, because only unbound drug in the plasma can equilibrate with intracellular compartments. This is particularly relevant for PIs, the activity of which is likely to take place intracellularly during assembly and budding of new virions. Several in vitro studies have shown that physiological concentrations of AAG substantially affect the antiviral potency of several PIs. An elevated AAG concentration can reduce uptake and decrease intracellular antiviral activity of various PIs, such as saquinavir, ritonavir, indinavir, nelfinavir, and amprenavir (36,38–40).

Genetic polymorphism of *ORM* (encoding AAG) and various alleles corresponding to the two loci have been reported (41). The first locus has two main variants (*ORM1 S* and *ORM1 F1*), whereas the second locus (*ORM2*) is mainly monomorphic (*ORM2 M*, originally called *ORM2 A*). These variants determine three main phenotypes for AAG in the human population, ORM1 F1S/ORM2 M, ORM1 F1/ORM2 M, and ORM1 S/ORM2 M. The two genes differ by 32 nucleotide substitutions in the coding sequence, resulting in 21 amino acid substitutions (42). Three common *ORM1* alleles result from A to G transitions at the codons for amino acid positions 20 and 156 in exons 1 and 5, respectively (43).

Control of AAG expression is both at the transcriptional and posttranscriptional level (44–47). One study showed that the proportion of *ORM2* varies threefold, representing 17% to 48% of the total AAG variants, whereas *ORM1 S* and *ORM1 F1* represent 0% to 65% and 0% to 89%, respectively (48). Important differences in polymorphisms of the *AAG* gene have been found in different ethnic populations. In African American populations, up to 14% of the subjects did not express the *ORM2 A* allele (49), whereas this allele is virtually present in all Caucasian subjects (41,48,49). On the other hand, in the Japanese population, *ORM* duplication occurs at a frequency as high as 20% (50). No study to date has assessed the relevance of these polymorphisms to the clinical management of HIV disease.

Tuberculosis

Tuberculosis (TB) kills approximately two million people each year. It has been estimated that between 2002 and 2020, approximately 1000 million people will be newly infected, more than 150 million people will get sick, and 36 million will die of TB—if control is not further strengthened. Treatment requires combination therapy generally including isoniazid, rifampin, ethambutol, and pyrazinamide for six to nine months. The success of therapy is greatly influenced by adherence, and by avoidance of toxicity, including the occurrence of fatal and severe liver injury associated with the combination of isonizid, rifampin, and pyrazinamide. Unfortunately, little is known about genetic predictors of toxicity with the exception of the association between the acetylator polymorphism and the neurological toxicity of isoniazid.

Isoniazid continues to play an important role in the management of TB. The metabolism of isoniazid takes place in the liver by two metabolic pathways: phase I oxidative metabolism by the cytochrome P450 enzymes, and phase II *N*-acetylation mediated by NAT (51,52). *N*-acetylation is important in the biotransformation of drugs, such as isoniazid, sulfonamides, and dapsone. The human acetylator polymorphism was one of the first hereditary traits affecting drug response to be discovered (5). This trait was found in patients who developed numbness and tingling in the fingers and toes after responding to isoniazid treatment (53). Further studies demonstrated that patients who were slow acetylators and excreted less acetyl-isoniazid were more prone to develop neurologic toxicity.

It is now known that the population ratio of rapid versus slow acetylators varies widely among different ethnic groups. The highest proportion of slow acetylators is found in Egyptians (80%), whereas 40% to 60% of the Caucasians and African Americans, and only 10% to 20% of the Japanese and Canadian Eskimos are slow acetylators. With some exceptions, the clinical consequences are that slow acetylators develop more adverse reactions, whereas rapid acetylators are more prone to have an inadequate response when prescribed a standard dose of the acetylated drug. Slow acetylators have been shown to be at risk of developing hypersensitivity reactions to drugs, such as sulfonamides and dapsone, particularly in HIV-infected patients. In addition, recent studies have demonstrated that slow acetylators have a higher risk of isoniazid-induced hepatotoxicity than rapid acetylators (26.4% vs. 11.1%, respectively) (10). In slow acetylators, the amount of NAT found in the liver is reduced, and in rapid acetylators the level of NAT activity present is at least twice as high as that found in slow acetylators (54,55).

Earlier studies suggested that acetylation capacity was a heritable autosomal trait, where the slow acetylators carried the homozygous gene for slow acetylation and the rapid acetylators carried either the homozygous or heterozygous gene for rapid acetylation. In man, three *NAT* genes have been found, with only the *NAT1* and *NAT2* genes being expressed (56). *NAT1* shows kinetic selectivity for monomorphic substrates, such as *p*-aminobenzoic acid and *p*-aminosalicylic acid, whereas *NAT2* is more important for clinically relevant substrates, such as isoniazid and sulfamethazine.

The *NAT2* acetylation polymorphism is one of the most common polymorphisms known in human populations (57,58). The reference *NAT2*4* is associated with the rapid acetylator phenotype and at least 25 *NAT2* allelic variants have been identified that account for 95% or more of the alleles in Caucasians, Asians, Hispanics, and African Americans (59,60). These alleles contain 11 different single-nucleotide polymorphisms (SNPs) in the *NAT2* coding region. A recent study investigated the functional effects of each of the 11 SNPs on *NAT2* catalytic activity, protein expression, and stability (60). In this study, a reduction in catalytic activity for the *N*-acetylation of sulfamethazine was observed for *NAT2* variants possessing G191A (R64Q), T341C (I114T), A434C (E145P), G590A (R197Q), A845C (K282T), or G857A (G286T). A reduction in expression of *NAT2* immunoreactive protein was also observed for *NAT2* variants possessing T341C, A434C, or G590A. A reduction in protein stability was noted for *NAT2* variants possessing G191A, A845C, G857A, and G590A. No significant differences in mRNA expression or transformation efficiency were observed among any of the *NAT2* alleles. The investigators concluded that variations in stability and catalytic activity were the mechanisms responsible for the slow acetylator phenotype. In patients who are at high risk of developing adverse effects or inadequate response to therapy, assessing the acetylator status might be useful in tailoring drug therapy to ensure maximal response.

Malaria

Malaria causes at least 300 million cases of acute illness each year and is the leading cause of deaths in young children. Pregnant women are the main adult risk group in most endemic areas of the world. Malaria is one of the major public health challenges eroding development resources in the poorest countries in the world. Malaria costs Africa more than US$12 billion annually. The potential toxicity of most antimalarials will require special surveillance programs as they will be increasingly used for treatment and prophylaxis. As it is the case with antituberculous medications, there is little knowledge about the molecular basis of drug toxicity or of the genetic markers for prediction of toxicity or treatment efficacy, with the notable exception primaquine.

Primaquine was introduced approximately 50 years ago, and it has long been used for the management of the chronic liver stage of malaria (61). During War World II, primaquine sensitivity was first observed in black soldiers who developed sudden hemolytic reaction after using the 8-aminoquinolone antimalarial drugs. The cause of primaquine sensitivity is now known as a deficiency in the hereditary enzyme glucose 6-phosphate dehydrogenase (G6PD) that causes hemolytic anemia in susceptible individuals after exposure to certain dietary substances, numerous drugs including the 8-aminoquinolones, and also other oxidant chemicals.

The enzyme G6PD is present in most cells and tissues and is responsible for the oxidation of glucose-6-phosphate to 6-phosphogluconic acid. This reaction is necessary to produce NADPH, which functions as a proton donor in the glutathione reductase reaction. Reduced glutathione protects sulfhydryl-dependent enzymes and other cellular proteins against oxidation. Primaquine induces hemolysis by causing further reduction in the level of reduced glutathione in the red cells that already have an impaired mechanism for the regeneration of NADPH. The hemolysis seen in the reduced glutathione-deficient state is the result of increased susceptibility of the erythrocyte to mechanical breakage (62).

The gene that encodes G6PD is located on the long arm of chromosome Xq28 and spans approximately 20 kb with a coding sequence of 1548 bp. Using biochemical techniques, more than 400 variants have been characterized, but only approximately 30 different polymorphims have been identified, almost all of which are found in the coding region (63,64). Two types of mutations are commonly found in Africans: G6PD A and G6PD A-. The first produces normal levels of red cell activity, and the second is unstable and produces only about 10% of the normal activity. G6PD A- is caused due to the substitution of Val to Met at codon 68 (G202 to A) (65). In the African variant G6PD Santamaria, a second mutation (A542 to T) also causes G6PD deficiency. This mutation causes an Asp to Val substitution at codon 181. In Mediterranean individuals, a C563 to T change results in Ser to Phe substitution at codon 188. Little is known about the mutations in Asians than in Mediterraneans, but one of the more common Asians variants, G6PD Canton, has an Arg to Leu substitution at codon 459 (66).

Sepsis

Sepsis, best defined as a systemic infection generally accompanied by bacteremia, is a frequent diagnosis leading to hospitalization. It is associated with high mortality despite advances in medical care and the availability of a broad spectrum of antibiotic therapy, and it often complicates hospitalization. Its most severe manifestation—septic shock—is the end result of many different insults. This complicates understanding of the pathogenesis, diagnosis, and targeted treatment. Thus, host genetics should first of all allow redefinition of the sepsis syndrome leading to a more rational approach in clinical trials. To date, host factors associated with sepsis have included polymorphic genes involved in pathogen recognition, inflammation, and coagulation cascades (Table 1). The required studies will entail the identification of new and additional SNPs associated with predisposition to severe sepsis, septic shock, and death from sepsis.

The controversy surrounding immune intervention using anticytokine therapy in sepsis illustrates this point. TNFα is one key mediator of sepsis, and this led to a number of studies that used anti-TNFα antibodies as therapy. Unfortunately, the complexity in the classification of sepsis described previously has probably limited the potential use of anti-TNFα as a therapeutic agent. The basic observation is that there is a marked difference in production of TNFα among individuals, and 60% of the differences can be attributed to genetic factors (Table 1) (67). A correct classification of the sepsis syndrome into separate distinct entities may help identify those individuals most likely to benefit from better targeting of anti-TNFα therapies (68).

In addition to SNP analyses, large scale analysis of gene expression using micro-array techniques may help characterize sepsis in a more pathogenesis-oriented classification with prognostic and therapeutic consequences (69–71). Finally, identification of specific polymorphisms in drug metabolism, transporter, and receptor genes may help limit the occurrence of adverse events that complicate intensive care management.

OTHER PHARMACOGENETIC MARKERS OF INTEREST

Drug Transporter Polymorphism

Uptake, distribution, and excretion of endogenous and exogenous compounds including antibiotics is controlled by polyspecific membrane transporters expressed in intestine, liver, kidney, placenta, testis, blood cells and the endothelial cell lining of brain capillaries, where they constitute the blood–brain barrier. Increasingly, membrane-spanning proteins involved in the inward or outward transport of a large variety of drugs have been recognized and characterized over the past years in almost all tissues (Table 2). Drug transporters can be viewed as completing the enzyme-based detoxification systems to achieve efficient protection against chemical toxins. Both systems show similar broad specificity and may even work in synergy. Drug uptake delivers the drug to the detoxification system facilitating metabolism, and drug efflux decreases the load on detoxification enzymes, thereby avoiding their saturation, while chemical modification, which usually increases the amphiphilicity of drugs, provides drug pumps with better substrates.

Although P-gp (*MDR1*, *ABCB1*) is the well-characterized ABC transporter, new polyspecific drug transporters are being investigated and have the potential for overlapping substrate specificities and for tissue-selective expression. These are the multidrug resistance1 MDR-related proteins, multidrug resistance-associated proteins (MRPs) (*ABCC*-family), the OATP-family (*SLC21A*) of organic anion transport proteins, the PEPT-family of peptide transporter, and a family of transporters (*SLC22A*) for cations (OCTs), anions (OATs), and carnitine and cations (OCTNs) (72–78). This section will focus on transport proteins for anti-infective drugs or transport proteins, which are otherwise functionally involved with infectious diseases.

The concerted action of different pumps located both in the basolateral and apical membranes of epithelial cells accounts for the preferential transfer of drugs from the gut into the systemic circulation and from the blood to the excretory pathways of the liver and kidneys. This cooperation is best evidenced in the liver, where OATPs, OCT1 (basolateral uptake) and MDR1 and MRP2 (apical efflux) ensure the unidirectional transfer of drugs into the bile (79). This is also present in the kidney proximal tubules with OATs, OCTs, MRP1, and OATP-B (basolateral uptake) and MDR1, and MRP2 (apical efflux) (74). It has also been demonstrated for the transepithelial transport of antibiotics in the intestine and airway epithelia (80,81).

The activity of pumps can explain the poor bioavailability of several antibiotics (80,82) and the increased clearance of β-lactam antibiotics modulated by certain compounds (74). Moreover, drug transporters determine the distribution of a drug within the body, that is, whether the drug levels are high enough for therapeutic effect at their site of action. The identification of efflux pumps in macrophages (83,84) and the reduced activity of macrolides, tetracyclines, lincosamides, and rifamycins in transporter overexpressing multidrug-resistant cells explains the potentially reduced intracellular activity of antibiotics (85). Drug efflux pumps reduce the amount of antibiotics to a point where it may no longer exceed the minimal inhibitory concentration.

The consequences of genetic polymorphisms of transporter proteins for the disposition and action of drugs have been appreciated only recently (75). As pointed out previously, a silent exonic C3435T mutation in exon 26 of the *MDRl* gene has been associated with diminished intestinal P-gp levels, increased uptake of digoxin from the gut (31), and reduced rhodamine efflux from lymphocytes (86) (Table 3). Although P-gp is the well-characterized transporter (see HIV section earlier), new members are being investigated (Table 2) and have the potential for overlapping substrate specificities and for cell-selective expression.

The identification of genetic variants with decreased transport function has several implications for drug development and therapy. However, the extrapolation of the function, in particular of in vitro data, of a single transporter to clinical in vivo consequences is difficult. In most cases, the overlap in substrates between drug transporters is extensive, and other transporters can most likely compensate for the absence of one transporting system. Otherwise, knockout mice with a full transporter deficiency would not be viable and fertile (87–89). Aside from drug clearance and oral bioavailability, the most important role of transporters for anti-infective treatments is the disposition and tissue penetration to achieve sufficiently high drug concentrations at the site of action (e.g., intracellularly) for effective treatment. Whether these processes are practically relevant remains to be investigated and confirmed in clinical studies.

Multidrug Resistance–Associated Proteins

MRP1–9 are all organic anion pumps, but they differ in substrate specificity, tissue distribution, and intracellular localization. MRP1 and MRP2 transport a similar large range of organic anions, including quinolones (90,91), macrolides (92), and HIV PIs (93). MRP1 is located in most organs including lung, muscle, kidney, testis, and peripheral mononuclear blood cells. The tissue distribution of MRP2 is much more restricted than that of MRP1 and is found in hepatic, intestinal, renal cells, brain, and placenta (94). MRP1 is basolateral and secretes drugs into the body, whereas MRP2 is located in the apical membrane and moves drugs out of the body (72).

Multidrug resistance–associated proteins (MRPs) have been implicated in the treatment failure of infectious diseases. An increased expression of the P-gp and MRP proteins has been suggested as a potential mechanism for decreased PI availability at certain intracellular sites that provide sanctuary for HIV (95,96). The expression and activity of MRPs can also be altered by certain drugs and disease states. MRP2 mRNA levels are reduced to 30% in hepatitis C virus-infected liver (97), and inhibition of MRP2 and reduction of the MRP2 expression level has been suggested to cause fusidate-induced hyperbilirubinemia (98), leading to the conclusion that subjects with hereditary MRP2 deficiency, such as patients with the Dubin-Johnson syndrome, are particularly likely to suffer complications.

MRP1 protein protects mice from TB (99) and augments HIV productive infection in CEM cells (100), and the antimalarial action of trimethoprim-sulfamethoxazole has partly been attributed to its inhibitory effect on MRP1 (101). Another interesting function of MRP1 is its ability to act as the major high-affinity transporter of leukotriene C4, which could influence susceptibility to, and the course of, infectious diseases. *MRP1* knockout mice show a diminished response to a nonspecific inflammatory stimulus (102), as expected, but they are nevertheless more resistant to an experimental *Streptococcus pneumoniae* infection than wild-type mice, presumably because the inability of macrophages, mast cells, and granulocytes to secrete LTC4 secondarily leads to increased leukotriene B4 excretion and more effective recruitment of phagocytic cells (87).

The *MRP1* and *MRP2* genes have been screened in healthy Japanese subjects and a number of SNPs, including nonsynonymous amino acid mutations, were detected, although these were not validated functionally (103–105). The *MRP1* G2168A and *MRP2* C-24T SNPs failed to show any correlation with duodenal mRNA levels (106). Conrad et al. (107,108) identified two rare mutations, of which Gly671Val showed no difference in organic anion transport, whereas Arg433Ser showed a twofold transport reduction and a twofold increased sensitivity to doxorubicin. In contrast to MRP1, mutations in the *MRP2* (*ABCC2*) gene result in the absence of protein from the canalicular membrane (105,109–112). These rare mutations cause the conjugated hyperbilirubinemia of Dubin-Johnson syndrome (113).

MRP4 and MRP5 are both organic anion pumps with the ability to transport cyclic nucleotides and nucleotide analogs, a class of organic anions apparently not transported by MRP1 to 3 or 6. The tissue distribution of MRP4 and MRP5 is still not well known. Recent studies suggest that *MRP4* is more widely expressed than was initially thought, with the highest levels in the kidney and prostate. In contrast, *MRP5* is ubiquitously expressed with the highest levels found in skeletal muscle, brain, and erythrocytes (72). The transport of nucleotide analogs by *MRP4* and *5* can result in resistance to clinically used base, nucleoside, and nucleotide analogs (114–117). Cells with high concentrations of *MRP4* are highly resistant to PMEA and AZT but much less resistant to other nucleoside analogs used in antiviral therapy, such as lamivudine, ddC, and d4T (118). As nucleobase and nucleoside analogs are used extensively in anticancer and antiviral therapies, there is a potential for *MRP4/5* to mediate resistance to these compounds. Screening of DNAs from 48 Japanese individuals revealed a number of SNPs in *MRP4* and *MRP5* (104). However, these have not been validated by in vitro experiments or in clinical studies with disease-susceptibility and drug response phenotypes.

Organic Anion Transporters

Most β-lactam antibiotics and antiviral drugs are amphiphilic organic anions, which are actively secreted into renal proximal tubules. Organic anion transporters (OATs) OAT1 (*SLC22A6*), OAT2 (*SLC22A7*), and to a lesser extent OAT3 (*SLC22A8*), have been suggested to be responsible for most of the uptake of organic anions, including cephalosporins into proximal tubule cells (119,120). Due to their role in renal drug excretion, they have an important impact on drug pharmacokinetics and pharmacodynamics. Competition may lead to decreased renal drug excretion and cause severe side effects with the potential for drug–drug interactions. For example, the cytotoxicity of adefovir and cidofovir was prevented by using probenecid, the OAT1 inhibitor, with hOAT1 expressing cells (121). The genetic variability of OATs, and their relevance for drug response, has however not yet been established.

Organic Cation Transporters

hOCT1 (*SLC22A1*) is primarily found in the sinusoidal (basolateral) membrane of hepatocytes and, to a lesser extent, in intestinal epithelial cells. Three polymorphisms have been identified to severely affect hOCT1 function in oocytes. These are Arg61Cys, Cys88Arg, and Gly401Ser, which result in a reduction of transport of various classical but structurally diverse organic cation transporter (OCT) substrates by 70%, 87%, and 98%, respectively

(122). Given the frequency of these alleles, 9%, 0.6%, and 3.2%, respectively, homozygotes and compound heterozygotes for these alleles would be expected to arise in Caucasian populations with a frequency of approximately 1.5%. Whether these are clinically relevant remains to be investigated. Based on what we know, probably the most important role of hOCT1 involves the disposition of substrate drugs (or toxins) for which the relevant pharmacodynamic (therapeutic or side effect) target lies within the liver. An interesting example is the PI, which is inactivated inside the liver by CYP-mediated metabolism. For example, plasma levels of desipramine or terfenadine, increased significantly when coadministrated with ritonavir, an interaction, which has mainly been explained by inhibition of CYP3A4 (73). However, PIs are only weak substrates but strong inhibitors of hOCT1 (123), and the organic cation desipramine is a substrate for hOCT1 (124). Inhibition of uptake leads to a poorer access of desipramine to metabolizing enzymes inside the liver. In these cases, even a moderate reduction in hepatic uptake might make an important difference, and people with genetically reduced hOCT1 levels might display an increased risk to PI-mediated drug–drug interactions. hOCT2 (*SLC22A2*) is mainly found in the kidney, most likely in the basolateral membrane of the renal tubules (74,125,126).

Recently, five rare mutations in hOCT2 have been reported that affect the transport function of hOCT2 in vitro. Collectively, variants P54S, M165I, R400C, K432Q and one insertion mutation that results in a prematurely truncated protein were present at allelic frequencies of 1% (5/494) only in African Americans, 0.6% (3/494) in African Americans and Mexican Americans, and 0.2% (1/494) in Caucasians, respectively (127). All four nonsynonymous mutations altered transporter function as assayed in oocytes, and the insertion mutation results in a prematurely truncated protein of 47 amino acids that almost certainly abolishes transporter function. The extrapolation of this in vitro data to in vivo renal clearance is currently not known.

Organic Anion-Transporting Polypeptides

OATP-C (*SLC21A6*), OATP8 (*SLC21A8*), and OATP-B (*SLC21A9*) have been established as the major organic anion-transporting polypetides (OATPs) at the basolateral membrane of the liver (128,129), although OATP-B is also expressed in placenta, intestine, kidney, and lung (77). They are the most important carriers for hepatic uptake of amphiphilic organic anions, such as sulfobromophthalein, bile salts, thyroid hormone, and unconjugated bilirubin (78), and antibiotics including rifampicin and rifamycin (128–131).

Tirona et al. (131) described six mutations in five alleles in the *SLC21A6* gene, which resulted in altered substrate transport in vitro. Variants Phe73Ala (**2* allele), Val82Ala and Glu156Gly (**3* allele), and Ile353Thr (**6* allele) were present with allelic frequencies of 2% in the Caucasians. Two variants, Val174Ala and Gly488Ala, had relatively high frequencies of 14% in the Caucasians and 9% in the African Americans, respectively (131). Two novel mutations in OATP-B, one rare (T392I) and one common variant (S486F), which occurred with a frequency of 31%, were detected in the Japanese (132). Interestingly, this common polymorphism led to a decrease in the V_{max} of [(3)H]estrone-3-sulfate uptake to 43% of that seen with the common variant.

Whether any of the mutations that are associated with impaired transport function in vitro have any consequences in vivo remains a subject of future investigations. However, Michalski et al. (133) identified a mutation (L193R), which reduced the amount of OATP-C protein in a heterozygous liver sample. In vitro validation of this variant revealed impaired protein maturation with a complete loss of transport function (133). It is known that hepatic bile salt and bilirubin elimination by human liver

OATPs can be inhibited by rifampicin or rifamycin (130). Therefore, even with a moderate reduction in hepatic uptake, the excretory system can be quickly pushed to its limits with an increased risk of toxic liver injury.

Aminoglycoside-Induced Deafness

Aminoglycoside antibiotic-induced ototoxicity is a major cause of irreversible deafness in many parts of the world (134,135). In China, because of the widespread use of aminoglycosides, in some areas, up to 25% of the cases of deafness were found to be caused by aminoglycosides (136). The pathogenesis of aminoglycoside-induced ototoxicity is divided into two types. One is prolonged or high-level drug exposure, and the other is idiosyncratic reaction resulting from minimal or regular exposure. The latter individuals are observed to be clustered in certain families, suggesting that genetic factors play a role in the susceptibility to aminoglycoside-induced ototoxicity. Studies in the Chinese and Japanese families have shown that the inheritance is exclusively through the maternal line (137–139).

The mechanism of the antimicrobial action of aminoglycosides is to bind to the 30S subunit of the bacterial ribosome, which ultimately leads to the inhibition of protein synthesis. It interferes with the initiation complex of peptide formation, which induces misreading of the code on the mRNA template and causes a breakup of polysomes into nonfunctional monosomes. Recent evidence suggests that the A1555G mutation in the mitochondrial 12S rRNA gene leads to susceptibility to aminoglycoside ototoxcity (140). The mutation causes the human mitochondrial rRNA to be more structurally similar to the bacterial rRNA that is the target of aminoglycoside action (141). The A1555G mutation has indeed been shown to cause an increase in the binding of aminoglycoside to the mitochondrial rRNA (142), and there is a decrease in mitochondrial protein synthesis in cells carrying the A1555G mutation (143). A T961C has now been discovered in an Italian family and in a Japanese patient (135,140).

The neuro-otological characteristics in patients with the A1555G mutation have been described (134). First, these patients exhibit a progressive loss of hearing. In most patients, the interval between the first complaint of hearing loss after aminoglycoside exposure and complete deafness was more than 10 years. Second, a better residual pure-tone threshold was found in these patients, suggesting that the organ of Corti was more or less preserved. Third, there was a lower threshold for electrical promontory stimulation in patients with the mutation than in those without. Fourth, the vestibular function was well preserved in these patients suggesting that increased susceptibility to aminoglycosides seems to occur mainly in the cochlea. It has been thought that the progressive hearing loss associated with this mutation is partly due to progressive reduction of the endocochlear potential production from the stria vascularis, which is known to contain many mitochondria in the intermediate cells (134). Screening for these mutations may lead to a reduction in the number of victims of progressive deafness induced by aminoglycosides.

Helicobacter pylori Infection and PPI

H. pylori is a major cause of gastritis, peptic ulcer disease, and gastric carcinoma. Eradication of *H. pylori* with a triple therapy involving a combination of antibiotics (amoxicillin, clarithromycin, metronidazole) and a proton pump inhibitor (PPI) (omeprazole, lansoprazole, rabeprazole) is effective in the treatment of these diseases. Suppression of acid secretion by PPIs increases the concentration of antibiotics and allows *H. pylori* to reach the growth phase and thus become more sensitive to antibiotics, and PPIs alone have an anti-*H. pylori* effect (144).

Omeprazole, lansoprazole, and to a lesser extent rabeprazole, are metabolized by CYP2C19 (143). The CYP2C19 PM phenotype comprises 2% to 5% of the Caucasians and 3% to 23% of the Asians, resulting from a single base pair mutation (A to G) in exon 5 of the coding region 7. The truncated mutant protein lacks the heme-binding region and is enzymatically inactive.

Some studies have shown that the therapeutic effects of PPIs and therefore the cure rates for *H. pylori* infection are significantly dependent on the CYP2C19 genotype status [PM, heterozygous extensive metabolizers (hetEM), and homozygous extensive metabolizers (homEM)]. A better cure rate was achieved with dual therapy rabeprazole and amoxicillin in patients with the PM genotype (93.8%) than the hetEM (91.7%) or the homEM (60.6%) genotype (145). In a second study using triple therapy including a PPI and amoxicillin and clarithromycin, the majority of patients without initial eradication of *H. pylori* were all EM of CYP2C19 (146). Some studies have failed to document an influence of CYP2C19 genetic polymorphism on the efficacy of PPI with amoxicillin and clarithromycin in eradicating *H. pylori* (147–149). These conflicting reports can be partially explained by the differences in patient inclusion criteria (some included only patients with gastric ulcer disease) (148), patient characteristics (one study included disproportionate number of smokers) (147), and dosage differences in the PPI (150). The inclusion of clarithromycin in the triple therapy regimen can also influence the response, because clarithromycin can interact with the other drugs, leading to an altered response. Despite these conflicting reports, some authors have suggested that genotyping for CYP2C19 prior to treatment with a PPI might be a clinically useful and cost-effective tool for optimal treatment of *H. pylori* infection (151).

Cephalosporin-Induced Bleeding Disorder

Cephalosporins are important antibiotics that are commonly used in the treatment of various infections and in the prophylaxis of surgical patients. Some cephalosporins (moxalactam, cefamandole, and cefoperazone) have been reported to cause life-threatening hypoprothrombinemia and hemorrhage (152,153). The cause of cephalosporin-induced bleeding lies within the chemical structure of these drugs. Cephalosporins contain an 1-methyltetrazole-5-thiol (MTT) leaving group that undergoes *S*-methylation, which is catalyzed by thiopurine *S*-methyltranferase (TPMT). MTT has been shown to be the cause of hypoprothrombinemia and hemorrhage. MTT inhibits the gamma-carboxylation of glutamic acid, a vitamin K-dependent reaction required for the formation of active clotting factors (153–155). A recent study showed that 2-methyl-1,3,4-thiadiazole-5-thiol (MTD), a thiol found in the structure of cefazolin, is found in tissues of patients who were treated with cefazolin (156). MTD is also a substrate for *S*-methylation catalyzed by TPMT, and it is also an inhibitor of gamma carboxylation of glutamate in vitro (152).

TPMT is a genetically polymorphic drug-metabolizing enzyme specifically catalyzing the conjugation of aromatic and heterocyclic sulfhydryl compounds. Individual variation in *S*-methylation catalyzed by TPMT may be responsible for differences in susceptibility to cephalosporin-induced hypoprothrombinemia (153). Those individuals who have genetically low or absent TPMT and can therefore not effectively catalyze *S*-methylation may be more prone to develop adverse events. A trimodal distribution of TPMT activity has been shown in a large randomly selected population, with 89% of the subjects having the homozygous trait with high TPMT activity, 11% heterozygous with intermediate activity, and approximately 1 in 300 subjects homozygous for the trait of low or absent TPMT activity (157). Similar TPMT polymorphic patterns have been observed in Caucasians and Black subjects, with 17% lower TPMT activity in Blacks (158). The functional gene of TPMT has now been cloned and was localized on chromosome 6. At least eight variant alleles that are associated with low levels of TPMT enzyme activity have been characterized (*TPMT**2*, *TPMT**3A*, *TPMT**3B*, *TPMT**3C*, *TPMT**3D*, *TPMT**4*, *TMPT**5*, and *TPMT**6*). *TPMT**2* is a relatively rare allele (159,160), and *TPMT**3A* is the most common variant allele in Caucasians, accounting for 55–57% of all variant forms of TPMT. The mechanism responsible for low TPMT activity in variant alleles **2*, **3A*, **3B*, and **3C* has been shown to be the reduced levels of TPMT immunoreactive protein due to enhanced protein degradation (161), and for *TPMT**4* it is due to very low mRNA levels (162). Differences in the level of TPMT activity have also been found to depend on ethnicity, gender, and age; however, the mechanisms underlying these findings are not clear (163). Patients with genetically low or absent TPMT who are treated with cephalosporin antibiotics may be at risk of developing hypoprothrombinemia and hemorrhage as a result of the inability to *S*-methylate MTT and MTD.

IMMUNOGENETICS IN INFECTIOUS DISEASES

Drug Hypersensitivity

Many hypersensitivity reactions appear to be the result of direct activation of the immune system. There is strong evidence for a role of drugs or drug metabolites as antigens or haptens in major histocompatibility complex (MHC)-restricted T-cell activation. Drugs may be conjugated to intracellular proteins and presented by MHC class I or class II molecules to $CD8^+$ or $CD4^+$ T-cells (164). They may also directly alter the MHC-associated peptide complex with subsequent recognition and activation of peptide-specific $CD8^+$ T-cells (165). *MHC* alleles have been associated with idiosyncratic reactions to nonsteroidal anti-inflammatory agents, pyrazolone derivatives, trimethoprim-sulfamethoxazole, and contact allergens (166–169). Two recent studies used immunogenetics to approach the problem of early, and some times deadly, hypersensitivity reactions to the reverse transcriptase inhibitor abacavir used in the treatment of HIV infection (170,171). The genetic susceptibility to abacavir hypersensitivity was shown to be associated with the *MHC 57.1* ancestral haplotype. However, the genetic approach to drug hypersensitivity is not new, and it has so far not led to a dramatic breakthrough in the prevention of immune-mediated drug reactions, in particular because MHC associations were difficult to reproduce. Thus, immunogenetics may complement and add to alternative diagnostic approaches, such as T-cell proliferation assays and epicutaneous tests, as none of these have much predictive value in unexposed subjects (3).

Response to Vaccination

Hepatitis B vaccination continues to be the best available means of preventing and controlling hepatitis B infection. Current recombinant hepatitis B vaccines achieve seroprotection in greater than 95% of the vaccinated adult population (172). However, approximately 5% of the adults respond inadequately to the standard three doses of hepatitis B vaccine. Those adults who have an antihepatitis B (anti-HBs) titer of less than 10 mIU/mL are defined as poor- and nonresponders. The lack of anti-HBs antibody response has been attributed to many factors and these include improper storage, advanced age, gender, obesity, renal failure, and smoking (172,173). In addition, genetic factors, specifically the histocompatibility leucocyte antigens (HLA)-linked immune response genes may control the response to hepatitis B vaccine, and a poor antibody response is associated with certain *HLA* haplotypes. Earlier studies have found that immune response to hepatitis B vaccine is largely determined by the *HLA-DR*, *-DP*, and *-DQ* genes. Specifically haplotypes *DRB1*1101*, and *-DQB1*020* were associated with poor responsiveness. There were also interactions between the *HLA* factors contributing to poor responsiveness. For example, *HLA-DPB1*02* was negatively associated with responsiveness when it occurred in association with haplotypes *DRB1*0701/DRB4*0101-DQB1*020**, and *DRB4*0101* was negatively associated with responsiveness when it occurred in association with the haplotype *DRB1*0301/DRB3*0101-DQB1*020** (174).

More recent studies have shown that different HLA products seem to act as agonists (*C4AQ0* and *HLA-DQB1*02*) or antagonists (*C4AQ0*, *HLA-DQB1*02*, and *HLA-DRB1*11*, *DQB1*0301*) in lowering the humoral response to hepatitis B vaccine (175). It was found that responders were characterized more for lacking "nonresponder" alleles than for having specific "responder" ones. Investigations into the associations of HLA alleles and antibody nonresponse in the Caucasian population have also identified other *HLA*-genotypes including *C4A3*, *B44*, *DR7*, *FC31*, *B8*, *DR3*, and *SC01* (176–178). Because genes present in the major histocompatibility complex modulate the immune response to hepatitis B vaccine, poor- and nonresponders may benefit from a course of revaccination (176). In fact one study showed that revaccination could enable persistently nonresponder individuals to produce an anti-HBs antibody response; however, the response was dependent on HLA haplotype and the dose of vaccine (179).

VALIDATION OF PHARMACOGENETIC MARKERS

The treatment of diseases, such as TB, malaria, and HIV, is highly standardized and would thus allow acquisition of genetic information at a rapid pace. Similarly, the abundance of clinical trials in infectious diseases could contribute to a critical resource of response and toxicity data. In clinical trials, genotype can be used as an exclusion criterion (180,181). Thus, the study group can be smaller and more homogeneous, although less representative of the population at large. This approach would be of particular interest in the study of sepsis, given the great heterogeneity of the syndrome. The genotype can also be used a posteriori as a stratification factor.

In some diseases, such as HIV infection, patients are expected to be on life-long treatment. Treatment is frequently changed because of toxicity or failure (182), and patients will possibly participate in multiple trials over the years. In this circumstance, certain authors propose the use of a "CYP passport" for volunteers who participate regularly in clinical trials (183). Trials will have to take into account the ethnic origin of the individuals because of its association with genetic polymorphisms (2). However, ethnic denominations may only partially reflect the genetic make-up, and genotyping may reveal more precisely specific associations. A number of X-linked microsatellites and SNP markers are used for the comprehensive analysis of the ethnical structure of the populations (1).

Adequate cohorts and studies have to be developed to allow a very clear definition of a clinical phenotype. This should lead to an integrated database allowing segregation, linkage, and association analysis. Acceptance by participants will be critical in such endeavors. However, in our own experience of offering participation to genetic testing to 1000 HIV-infected patients, the rate of approval has been extremely high at 97%.

These issues (Table 4) are critical, as there is a paucity of in vivo validation of the value of pharmacogenetic markers in predicting treatment response or toxicity of anti-infective agents. Antiretroviral agents are excellent targets for the validation of

Table 4 Validation of Pharmacogenetic Markers in Infectious Diseases

Issues	Comments
Standardized treatment for many diseases	Allows coherent collection of data. Phenotype should be carefully defined
Abundance of clinical trials	Allows rapid collection of data. Genotype can be used to better define the target population (smaller and more homogeneous study population) or for stratification for analysis
Regular participation to consecutive trials (volunteers, HIV-infected)	Creation of a "genetic passport"
Use of anti-infective agents in different ethnic groups	Ethnic denominations may only partially reflect the genetic make-up. Genotyping could reveal specific associations

pharmacogenetic markers in the clinical arena. In one of the first attempts at evaluating known genetic and functional polymorphism of the proteins involved in drug metabolism and disposition, Fellay et al. (20) performed a pilot evaluation in a cohort of well-defined HIV-infected patients receiving protease- or non-nucleoside reverse transcriptase inhibitor-containing regimens. Genetic analysis included the investigation of key polymorphisms of *CYP3A4*, *3A5*, *2D6*, *2C19*, *MDR1*, *CCR5* (a viral receptor that modifies susceptibility to infection and possibly response to therapy), and also expression of P-gp, MRP1, and MRP2 in lymphocytes. Polymorphisms in *MDR1* (C3435T, Exon 26) and *CYP2D6* genes were associated with differences in plasma drug levels. *MDR1* C3435T was also associated with better immune recovery over the first 6 months of treatment. However, this attempt in evaluating the usefulness of pharmacogenetic markers in vivo generated paradoxical results and considerable controversy. *MDR1* 3435 TT polymorphism, associated with this and with other studies with a reduction in *MDR1* expression (Table 3), was associated with low rather that high drug plasma levels. The association was observed both for the P-gp substrate nelfinavir and surprisingly for efavirenz, which is recognized not to be a substrate of this transporter. The issue is also confounded by a potential role of PIs as inducers or inhibitors of P-gp and by evidence for tissue- and developmental-specific expression of many transporters. Unfortunately, this paradox, possibly explained by the existence of complex compensatory mechanisms (184), underscores the difficulties that will be encountered when applying knowledge obtained from in vitro studies to the clinical field.

CONCLUSIONS

The current state of knowledge of pharmacogenetics in the area of infectious diseases mainly includes the identification of genetic polymorphism leading to changes in the activity of phase I and phase II metabolic pathways and in transporters. These polymorphisms were the first to be recognized because research was specifically directed to relevant metabolic or transport genes. As a result of genome-wide investigations, a new generation of markers will be found associated with specific toxicities or lack-of-efficacy phenotypes. These labor-intensive analyses will lead to identification of additional polymorphisms with potential functional relevance. Polymorphisms may remain remote to the gene of interest (e.g., regulators, suppressor genes) or be present in noncoding regions (promoter, intron, 3′ untranslated region), contributing to modified expression, splicing, or protein stability. Transcriptome analysis using microarrays also promises to deliver information about individual expression profiles that may lead to genes participating in complex regulatory or signaling cascades. These cascades may be investigated in detail to identify polymorphims and modification of function distant to the key metabolic or transport genes.

Understanding of the genetics of disease susceptibility may also help in the development of new drugs. Identification of a polymorphism of the HIV cellular receptor CCR5 that resulted in the absence of a functional protein and high-level protection from HIV infection led to the initiation of an intense research in drug development, including that of an orally active CCR5 receptor antagonist that blocks the entry of HIV-1, currently in clinical trial.

Importantly, pharmacogenetics and immunogenetics of anti-infective chemotherapy will complement the field of genetics of susceptibility to a pathogen. For major pathogens, such as HIV, malaria, and TB, this has the potential to dramatically improve management and limit the number of patients requiring therapy. Fortunately, knowledge acquired on inherited differences in the metabolism, transport, and disposition of anti-infective drugs will be to a significant extent shared by drugs used in other disciplines. The fields will thus move forward together.

ACKNOWLEDGMENT

This work was supported by the Swiss National Science Foundation and by the Santos Suarez Foundation.

REFERENCES

1. Wilson JF, Weale ME, Smith AC, et al. Population genetic structure of variable drug response. Nat Genet 2001; 29:265–269.
2. Risch N, Burchard E, Ziv E, Tang H. Categorization of humans in biomedical research: genes, race and disease. Genome Biol 2002; 3; comment 2007.
3. Telenti A, Aubert V, Spertini F. Individualising HIV treatment–pharmacogenetics and immunogenetics. Lancet 2002; 359:722–723.
4. Penn DJ, Damjanovich K, Potts WK. MHC heterozygosity confers a selective advantage against multiple-strain infections. Proc Natl Acad Sci USA 2002; 99:11260–11264.
5. Bönicke R, Reif W. Enzymatic inactivation of isonicotinic acid hydrazide in humans and animals. Arch Exp Pathol Pharmacol 1953; 220:321–333.
6. Marzolini C, Telenti A, Decosterd L, Biollaz J, Buclin T. 'Efavirenz plasma levels can predict treatment failure and central nervous system side effects in HIV-1-infected patients.' AIDS 2001; 15:1193–1194.
7. Marzolini C, Buclin T, Decosterd LA, Biollaz J, Telenti A. Nelfinavir plasma levels under twice-daily and three-times-daily regimens: high interpatient and low intrapatient variability. Ther Drug Monit 2001; 23:394–398.
8. Fellay J, Boubaker K, Ledergerber B, et al. Prevalence of adverse events associated with potent antiretroviral treatment: Swiss HIV Cohort Study. Lancet 2001; 358:1322–1327.
9. Lee BL, Wong D, Benowitz NL, Sullam PM. Altered patterns of drug metabolism in patients with acquired immunodeficiency syndrome. Clin Pharmacol Ther 1993; 53:529–535.
10. Gronhagen-Riska C, Hellstrom PE, Froseth B. Predisposing factors in hepatitis induced by isoniazid-rifampin treatment of tuberculosis. Am Rev Respir Dis 1978; 118:461–466.

11. Rieder MJ, Shear NH, Kanee A, Tang BK, Spielberg SP. Prominence of slow acetylator phenotype among patients with sulfonamide hypersensitivity reactions. Clin Pharmacol Ther 1991; 49:13–17.
12. Huang YS, Chern HD, Su WJ, et al. Polymorphism of the N-acetyltransferase 2 gene as a susceptibility risk factor for antituberculosis drug-induced hepatitis. Hepatology 2002; 35:883–889.
13. Barry M, Mulcahy F, Merry C, Gibbons S, Back D. Pharmacokinetics and potential interactions amongst antiretroviral agents used to treat patients with HIV infection. Clin Pharmacokinet 1999; 36:289–304.
14. Erickson DA, Mather G, Trager WF, Levy RH, Keirns JJ. Characterization of the in vitro biotransformation of the HIV-1 reverse transcriptase inhibitor nevirapine by human hepatic cytochromes P-450. Drug Metab Dispos 1999; 27:1488–1495.
15. Hesse LM, von Moltke LL, Shader RI, Greenblatt DJ. Ritonavir, efavirenz, and nelfinavir inhibit CYP2B6 activity in vitro: potential drug interactions with bupropion. Drug Metab Dispos 2001; 29:100–102.
16. Malaty LI, Kuper JJ. Drug interactions of HIV protease inhibitors. Drug Saf 1999; 20:147–169.
17. Eagling VA, Back DJ, Barry MG. Differential inhibition of cytochrome P450 isoforms by the protease inhibitors, ritonavir, saquinavir and indinavir. Br J Clin Pharmacol 1997; 44:190–194.
18. von Moltke LL, Greenblatt DJ, Grassi JM, et al. Protease inhibitors as inhibitors of human cytochromes P450: high risk associated with ritonavir. J Clin Pharmacol 1998; 38:106–111.
19. O'Neil WM, Gilfix BM, Markoglou N, et al. Genotype and phenotype of cytochrome P450 2D6 in human immunodeficiency virus-positive patients and patients with acquired immunodeficiency syndrome. Eur J Clin Pharmacol 2000; 56:231–240.
20. Fellay J, Marzolini C, Meaden ER, et al. Response to antiretroviral treatment in HIV-1-infected individuals with allelic variants of the multidrug resistance transporter 1: a pharmacogenetics study. Lancet 2002; 359:30–36.
21. Sata F, Sapone A, Elizondo G, et al. CYP3A4 allelic variants with amino acid substitutions in exons 7 and 12: evidence for an allelic variant with altered catalytic activity. Clin Pharmacol Ther 2000; 67:48–56.
22. Heim M, Meyer UA. Genotyping of poor metabolisers of debrisoquine by allele-specific PCR amplification. Lancet 1990; 336:529–532.
23. Griese EU, Zanger UM, Brudermanns U, et al. Assessment of the predictive power of genotypes for the in-vivo catalytic function of CYP2D6 in a German population. Pharmacogenetics 1998; 8:15–26.
24. Johansson I, Lundqvist E, Dahl ML, Ingelman-Sundberg M. PCR-based genotyping for duplicated and deleted CYP2D6 genes. Pharmacogenetics 1996; 6:351–355.
25. Bardsley-Elliot A, Plosker GL. Nelfinavir: an update on its use in HIV infection. Drugs 2000; 59:581–620.
26. Kuehl P, Zhang J, Lin Y, et al. Sequence diversity in CYP3A promoters and characterization of the genetic basis of polymorphic CYP3A5 expression. Nat Genet 2001; 27:383–391.
27. www.imm.ki.se/CYPalleles/
28. Jones K, Hoggard PG, Sales SD, et al. Differences in the intracellular accumulation of HIV protease inhibitors in vitro and the effect of active transport. AIDS 2001; 15:675–681.
29. Jones K, Bray PG, Khoo SH, et al. P-Glycoprotein and transporter MRP1 reduce HIV protease inhibitor uptake in CD4 cells: potential for accelerated viral drug resistance? AIDS 2001; 15:1353–1358.
30. Kim RB. MDR1 single nucleotide polymorphisms: multiplicity of haplotypes and functional consequences. Pharmacogenetics 2002; 12:425–427.
31. Hoffmeyer S, Burk O, von Richter O, et al. Functional polymorphisms of the human multidrug-resistance gene: multiple sequence variations and correlation of one allele with P-glycoprotein expression and activity in vivo. Proc Natl Acad Sci USA 2000; 97:3473–3478.

32. Sakaeda T, Nakamura T, Horinouchi M, et al. MDR1 genotype-related pharmacokinetics of digoxin after single oral administration in healthy Japanese subjects. Pharm Res 2001; 18:1400–1404.
33. Nakamura T, Sakaeda T, Horinouchi M, et al. Effect of the mutation (C3435T) at exon 26 of the MDR1 gene on expression level of MDR1 messenger ribonucleic acid in duodenal enterocytes of healthy Japanese subjects. Clin Pharmacol Ther 2002; 71: 297–303.
34. Kim RB, Leake BF, Choo EF, et al. Identification of functionally variant MDR1 alleles among European Americans and African Americans. Clin Pharmacol Ther 2001; 70:189–199.
35. Goto M, Masuda S, Saito H, et al. C3435T polymorphism in the MDR1 gene affects the enterocyte expression level of CYP3A4 rather than Pgp in recipients of living-donor liver transplantation. Pharmacogenetics 2002; 12:451–457.
36. Jones K, Hoggard PG, Khoo S, Maher B, Back DJ. Effect of alpha1-acid glycoprotein on the intracellular accumulation of the HIV protease inhibitors saquinavir, ritonavir and indinavir in vitro. Br J Clin Pharmacol 2001; 51:99–102.
37. Holladay JW, Dewey MJ, Michniak BB, et al. Elevated alpha-1-acid glycoprotein reduces the volume of distribution and systemic clearance of saquinavir. Drug Metab Dispos 2001; 29:299–303.
38. Bilello JA, Bilello PA, Stellrecht K, et al. Human serum alpha 1 acid glycoprotein reduces uptake, intracellular concentration, and antiviral activity of A-80987, an inhibitor of the human immunodeficiency virus type 1 protease. Antimicrob Agents Chemother 1996; 40:1491–1497.
39. Bryant M, Getman D, Smidt M, et al. SC-52151, a novel inhibitor of the human immunodeficiency virus protease. Antimicrob Agents Chemother 1995; 39:2229–2234.
40. Zhang XQ, Schooley RT, Gerber JG. The effect of increasing alpha1-acid glycoprotein concentration on the antiviral efficacy of human immunodeficiency virus protease inhibitors. J Infect Dis 1999; 180:1833–1837.
41. Eap CB, Cuendet C, Baumann P. Orosomucoid (alpha-1 acid glycoprotein) phenotyping by use of immobilized pH gradients with 8 M urea and immunoblotting. A new variant encountered in a population study. Hum Genet 1988; 80:183–185.
42. Dente L, Pizza MG, Metspalu A, Cortese R. Structure and expression of the genes coding for human alpha 1-acid glycoprotein. EMBO J 1987; 6:2289–2296.
43. Yuasa I, Umetsu K, Vogt U, et al. Human orosomucoid polymorphism: molecular basis of the three common ORM1 alleles, ORM1*F1, ORM1*F2, and ORM1*S. Hum Genet 1997; 99:393–398.
44. Hunziker K, Schmid K. A brief method for the identification of the alpha-1-acid glycoprotein variants. Anal Biochem 1967; 20:495–501.
45. Schmid K, Field RA, Yoshizaki H. Constancy of alpha-1-acid glycoprotein variants of Caucasian patients under conditions of severe stress. J Med Genet 1968; 5:36–39.
46. Herve F, Duche JC, Jaurand MC. Changes in expression and microheterogeneity of the genetic variants of human alpha1-acid glycoprotein in malignant mesothelioma. J Chromatogr B Biomed Sci Appl 1998; 715:111–123.
47. Duche JC, Herve F, Tillement JP. Study of the expression of the genetic variants of human alpha1-acid glycoprotein in healthy subjects using isoelectric focusing and immunoblotting. J Chromatogr B Biomed Sci Appl 1998; 715:103–109.
48. Eap CB, Cuendet C, Baumann P. Binding of d-methadone, l-methadone, and dl-methadone to proteins in plasma of healthy volunteers: role of the variants of alpha 1-acid glycoprotein. Clin Pharmacol Ther 1990; 47:338–346.
49. McCollam PL, Crouch MA, Arnaud P. Caucasian versus African-American differences in orosomucoid: potential implications for therapy. Pharmacotherapy 1998; 18:620–626.
50. Nakamura H, Yuasa I, Umetsu K, et al. The rearrangement of the human alpha(1)-acid glycoprotein/orosomucoid gene: evidence for tandemly triplicated genes consisting of two AGP1 and one AGP2. Biochem Biophys Res Commun 2000; 276:779–784.

51. Shear NH, Spielberg SP, Grant DM, Tang BK, Kalow W. Differences in metabolism of sulfonamides predisposing to idiosyncratic toxicity. Ann Intern Med 1986; 105:179–184.
52. Weber WW, Hein DW. N-Acetylation pharmacogenetics. Pharmacol Rev 1985; 37:25–79.
53. Hein DW, McQueen CA, Grant DM, et al. Pharmacogenetics of the arylamine N-acetyltransferases: a symposium in honor of Wendell W. Weber. Drug Metab Dispos 2000; 28:1425–1432.
54. La Du BN. Isoniazid and psuedocholinesterase polymorphisms. Fed Proc 1972; 31:1276–1285.
55. Grant DM, Blum M, Meyer UA. Polymorphisms of N-acetyltransferase genes. Xenobiotica 1992; 22:1073–1081.
56. Grant DM. Molecular genetics of the N-acetyltransferases. Pharmacogenetics 1993; 3:45–50.
57. Cascorbi I, Drakoulis N, Brockmoller J, et al. Arylamine N-acetyltransferase (NAT2) mutations and their allelic linkage in unrelated Caucasian individuals: correlation with phenotypic activity. Am J Hum Genet 1995; 57:581–592.
58. Grant DM, Hughes NC, Janezic SA, et al. Human acetyltransferase polymorphisms. Mutat Res 1997; 376:61–70.
59. Vatsis KP, Weber WW, Bell DA, et al. Nomenclature for N-acetyltransferases. Pharmacogenetics 1995; 5:1–17.
60. Fretland AJ, Leff MA, Doll MA, Hein DW. Functional characterization of human N-acetyltransferase 2 (NAT2) single nucleotide polymorphisms. Pharmacogenetics 2001; 11:207–215.
61. Shanks GD, Kain KC, Keystone JS. Malaria chemoprophylaxis in the age of drug resistance. II. Drugs that may be available in the future. Clin Infect Dis 2001; 33:381–385.
62. Kletzien RF, Harris PK, Foellmi LA. Glucose-6-phosphate dehydrogenase: a "housekeeping" enzyme subject to tissue-specific regulation by hormones, nutrients, and oxidant stress. FASEB J 1994; 8:174–181.
63. Vulliamy TJ, D'Urso M, Battistuzzi G, et al. Diverse point mutations in the human glucose-6-phosphate dehydrogenase gene cause enzyme deficiency and mild or severe hemolytic anemia. Proc Natl Acad Sci USA 1988; 85:5171–5175.
64. Beutler E. The molecular biology of G6PD variants and other red cell enzyme defects. Annu Rev Med 1992; 43:47–59.
65. Hirono A, Beutler E. Molecular cloning and nucleotide sequence of cDNA for human glucose-6-phosphate dehydrogenase variant A(-). Proc Natl Acad Sci USA 1988; 85:3951–3954.
66. Weber WW. Populations and genetic polymorphisms. Mol Diagn 1999; 4:299–307.
67. Westendorp RG, Langermans JA, Huizinga TW, Verweij CL, Sturk A. Genetic influence on cytokine production in meningococcal disease. Lancet 1997; 349:1912–1913.
68. Cariou A, Chiche JD, Charpentier J, Dhainaut JF, Mira JP. The era of genomics: impact on sepsis clinical trial design. Crit Care Med 2002; 30:S341–S348.
69. Chinnaiyan AM, Huber-Lang M, Kumar-Sinha C, et al. Molecular signatures of sepsis: multiorgan gene expression profiles of systemic inflammation. Am J Pathol 2001; 159:1199–1209.
70. Kato-Maeda M, Gao Q, Small PM. Microarray analysis of pathogens and their interaction with hosts. Cell Microbiol 2001; 3:713–719.
71. Huang Q, Liu D, Majewski P, et al. The plasticity of dendritic cell responses to pathogens and their components. Science 2001; 294:870–875.
72. Borst P, Elferink RO. Mammalian ABC transporters in health and disease. Annu Rev Biochem 2002; 71:537–592.
73. Dresser GK, Spence JD, Bailey DG. Pharmacokinetic-pharmacodynamic consequences and clinical relevance of cytochrome P450 3A4 inhibition. Clin Pharmacokinet 2000; 38:41–57.
74. Inui KI, Masuda S, Saito H. Cellular and molecular aspects of drug transport in the kidney. Kidney Int 2000; 58:944–958.
75. Kerb R, Hoffmeyer S, Brinkmann U. ABC drug transporters: hereditary polymorphisms and pharmacological impact in MDR1, MRP1 and MRP2. Pharmacogenomics 2001; 2:51–64.

76. Koepsell H. Organic cation transporters in intestine, kidney, liver, and brain. Annu Rev Physiol 1998; 60:243–266.
77. Kullak-Ublick GA, Ismair MG, Stieger B, et al. Organic anion-transporting polypeptide B (OATP-B) and its functional comparison with three other OATPs of human liver. Gastroenterology 2001; 120:525–533.
78. Meier PJ, Stieger B. Bile salt transporters. Annu Rev Physiol 2002; 64:635–661.
79. Ayrton A, Morgan P. Role of transport proteins in drug absorption, distribution and excretion. Xenobiotica 2001; 31:469–497.
80. Saitoh H, Fujisaki H, Aungst BJ, Miyazaki K. Restricted intestinal absorption of some beta-lactam antibiotics by an energy-dependent efflux system in rat intestine. Pharm Res 1997; 14:645–649.
81. Cavet ME, West M, Simmons NL. Transepithelial transport of the fluoroquinolone ciprofloxacin by human airway epithelial Calu-3 cells. Antimicrob Agents Chemother 1997; 41:2693–2698.
82. Saitoh H, Gerard C, Aungst BJ. The secretory intestinal transport of some beta-lactam antibiotics and anionic compounds: a mechanism contributing to poor oral absorption. J Pharmacol Exp Ther 1996; 278:205–211.
83. Cao CX, Silverstein SC, Neu HC, Steinberg TH. J774 macrophages secrete antibiotics via organic anion transporters. J Infect Dis 1992; 165:322–328.
84. Rudin DE, Gao PX, Cao CX, Neu HC, Silverstein SC. Gemfibrozil enhances the listeriacidal effects of fluoroquinolone antibiotics in J774 macrophages. J Exp Med 1992; 176:1439–1447.
85. Nichterlein T, Kretschmar M, Schadt A, et al. Reduced intracellular activity of antibiotics against Listeria monocytogenes in multidrug resistant cells. Int J Antimicrob Agents 1998; 10:119–125.
86. Hitzl M, Drescher S, van der KH, et al. The C3435T mutation in the human MDR1 gene is associated with altered efflux of the P-glycoprotein substrate rhodamine 123 from CD56+ natural killer cells. Pharmacogenetics 2001; 11:293–298.
87. Schultz MJ, Wijnholds J, Peppelenbosch MP, et al. Mice lacking the multidrug resistance protein 1 are resistant to Streptococcus pneumoniae-induced pneumonia. J Immunol 2001; 166:4059–4064.
88. Schinkel AH. Pharmacological insights from P-glycoprotein knockout mice. Int J Clin Pharmacol Ther 1998; 36:9–13.
89. Jonker JW, Wagenaar E, Mol CA, et al. Reduced hepatic uptake and intestinal excretion of organic cations in mice with a targeted disruption of the organic cation transporter 1 (Oct1 [Slc22a1]) gene. Mol Cell Biol 2001; 21:5471–5477.
90. Lowes S, Simmons NL. Multiple pathways for fluoroquinolone secretion by human intestinal epithelial (Caco-2) cells. Br J Pharmacol 2002; 135:1263–1275.
91. Ruiz-GarcIa A, Lin H, Pl ADJM, Hu M. Kinetic characterization of secretory transport of a new ciprofloxacin derivative (CNV97100) across Caco-2 cell monolayers. J Pharm Sci 2002; 91:2511–2519.
92. Terashi K, Oka M, Soda H, et al. Interactions of ofloxacin and erythromycin with the multidrug resistance protein (MRP) in MRP-overexpressing human leukemia cells. Antimicrob Agents Chemother 2000; 44:1697–1700.
93. Huisman MT, Smit JW, Schinkel AH. Significance of P-glycoprotein for the pharmacology and clinical use of HIV protease inhibitors [Review]. AIDS 2000; 14:237–242.
94. Scheffer GL, Kool M, Heijn M, et al. Specific detection of multidrug resistance proteins MRP1, MRP2, MRP3, MRP5, and MDR3 P-glycoprotein with a panel of monoclonal antibodies. Cancer Res 2000; 60:5269–5277.
95. Meaden ER, Hoggard PG, Newton P, et al. P-glycoprotein and MRP1 expression and reduced ritonavir and saquinavir accumulation in HIV-infected individuals. J Antimicrob Chemother 2002; 50:583–588.
96. Meaden ER, Hoggard PG, Maher B, Khoo SH, Back DJ. Expression of P-glycoprotein and multidrug resistance-associated protein in healthy volunteers and HIV-infected patients. AIDS Res Hum Retroviruses 2001; 17:1329–1332.

97. Hinoshita E, Taguchi K, Inokuchi A, et al. Decreased expression of an ATP-binding cassette transporter, MRP2, in human livers with hepatitis C virus infection. J Hepatol 2001; 35:765–773.
98. Bode KA, Donner MG, Leier I, Keppler D. Inhibition of transport across the hepatocyte canalicular membrane by the antibiotic fusidate. Biochem Pharmacol 2002; 64:151–158.
99. Verbon A, Leemans JC, Weijer S, Florquin S, Van Der Poll T. Mice lacking the multidrug resistance protein 1 have a transiently impaired immune response during tuberculosis. Clin Exp Immunol 2002; 130:32–36.
100. Speck RR, Yu XF, Hildreth J, Flexner C. Differential effects of p-glycoprotein and multidrug resistance protein-1 on productive human immunodeficiency virus infection. J Infect Dis 2002; 186:332–340.
101. Klokouzas A, Barrand MA, Hladky SB. Effects of clotrimazole on transport mediated by multidrug resistance associated protein 1 (MRP1) in human erythrocytes and tumour cells. Eur J Biochem 2001; 268:6569–6577.
102. Wijnholds J, Evers R, van Leusden MR, et al. Increased sensitivity to anticancer drugs and decreased inflammatory response in mice lacking the multidrug resistance-associated protein. Nat Med 1997; 3:1275–1279.
103. Ito S, Ieiri I, Tanabe M, et al. Polymorphism of the ABC transporter genes, MDR1, MRP1 and MRP2/cMOAT, in healthy Japanese subjects. Pharmacogenetics 2001; 11:175–184.
104. Saito S, Iida A, Sekine A, et al. Identification of 779 genetic variations in eight genes encoding members of the ATP-binding cassette, subfamily C (ABCC/MRP/CFTR). J Hum Genet 2002; 47:147–171.
105. Itoda M, Saito Y, Soyama A, et al. Polymorphisms in the ABCC2 (cMOAT/MRP2) gene found in 72 established cell lines derived from Japanese individuals: an association between single nucleotide polymorphisms in the 5′-untranslated region and exon 28. Drug Metab Dispos 2002; 30:363–364.
106. Moriya Y, Nakamura T, Horinouchi M, et al. Effects of polymorphisms of MDR1, MRP1, and MRP2 genes on their mRNA expression levels in duodenal enterocytes of healthy Japanese subjects. Biol Pharm Bull 2002; 25:1356–1359.
107. Conrad S, Kauffmann HM, Ito K, et al. Identification of human multidrug resistance protein 1 (MRP1) mutations and characterization of a G671V substitution. J Hum Genet 2001; 46:656–663.
108. Conrad S, Kauffmann HM, Ito K, et al. A naturally occurring mutation in MRP1 results in a selective decrease in organic anion transport and in increased doxorubicin resistance. Pharmacogenetics 2002; 12:321–330.
109. Konig J, Nies AT, Cui Y, Leier I, Keppler D. Conjugate export pumps of the multidrug resistance protein (MRP) family: localization, substrate specificity, and MRP2-mediated drug resistance. Biochim Biophys Acta 1999; 1461:377–394.
110. Keitel V, Nies AT, Brom M, et al. A common Dubin-Johnson syndrome mutation impairs protein maturation and transport activity of MRP2 (ABCC2). Am J Physiol Gastrointest Liver Physiol 2002; 2:2.
111. Keitel V, Kartenbeck J, Nies AT, et al. Impaired protein maturation of the conjugate export pump multidrug resistance protein 2 as a consequence of a deletion mutation in Dubin-Johnson syndrome. Hepatology 2000; 32:1317–1328.
112. Mor-Cohen R, Zivelin A, Rosenberg N, et al. Identification and functional analysis of two novel mutations in the multidrug resistance protein 2 gene in Israeli patients with Dubin-Johnson syndrome. J Biol Chem 2001; 276:36923–36930.
113. Tsujii H, Konig J, Rost D, et al. Exon-intron organization of the human multidrug-resistance protein 2 (MRP2) gene mutated in Dubin-Johnson syndrome. Gastroenterology 1999; 117:653–660.
114. Chen ZS, Lee K, Walther S, et al. Analysis of methotrexate and folate transport by multidrug resistance protein 4 (ABCC4): MRP4 is a component of the methotrexate efflux system. Cancer Res 2002; 62:3144–3150.
115. Chen ZS, Lee K, Kruh GD. Transport of cyclic nucleotides and estradiol 17-beta-D-glucuronide by multidrug resistance protein 4. Resistance to 6-mercaptopurine and 6- thioguanine. J Biol Chem 2001; 276:33747–33754.

116. Schuetz JD, Connelly MC, Sun D, et al. MRP4: A previously unidentified factor in resistance to nucleoside-based antiviral drugs. Nat Med 1999; 5:1048–1051.
117. Wijnholds J, Mol CA, van Deemter L, et al. Multidrug-resistance protein 5 is a multispecific organic anion transporter able to transport nucleotide analogs. Proc Natl Acad Sci USA 2000; 97:7476–7481.
118. Lee K, Klein-Szanto AJ, Kruh GD. Analysis of the MRP4 drug resistance profile in transfected NIH3T3 cells. J Natl Cancer Inst 2000; 92:1934–1940.
119. Sekine T, Cha SH, Endou H. The multispecific organic anion transporter (OAT) family. Pflugers Arch 2000; 440:337–350.
120. Takeda M, Khamdang S, Narikawa S, et al. Characterization of methotrexate transport and its drug interactions with human organic anion transporters. J Pharmacol Exp Ther 2002; 302:666–671.
121. Ho ES, Lin DC, Mendel DB, Cihlar T. Cytotoxicity of antiviral nucleotides adefovir and cidofovir is induced by the expression of human renal organic anion transporter 1. J Am Soc Nephrol 2000; 11:383–393.
122. Kerb R, Brinkmann U, Chatskaia N, et al. Identification of genetic variations of the human organic cation transporter hOCT1 and their functional consequences. Pharmacogenetics 2002; 12:591–595.
123. Zhang L, Gorset W, Washington CB, et al. Interactions of HIV protease inhibitors with a human organic cation transporter in a mammalian expression system. Drug Metab Dispos 2000; 28:329–334.
124. van Montfoort JE, Müller M, Groothuis GM, et al. Comparison of "type I" and "type II" organic cation transport by organic cation transporters and organic anion-transporting polypeptides. J Pharmacol Exp Ther 2001; 298:110–115.
125. Dresser MJ, Leabman MK, Giacomini KM. Transporters involved in the elimination of drugs in the kidney: organic anion transporters and organic cation transporters. J Pharm Sci 2001; 90:397–421.
126. Gorboulev V, Ulzheimer JC, Akhoundova A, et al. Cloning and characterization of two human polyspecific organic cation transporters. DNA Cell Biol 1997; 16:871–881.
127. Leabman MK, Huang CC, Kawamoto M, et al. Polymorphisms in a human kidney xenobiotic transporter, OCT2, exhibit altered function. Pharmacogenetics 2002; 12:395–405.
128. Cui Y, Konig J, Keppler D. Vectorial transport by double-transfected cells expressing the human uptake transporter SLC21A8 and the apical export pump ABCC2. Mol Pharmacol 2001; 60:934–943.
129. Tamai I, Nezu J, Uchino H, et al. Molecular identification and characterization of novel members of the human organic anion transporter (OATP) family. Biochem Biophys Res Commun 2000; 273:251–260.
130. Vavricka SR, Van Montfoort J, Ha HR, Meier PJ, Fattinger K. Interactions of rifamycin SV and rifampicin with organic anion uptake systems of human liver. Hepatology 2002; 36:164–172.
131. Tirona RG, Leake BF, Merino G, Kim RB. Polymorphisms in OATP-C: identification of multiple allelic variants associated with altered transport activity among European- and African-Americans. J Biol Chem 2001; 276:35669–35675.
132. Nozawa T, Nakajima M, Tamai I, et al. Genetic polymorphisms of human organic anion transporters OATP-C (SLC21A6) and OATP-B (SLC21A9): allele frequencies in the Japanese population and functional analysis. J Pharmacol Exp Ther 2002; 302:804–813.
133. Michalski C, Cui Y, Nies AT, et al. A naturally occurring mutation in the SLC21A6 gene causing impaired membrane localization of the hepatocyte uptake transporter. J Biol Chem 2002; 277:43058–43063.
134. Tono T, Kiyomizu K, Matsuda K, et al. Different clinical characteristics of aminoglycoside-induced profound deafness with and without the 1555 A–>G mitochondrial mutation. ORL J Otorhinolaryngol Relat Spec 2001; 63:25–30.
135. Casano RA, Johnson DF, Bykhovskaya Y, et al. Inherited susceptibility to aminoglycoside ototoxicity: genetic heterogeneity and clinical implications. Am J Otolaryngol 1999; 20:151–156.

136. Hu DN, Qui WQ, Wu BT, et al. Genetic aspects of antibiotic induced deafness: mitochondrial inheritance. J Med Genet 1991; 28:79–83.
137. Usami S, Abe S, Shinkawa H, Kimberling WJ. Sensorineural hearing loss caused by mitochondrial DNA mutations: special reference to the A1555G mutation. J Commun Disord 1998; 31:423–434.
138. Fischel-Ghodsian N. Genetic factors in aminoglycoside toxicity. Ann NY Acad Sci 1999; 884:99–109.
139. Hutchin T. Sensorineural hearing loss and the 1555G mitochondrial DNA mutation. Acta Otolaryngol 1999; 119:48–52.
140. Yoshida M, Shintani T, Hirao M, et al. Aminoglycoside-induced hearing loss in a patient with the 961 mutation in mitochondrial DNA. ORL J Otorhinolaryngol Relat Spec 2002; 64:219–222.
141. Hutchin T, Haworth I, Higashi K, et al. A molecular basis for human hypersensitivity to aminoglycoside antibiotics. Nucleic Acids Res 1993; 21:4174–4179.
142. Hamasaki K, Rando RR. Specific binding of aminoglycosides to a human rRNA construct based on a DNA polymorphism which causes aminoglycoside-induced deafness. Biochemistry 1997; 36:12323–12328.
143. Guan MX, Fischel-Ghodsian N, Attardi G. A biochemical basis for the inherited susceptibility to aminoglycoside ototoxicity. Hum Mol Genet 2000; 9:1787–1793.
144. Furuta T, Shirai N, Xiao F, Ohashi K, Ishizaki T. Effect of high-dose lansoprazole on intragastic pH in subjects who are homozygous extensive metabolizers of cytochrome P4502C19. Clin Pharmacol Ther 2001; 70:484–492.
145. Furuta T, Shirai N, Takashima M, et al. Effects of genotypic differences in CYP2C19 status on cure rates for Helicobacter pylori infection by dual therapy with rabeprazole plus amoxicillin. Pharmacogenetics 2001; 11:341–348.
146. Furuta T, Shirai N, Watanabe F, et al. Effect of cytochrome P4502C19 genotypic differences on cure rates for gastroesophageal reflux disease by lansoprazole. Clin Pharmacol Ther 2002; 72:453–460.
147. Miyoshi M, Mizuno M, Ishiki K, et al. A randomized open trial for comparison of proton pump inhibitors, omeprazole versus rabeprazole, in dual therapy for Helicobacter pylori infection in relation to CYP2C19 genetic polymorphism. J Gastroenterol Hepatol 2001; 16:723–728.
148. Hokari K, Sugiyama T, Kato M, et al. Efficacy of triple therapy with rabeprazole for Helicobacter pylori infection and CYP2C19 genetic polymorphism. Aliment Pharmacol Ther 2001; 15:1479–1484.
149. Dojo M, Azuma T, Saito T, et al. Effects of CYP2C19 gene polymorphism on cure rates for Helicobacter pylori infection by triple therapy with proton pump inhibitor (omeprazole or rabeprazole), amoxycillin and clarithromycin in Japan. Dig Liver Dis 2001; 33: 671–675.
150. Inaba T, Mizuno M, Kawai K, et al. Randomized open trial for comparison of proton pump inhibitors in triple therapy for Helicobacter pylori infection in relation to CYP2C19 genotype. J Gastroenterol Hepatol 2002; 17:748–753.
151. Desta Z, Zhao X, Shin JG, Flockhart DA. Clinical significance of the cytochrome P450 2C19 genetic polymorphism. Clin Pharmacokinet 2002; 41:913–958.
152. Kerremans AL, Lipsky JJ, Van Loon J, Gallego MO, Weinshilboum RM. Cephalosporin-induced hypoprothrombinemia: possible role for thiol methylation of 1-methyltetrazole-5-thiol and 2-methyl-1,3,4-thiadiazole-5-thiol. J Pharmacol Exp Ther 1985; 235: 382–388.
153. Lipsky JJ. Antibiotic-associated hypoprothrombinaemia. J Antimicrob Chemother 1988; 21:281–300.
154. Suttie JW. The vitamin K-dependent carboxylation of glutamyl residues in a prothrombin precursor. World Rev Nutr Diet 1978; 31:196–201.
155. Lipsky JJ, Lewis JC, Novick WJ Jr. Production of hypoprothrombinemia by moxalactam and 1-methyl-5-thiotetrazole in rats. Antimicrob Agents Chemother 1984; 25:380–381.

156. Wood TC, Johnson KL, Naylor S, Weinshilboum RM. Cefazolin administration and 2-methyl-1,3,4-thiadiazole-5-thiol in human tissue: possible relationship to hypoprothrombinemia. Drug Metab Dispos 2002; 30:1123–1128.
157. Weinshilboum RM, Sladek SL. Mercaptopurine pharmacogenetics: monogenic inheritance of erythrocyte thiopurine methyltransferase activity. Am J Hum Genet 1980; 32:651–662.
158. McLeod HL, Lin JS, Scott EP, Pui CH, Evans WE. Thiopurine methyltransferase activity in American white subjects and black subjects. Clin Pharmacol Ther 1994; 55:15–20.
159. Otterness D, Szumlanski C, Lennard L, et al. Human thiopurine methyltransferase pharmacogenetics: gene sequence polymorphisms. Clin Pharmacol Ther 1997; 62:60–73.
160. Yates CR, Krynetski EY, Loennechen T, et al. Molecular diagnosis of thiopurine S-methyltransferase deficiency: genetic basis for azathioprine and mercaptopurine intolerance. Ann Intern Med 1997; 126:608–614.
161. Tai HL, Krynetski EY, Schuetz EG, Yanishevski Y, Evans WE. Enhanced proteolysis of thiopurine S-methyltransferase (TPMT) encoded by mutant alleles in humans (TPMT*3A, TPMT*2): mechanisms for the genetic polymorphism of TPMT activity. Proc Natl Acad Sci USA 1997; 94:6444–6449.
162. Otterness DM, Szumlanski CL, Wood TC, Weinshilboum RM. Human thiopurine methyltransferase pharmacogenetics. Kindred with a terminal exon splice junction mutation that results in loss of activity. J Clin Invest 1998; 101:1036–1044.
163. Weinshilboum RM, Otterness DM, Szumlanski CL. Methylation pharmacogenetics: catechol O-methyltransferase, thiopurine methyltransferase, and histamine N-methyltransferase. Annu Rev Pharmacol Toxicol 1999; 39:19–52.
164. von Greyerz S, Zanni MP, Frutig K, et al. Interaction of sulfonamide derivatives with the TCR of sulfamethoxazole-specific human alpha beta+ T cell clones. J Immunol 1999; 162:595–602.
165. Pichler WJ. Predictive drug allergy testing: an alternative viewpoint. Toxicology 2001; 158:31–41.
166. Pellicano R, Lomuto M, Ciavarella G, Di Giorgio G, Gasparini P. Fixed drug eruptions with feprazone are linked to HLA-B22. J Am Acad Dermatol 1997; 36:782–784.
167. Elmets CA, Athar M, Tubesing KA, et al. Susceptibility to the biological effects of polyaromatic hydrocarbons is influenced by genes of the major histocompatibility complex. Proc Natl Acad Sci USA 1998; 95:14915–14919.
168. Quiralte J, Sanchez-Garcia F, Torres MJ, et al. Association of HLA-DR11 with the anaphylactoid reaction caused by nonsteroidal anti-inflammatory drugs. J Allergy Clin Immunol 1999; 103:685–689.
169. Ozkaya-Bayazit E, Akar U. Fixed drug eruption induced by trimethoprim-sulfamethoxazole: evidence for a link to HLA-A30 B13 Cw6 haplotype. J Am Acad Dermatol 2001; 45:712–717.
170. Mallal SA, John M, Moore CB, James IR, McKinnon EJ. Contribution of nucleoside analogue reverse transcriptase inhibitors to subcutanous fat wasting in patients with HIV infection. AIDS 2000; 14:1309–1316.
171. Hetherington S, Hughes AR, Mosteller M, et al. Genetic variations in HLA-B region and hypersensitivity reactions to abacavir. Lancet 2002; 359:1121–1122.
172. Desombere I, Van der WM, Van Damme P, et al. Immune response of HLA DQ2 positive subjects, vaccinated with HBsAg/AS04, a hepatitis B vaccine with a novel adjuvant. Vaccine 2002; 20:2597–2602.
173. Alper CA, Kruskall MS, Marcus-Bagley D, et al. Genetic prediction of nonresponse to hepatitis B vaccine. N Engl J Med 1989; 321:708–712.
174. Desombere I, Willems A, Leroux-Roels G. Response to hepatitis B vaccine: multiple HLA genes are involved. Tissue Antigens 1998; 51:593–604.
175. Martinetti M, De Silvestri A, Belloni C, et al. Humoral response to recombinant hepatitis B virus vaccine at birth: role of HLA and beyond. Clin Immunol 2000; 97:234–240.
176. Craven DE, Awdeh ZL, Kunches LM, et al. Nonresponsiveness to hepatitis B vaccine in health care workers. Results of revaccination and genetic typings. Ann Intern Med 1986; 105:356–360.

177. McDermott AB, Zuckerman JN, Sabin CA, Marsh SG, Madrigal JA. Contribution of human leukocyte antigens to the antibody response to hepatitis B vaccination. Tissue Antigens 1997; 50:8–14.
178. Zuckerman JN, Sabin C, Craig FM, Williams A, Zuckerman AJ. Immune response to a new hepatitis B vaccine in healthcare workers who had not responded to standard vaccine: randomised double blind dose-response study. BMJ 1997; 314:329–333.
179. McDermott AB, Cohen SB, Zuckerman JN, Madrigal JA. Human leukocyte antigens influence the immune response to a pre-S/S hepatitis B vaccine. Vaccine 1999; 17:330–339.
180. Murphy MP, Beaman ME, Clark LS, et al. Prospective CYP2D6 genotyping as an exclusion criterion for enrollment of a phase III clinical trial. Pharmacogenetics 2000; 10:583–590.
181. Tribut O, Lessard Y, Reymann JM, Allain H, Bentue-Ferrer D. Pharmacogenomics. Med Sci Monit 2002; 8:RA152–RA163.
182. Ledergerber B, Egger M, Opravil M, et al. Highly active antiretroviral therapy: low rates of clinical disease progression despite high rates of virological failure. Lancet 1999; 353:863–868.
183. Norton RM. Clinical pharmacogenomics: applications in pharmaceutical R&D. Drug Discov Today 2001; 6:180–185.
184. Dietrich CG, Geier A, Matern S, Gartung C. Multidrug resistance and response to antiretroviral treatment. Lancet 2002; 359:2114–2115.
185. Kwiatkowski D. Science, medicine, and the future: susceptibility to infection. BMJ 2000; 321:1061–1065.
186. Cooke GS, Hill AV. Genetics of susceptibility to human infectious disease. Nat Rev Genet 2001; 2:967–977.
187. Nakamura T, Sakaeda T, Horinouchi M, et al. Effect of the mutation (C3435T) at exon 26 of the MDR1 gene on expression level of MDR1 messenger ribonucleic acid in duodenal enterocytes of healthy Japanese subjects. Clin Pharmacol Ther 2002; 71:297–303.
188. Kim RB, Leake BF, Choo EF, et al. Identification of functionally variant MDR1 alleles among European Americans and African Americans. Clin Pharmacol Ther 2001; 70:189–199.
189. Drescher S, Schaeffeler E, Hitzl M, et al. MDR1 gene polymorphisms and disposition of the P-glycoprotein substrate fexofenadine. Br J Clin Pharmacol 2002; 53:526–534.
190. von Ahsen N, Richter M, Grupp C, et al. No influence of the MDR-1 C3435T polymorphism or a CYP3A4 promoter polymorphism (CYP3A4-V allele) on dose-adjusted cyclosporin A trough concentrations or rejection incidence in stable renal transplant recipients. Clin Chem 2001; 47:1048–1052.
191. Min DI, Ellingrod VL. C3435T mutation in exon 26 of the human MDR1 gene and cyclosporine pharmacokinetics in healthy subjects. Ther Drug Monit 2002; 24:400–404.
192. Tanabe M, Ieiri I, Nagata N, et al. Expression of P-glycoprotein in human placenta: relation to genetic polymorphism of the multidrug resistance (MDR)-1 gene. J Pharmacol Exp Ther 2001; 297:1137–1143.
193. Roberts RL, Joyce PR, Mulder RT, Begg EJ, Kennedy MA. A common P-glycoprotein polymorphism is associated with nortriptyline-induced postural hypotension in patients treated for major depression. Pharmacogenomics J 2002; 2:191–196.
194. Kimchi-Sarfaty C, Gribar JJ, Gottesman MM. Functional characterization of coding polymorphisms in the human MDR1 gene using a vaccinia virus expression system. Mol Pharmacol 2002; 62:1–6.
195. Johne A, Kopke K, Gerloff T, et al. Modulation of steady-state kinetics of digoxin by haplotypes of the P- glycoprotein MDR1 gene. Clin Pharmacol Ther 2002; 72:584–594.
196. Kurata Y, Ieiri I, Kimura M, et al. Role of human MDR1 gene polymorphism in bioavailability and interaction of digoxin, a substrate of P-glycoprotein. Clin Pharmacol Ther 2002; 72:209–219.

10
Pharmacogenetics in Rheumatology

Samantha L. Hider, Catharine Morgan, Wendy Thomson, and Ian N. Bruce
arc Epidemiology Unit, University of Manchester, Manchester, U.K.

INTRODUCTION

Within rheumatic diseases, the therapeutic armamentarium has traditionally been limited to a relatively small number of drugs. When considering drugs used in rheumatology, it is useful to consider the therapeutic paradigm for rheumatoid arthritis (RA). RA is the most prevalent of the inflammatory rheumatic diseases encountered and therefore is a key example to consider. In this chapter, we briefly review the current therapies used in RA and consider their relative efficacy and toxicity. Evidence for the genetic basis underlying these outcomes is then reviewed, and areas of future research are highlighted.

THERAPEUTIC OPTIONS IN THE TREATMENT OF RHEUMATOID ARTHRITIS

RA is a chronic inflammatory disease of the joints that affects approximately 1% of the general population. It is characterized by swelling, stiffness, and pain in multiple joints, and particularly, symmetrical involvement of the small joints of the hands and feet. RA is a significant cause of disability, and the majority of patients experience progressive joint destruction, deformity, and functional decline over a 10- to 15-year period (1). The basic aim of RA management is to reduce pain, improve function, and prevent or retard long-term disease progression. The major groups of therapeutic agents used are summarized in Table 1. Symptomatic agents include simple analgesia and nonsteroidal anti-inflammatory drugs (NSAIDs). These drugs reduce pain and may improve function but do not fundamentally alter the underlying course of the disease. The second major class of agents are the disease-modifying antirheumatic drugs (DMARDs). This group of drugs usually takes several weeks or months to realize their full effect. They not only cause reduction in pain and swelling but, more importantly, also retard the rate of joint erosion, thus modulating the disease course. Corticosteroids are also frequently

Table 1 Classification of Drugs Commonly Used in the Treatment of Rheumatoid Arthritis

Drug group	Examples
Simple analgesia	Paracetamol, codeine
NSAIDs	Ibuprofen, diclofenac, celecoxib, rofecoxib
Corticosteroids	Prednisolone, prednisone, deflazocort
DMARDs	MTX, sulfasalazine, gold, sodium aurothiomalate, D-penicillamine, hydroxychloroquine, AZA, leflunomide
Biologic drugs[a]	Anti-TNF-α drugs: infliximab, etanercept, adalimumab; IL-1 receptor antagonists: anakinra

[a]Some are classified as disease-controlling antirheumatic drugs (DCARTs).
Abbreviations: NSAIDs, nonsteroidal anti-inflammatory drugs; DMARDs, disease-modifying antirheumatic drugs; TNF-α, tumor necrosis factor-α; IL-1, interleukin-1; MTX, methotrexate; AZA, azathioprine.

used in the management of RA. These drugs are anti-inflammatory and are employed as symptomatic agents. There is evidence, however, to support a disease-modifying role for corticosteroids in RA (2,3). More recently, biologic agents have been introduced for the treatment of RA (4,5). These drugs are specifically designed to block key mediators of the RA inflammatory pathway (6). They have considerable potential to retard the disease process, and the term "disease-controlling antirheumatic therapy (DCART)" has been coined to reflect the fact that certain of these biologic agents may halt further joint destruction in a majority of patients.

EFFICACY AND TOXICITY OF ANTIRHEUMATIC THERAPIES

There is evidence to support the efficacy of DMARDs in RA. These drugs are superior to placebo in reducing signs of inflammation and improving function (7). There is, however, variability in the response to these agents, and different drugs display different levels of efficacy. In general, drugs such as sulfasalazine and methotrexate (MTX) have been found to be more efficacious than such agents as auranofin and hydroxychloroquine (7). Recently, studies have employed more standardized measures of response. One such measure is the American College of Rheumatology 20% response criteria (ACR 20). This level of "response" is generally accepted as the minimum difference that is clinically noticeable by a patient (8). In randomized trials, an ACR 20 response is achieved by 45% to 65% of patients treated with sulfasalazine, MTX, and leflunomide (9–11). There are, therefore, a considerable number of patients who will fail to respond in a clinically important manner to any single agent. As a result of the limited efficacy of monotherapy, combinations of traditional DMARDs are increasingly being employed in the management of RA. Such combinations appear to have superior efficacy to individual monotherapy (3,12,13). The other approach to improving therapeutic responses has been to introduce biologic agents. Although these agents have a more specific mode of action, they are nevertheless not universally effective. Several trials of antitumor necrosis factor-alpha (TNF-α) agents have shown that 50% to 60% of the patients will achieve an ACR 20 response (4,5). Similarly 43% of the patients treated with anakinra, an interleukin-1 receptor antagonist (IL-1ra), achieved an ACR 20 response (14).

In addition to issues of limited efficacy, disease-modifying drugs are also associated with a significant range of adverse events, which again limit their use. In general, certain drugs have poor long-term tolerability, for example, the use of intramuscular gold salts and D-penicillamine (D-Pa) is often limited by the occurrence of rash and proteinuria. In long-term follow-up, "survival" on a particular drug is therefore limited by either lack of efficacy and/or adverse events. Pincus et al. found in a five-year follow-up study that 60% of the patients will remain on MTX over this time period. In contrast, <30% remained on D-Pa or oral gold, both being frequently stopped due to inefficacy and/or toxicity (15). Morgan et al. (16) have also noted similar trends. This study found that antimalarials were frequently stopped due to inefficacy, whereas 54% of the patients stopped IM gold salts due to toxicity. There were significant differences between different DMARDs in the proportion of courses ending in inefficacy. Interestingly, it was also noted that there were significant differences *between subjects* for the probability of failure on a particular drug. Overall, 35% of the variance of the probability of failure was due to these *between subject* differences. Although compliance and differences in inflammatory mechanisms between individual patients are likely to be important, individual variability in the metabolic pathways associated with each drug are also hypothesized to be important. Genetic variability in the absorption and handling of these agents is one aspect that might significantly influence the likelihood of response or toxicity. We will now consider several individual drugs and evidence for the influence of such genetic variability on the efficacy and safety of antirheumatic therapies.

NONSTEROIDAL ANTI-INFLAMMATORY DRUGS

Nonsteroidal anti-inflammatory drugs (NSAIDs) are symptomatic agents used in many rheumatic conditions, including RA. They have analgesic and also anti-inflammatory properties and are effective in the relief of inflammatory symptoms and signs, such as joint stiffness, swelling, and tenderness. They also have a widening range of uses outside of rheumatology: for example, these agents are used for dysmenorrhoea, renal colic, and postoperative pain. In contrast to many of the drugs that will be reviewed later, NSAIDs do not fundamentally alter the underlying course of such diseases as RA. A large number of NSAIDs are currently available and these agents are derivatives of different acidic compounds, such as salicylic acid, acetic acid, and propionic acid (17). As a result of their variable chemical structure, there is significant variability in many of the pharmacokinetic properties of NSAIDs. For example, the elimination of naproxen and ketoprofen is significantly reduced by renal impairment, whereas sulindac and piroxicam are less influenced by renal impairment (17).

Despite variability in their chemical structure and pharmacokinetics, NSAIDs mediate their principal anti-inflammatory effects by inhibiting the cyclo-oxygenase (*COX*) enzyme system. This is a key enzyme in the production of proinflammatory prostaglandins from phospholipids and arachadonic acid (Fig. 1). Recently, it has been noted that there are two distinct forms of the COX enzyme. COX-1 is a constitutive enzyme, which is important in the production of prostaglandins for physiological purposes, such as maintenance of the acid barrier in the stomach and also in the control of renal blood flow and sodium excretion. COX-2, in contrast, is an inducible enzyme, production of which is upregulated by proinflammatory cytokines, such as IL-1 and TNF-α (17). The production of prostaglandins by this mechanism is increased at sites of inflammation,

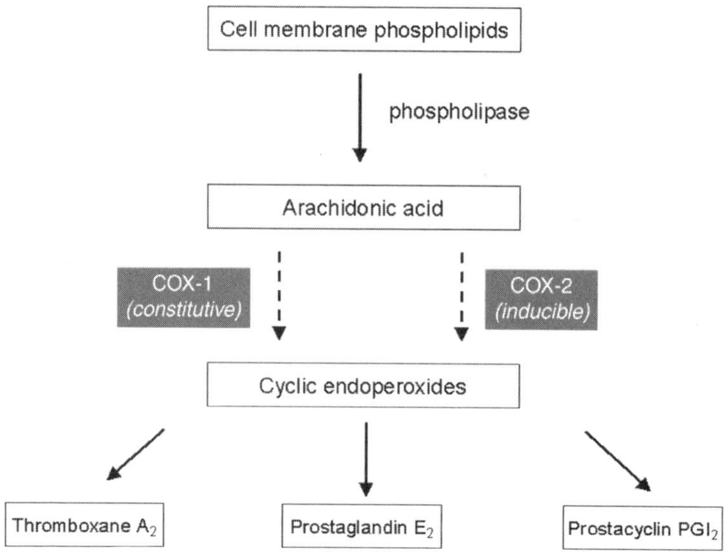

Figure 1 Summary of prostaglandin synthetic pathway and the role of COX enzymes. The COX-1 and COX-2 enzymes (*gray boxs*) are inhibited to a variable degree by most NSAIDs. *Abbreviations*: COX, cyclo-oxygenase; NSAIDs, nonsteroidal anti-inflammatory drugs.

such as the rheumatoid synovium. In recent years, several new NSAIDs have been developed, which selectively or specifically inhibit the inducible COX-2 enzyme. These agents are associated with a reduced risk of certain complications, particularly peptic ulceration and its consequences (18,19).

Pharmacogenetics of NSAIDs

There have been several studies exploring how genetic variability in pathways of relevance to NSAID metabolism and action may influence drug kinetics and/or the incidence of adverse effects. Recently, Kirchheiner et al. studied genetic variability of the cytochrome P450 (CYP) 2C9 enzyme and their influence on ibuprofen metabolism. *CYP2C9* polymorphisms were identified, and subjects with various combinations of the **1*, **2*, **3* genotypes were studied. Metabolism of the dextrorotatory *S*-ibuprofen was significantly reduced in subjects carrying at least one **3* allele. In subjects homozygous for the **3* allele, *S*-ibuprofen clearance was reduced by approximately 50%. These subjects also displayed more significant inhibition of COX-1 and COX-2 (20). It has therefore been hypothesized that *CYP2C9* genotypes may be associated with an increased risk of NSAID-associated adverse effects, such as upper GI haemorrhage. Although several other NSAIDs, including diclofenac and celecoxib, are also *CYP2C9* substrates, studies suggest that the *CYP2C9* genotype does not significantly affect the pharmacokinetics of either agent (21).

There is also a well-recognized risk of asthma being provoked or exacerbated in patients who use aspirin or NSAIDs. Approximately 10% to 11% of the asthmatics have been categorized as suffering from "aspirin-induced asthma" (22). The mechanism of worsening of asthma in this context appears to be mediated by alterations in eicosanoid metabolism. In particular, prostaglandin E2 (PGE2), produced by COX-1, acts to counterbalance proinflammatory leukotrienes especially cysteinyl leukotriene (Cys-LT). The addition of aspirin or other NSAIDs, which inhibit COX-1, results in rapid depletion of PGE2 and worsening of asthma and rhinitis symptoms. The enzyme, leukotriene C synthase (LTC4S) is upregulated in the bronchial mucosa of asthmatics. Patients with asthma who have an A–C transversion of nucleotide 444 in the LTC4S enzyme have increased expression of this enzyme in peripheral blood eosinophils. The *C444* allele is also observed more commonly in patients with aspirin-induced asthma, compared with the healthy controls or asthmatics who are not aspirin-sensitive (23). For a full discussion of this topic see Chapter 6.

METHOTREXATE

Pharmacology and Mechanism of Action

MTX is currently the cornerstone of drug treatment for RA. It is increasingly employed as the first DMARD used (24). It can be given orally or subcutaneously, because there is considerable variation in oral absorption (25). MTX was first used in RA and psoriatic arthritis in the early 1960s; however, the higher dose regimes used then were associated with significant and serious toxicity. As a result, it is now used in a low-dose weekly regime of 7.5–25 mg per week. MTX is taken up into cells via the reduced folate carrier and is polyglutamated. Polyglutamation prolongs the intracellular half-life (26). Although originally believed to mediate its effect by inhibition of folate metabolism, it has become increasingly clear that this is not its only mechanism of action (26,27). MTX inhibits a number of essential enzymes, such as thymidylate synthase, dihydrofolate reductase (leading to an inhibition of pyrimidine and purine metabolism), and aminoamidazole carboxamide ribonucleotide transformylase (AICAR) (Fig. 2) (28,29). This leads to release of adenosine, which inhibits leucocyte migration and, acting via the A2a and A3 receptors, has potent anti-inflammatory actions (30).

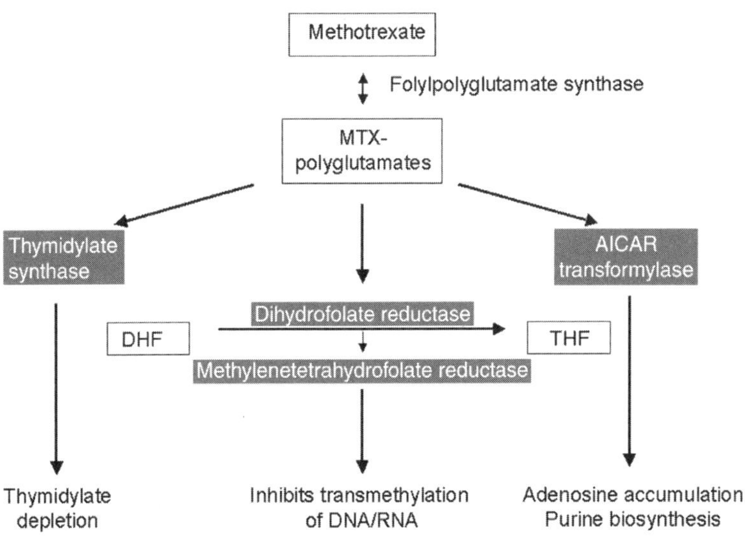

Figure 2 Overview of the mechanisms by which methotrexate mediates its anti-inflammatory effects in rheumatoid arthritis and related disorders. Key enzymes inhibited by MTX are highlighted in gray boxes. *Abbreviations*: DHF, dihydrofolate; MTX, methotrexate; THF, tehrahydrofolate; AICAR, 5-aminoimidazole-4-carboxamide ribonucleotide.

Clinically, MTX is capable of significantly reducing joint inflammation and retarding radiographic progression (31). Clinical trials confirm that ACR20 responses to low-dose MTX range from 44% to 65%, (9,10,32). In addition, MTX is relatively well tolerated, and many patients are able to remain on MTX for long periods of time. Wolfe et al. (33) found that the median time to discontinuation of MTX was 4.25 years, compared with two years for other DMARDs. Pincus et al. (15) also confirmed that over a five year period, "drug survival" times for MTX were superior to other DMARDs.

Pharmacogenetics

The effect of polymorphisms in the methylenetetrahydrofolate reductase (MTHFR) gene has been evaluated. Several polymorphisms have been identified, although two single-nucleotide polymorphisms (SNPs), *C677T* and *A1298C*, have been commonly linked to adverse drug events. The *C677T* is a common polymorphism, with mutant homozygotes representing around 8% of the Caucasian population. This polymorphism leads to an alanine $\rightarrow$ valine substitution that makes the enzyme more thermolabile; this variant has a 30% reduced enzymatic activity compared with the wild-type (29). Van Ede et al. (34) studied the *C677T* polymorphism with regard to toxicity and efficacy of MTX in 236 RA patients. They found that 48% of the patients carried at least one *T* allele and that the presence of the *C677CT* or *C677TT* genotype increased the risk of stopping MTX due to adverse events (RR 2.01, 95% CI 1.09–3.7), especially increased liver transaminases (RR 2.38, 95% CI 1.06–5.34). No difference in MTX efficacy was seen between the groups. In a Japanese cohort of 106 RA patients, Urano et al. (35) studied two polymorphisms of MTHFR, the *C677T* polymorphism and the *A1298C* polymorphism. The latter polymorphism results in a glutamine $\rightarrow$ alanine substitution and reduced enzyme activity. In this cohort, MTX toxicity was more frequent in patients with the *C677T* allele, compared with those without the *T* allele (27% vs. 8.6%, RR 1.25, $p < 0.05$). No correlation was observed between this polymorphism and treatment efficacy. In 80 patients, the *A1298C* polymorphism was also studied. Patients with the *C* allele required significantly lower doses of MTX than patients without the allele (RR 2.18, 95% CI 1.17–4.06, $p < 0.05$), and there was a trend towards improved efficacy in patients with the *C* allele, with greater improvements in the ESR and CRP. There was, however, a higher baseline ESR in the *C/C* group. No association was observed between *A1298C* polymorphism and toxicity. They concluded that the *C677T* polymorphism leads to increased toxicity, whereas *A1298C* improved efficacy of MTX. A second study, however, found no association between MTHFR *C677T* or *A1298C* genotypes and outcome of the MTX treatment in a Japanese cohort (36).

Clearly there are other potential candidate genes that may affect MTX efficacy and toxicity, including dihydrofolate reductase, thymidylate synthase, and folylpolyglutamate synthase (which mediates the polyglutamation of MTX). To date, only a single study (36) has examined the effect of polymorphisms in the thymidylate synthase gene (TYMS) and outcome of MTX treatment. Patients who were homozygous for the triple-repeat allele in the promoter region of the TYMS gene required higher doses of MTX than those carrying the double-repeat allele ($p = 0.033$), although all patients were on low doses of MTX. In addition patients who were homozygous for the deletion allele of the polymorphism in the 3′-untranslated region of the TYMS gene had a higher rate of improvement (measured by a 50% fall in the CRP level) than patients without this polymorphism ($p = 0.383$). Clearly these studies require replication, but it is likely that polymorphisms in these and other enzymes in the MTX pathway will be of importance in predicting efficacy and/or toxicity to MTX.

SULFASALAZINE

Pharmacology and Mechanism of Action

Sulfasalazine consists of sulfapyridine and 5-aminosalicylate (the active component in inflammatory bowel disease). Both components have anti-inflammatory effects (37). Sulfasalazine is highly protein-bound and undergoes *N*-acetylation in the liver before being excreted via the renal tract. The mechanism of action is unclear and may include effects on B cell, synoviocyte, and endothelial cell proliferation (37). Other mechanisms of action include reduction of cytokines, such as IL1β and TNFα (37,38). Sulfasalazine is commonly used for the treatment of RA. Recent studies comparing sulfasalazine with other DMARDs have shown efficacy comparable with leflunomide and MTX, with ACR20 responses of between 44% and 59% (10,11).

Pharmacogenetics

Studies to date have focused on the effect of acetylator status and side effects. Kitas et al. (39) found no effect of acetylator status on toxicity or efficacy. Pullar et al. (40) found that there was an increased risk of nausea and vomiting in slow acetylators but no difference in the rates of serious toxicity. Several studies have examined the effect of the *N*-acetyltransferase 2 (NAT2) polymorphism on treatment outcome. To date, at least 19 SNPs have been identified within the coding region of NAT2 (41). Tanaka et al. (42) studied a Japanese RA cohort and found that patients without the *NAT2*4* haplotype, which is associated with rapid acetylation status, had a significantly higher number of adverse events than patients with the *NAT2*4* haplotype (62.5% vs. 8.1%; OR 7.73). Sabbagh et al. (43) also found a higher rate of side effects with sulfasalazine in slow acetylators with chronic discoid lupus. However, a study by Ricart et al. (44) in ulcerative colitis patients found no association between NAT2 polymorphisms and sulfasalazine toxicity. Further studies are required to resolve these issues.

D-PENICILLAMINE

Pharmacology and Mechanism of Action

D-Penicillamine (D-Pa) is an amino acid with a thiol side-chain. The serum half-life is approximately two to four hours, although this increases to four to six days (45) in patients on long-term therapy. Its bioavailability is severely reduced if taken with food. The mechanism of action is unclear, although it is thought to act by inhibiting leucocyte myeloperoxidases and by effecting T-cell proliferation (37,45). It has also been postulated that the thiol side-chain acts as a metal chelator with subsequent effects on cell surface receptors (37). Although efficacious for the treatment of RA (45), it has been generally superseded by other DMARDs because of problems with side effects and toxicity.

Pharmacogenetics

Initial studies looked at the effect of sulfoxidation status and toxicity with D-Pa. Emery et al. (46) found a significant association with toxicity and impaired sulfoxidation status in 66 RA patients. Emery also looked at human leukocyte antigen (HLA) associations in these patients and found that HLA-DR3 was associated with toxicity independently of sulfoxidation status. Similarly, Madhok et al. (47) found in a study of 50 RA patients that those with poor sulfoxidation status were 3.9 times more likely to have an adverse event. There was no difference in the two groups in terms of clinical response to D-Pa. Layton et al. (48) investigated the effect of polymorphisms in the glutathione-*S*-transferase (GST superfamily) on therapeutic outcomes in 81 RA patients. The frequency of the *GSTM1* null allele was higher in treatment nonresponders ($n = 18$) than in responders (72.2% vs. 47.6%; OR 3.94). There was also an association between the haplotype *GSTM1*0/GSTM3*A* and poor response to D-Pa (OR 7.63).

GOLD

Pharmacology and Mechanism of Action

Gold may be prescribed either orally (auranofin) or parenterally (as aurothiomalate or aurothioglucose). Gold is highly protein-bound to albumin. Peak blood concentrations are reached after two to six hours. Plasma half-life is around seven days for a 50 mg dose (37). Again, the mechanism of action is unclear but is thought to be via effects on neutrophils and monocytes (37). Gold is considered to be as effective for RA as either sulfasalazine or MTX. It has, however, a higher rate of treatment withdrawal for side effects when compared with other drugs, such as sulfasalazine (49).

Pharmacogenetics

Early studies examined the influence of HLA type on the side effect profile. Singal et al. (50) showed an increased prevalence of *HLA-DR3* in patients with side effects from gold compared with patients without side effects, although Ten Wolde (51) and Alarcon (52) failed to replicate the association. Hakala et al. (53) suggested an increased prevalence of *HLA-B40* in patients with gold pneumonitis. Stockman et al. (54) also found an association between proteinuria and *HLA-DR3* and *HLA-B8* and thrombocytopenia with *HLA-A1* and *HLA-DR4*. Other genes within the major histocompatibility complex (MHC) have also been studied. One small study by Clarkson et al. (55) found that patients with the C4 null allele were more likely to develop side effects from either gold or D-Pa. Evans et al. (56) investigated the association between TNF microsatellite markers and gold intolerance and found that the haplotypes *TNFa5b5* and *TNFa6b5* had an increased risk of mucocutaneous side effects. These studies are suggestive of a role for gene(s) within the MHC in toxicity to gold, but this obviously requires further investigation.

AZATHIOPRINE

Pharmacology and Mechanism of Action

Azathioprine (AZA) is an immunosuppressive agent that is widely used in inflammatory rheumatic diseases, including RA, where there is evidence to support its role in suppression of disease activity (57). A typical dose for RA is 1 mg/kg/day increasing after four to six weeks to 2–3 mg/day. AZA is a prodrug, which is converted after absorption to the active agent, 6-mercaptopurine (6-MP). This is then converted by hypoxanthine-guanine phosporibosyl transferase (HGPRT) to 6-thioguanine nucleotides (6-TGNs). These play a major role in the development of cytotoxicity when incorporated into DNA and RNA (58). Two enzymes compete with HGPRT to reduce the intracellular levels of 6-TGNs. The first, xanthine oxidase, results in the formation of thiouric acid. This is an important route for the inactivation of 6-MP, and the xanthine oxidase inhibitor allopurinol significantly increases the risk of toxicity of AZA (59). Xanthine oxidase

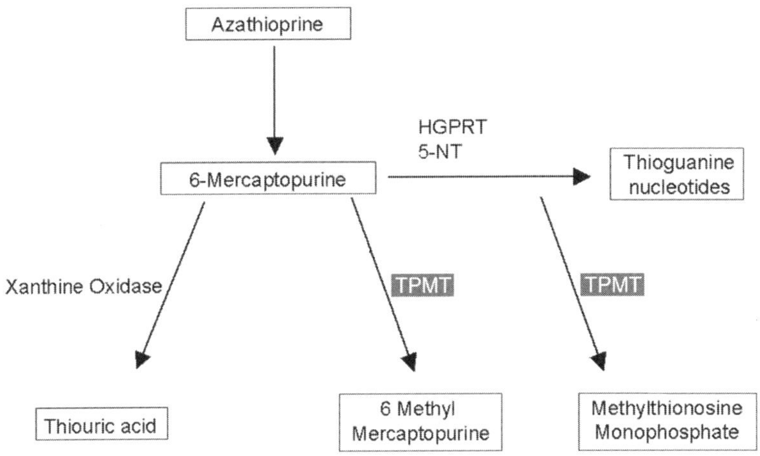

Figure 3 The metabolic pathway involved in the detoxification of azathioprine/6-MP. TPMT is a key enzyme (*gray boxes*) in which polymorphic variability can result in an increased risk of azathioprine toxicity. *Abbreviations*: HGPRT, hypoxanthine guanine phosphoribosyltransferase; MP, mercaptopurine; TPMT, thiopurine methyltransferase.

levels, however, do not appear to vary greatly between individuals. The second enzyme involved in 6-MP clearance is thiopurine methyltransferase (TPMT). TPMT inactivates 6-MP through the formation of methyl mercaptopurine (58) (Fig. 3).

Studies of TPMT in Rheumatology

Some of the variation in AZA metabolism can be accounted for by the fact that there is clear variation in TPMT enzyme activity between individuals; the genetic basis for this has been determined. The TPMT gene, localized to chromosome 6p22.3, displays at least eight polymorphisms associated with reduced enzyme activity. The nonmutant gene is designated *TPMT*1,* and mutated genes are assigned as *TPMT *2–*6*. In Caucasians the most common polymorphism associated with reduced enzyme activity is **3A* [point mutation 460 (G → A) and 719 (A → G)] (60). The isolated mutation at position 719 (**3C*) is a common cause of low activity in African populations (61,62). Approximately 89% of the white Caucasian subjects are homozygous (two wild-type alleles) for the inherited trait of high TPMT activity. Eleven percent are heterozygous (one wild type and one variant allele) and have intermediate TPMT activity, while approximately 0.3% are homozygous for the trait of very low or absent activity (two variant alleles) (63–65). There is a good correlation between genotype and functional enzymatic activity, and both approaches have been studied to assess the risk of toxicity in patients taking AZA. In a study of patients with RA, the risk of any adverse event was significantly associated with intermediate or low enzyme activity. In particular, all cases of myelosuppression and 50% of the GI adverse effects were associated with low enzyme activity. In contrast, there was no association with idiosyncratic reactions, such as hepatitis (64). Using genotyping alone in a cohort of patients with rheumatic diseases, Black et al. (66) found that bone marrow toxicity only occurred in patients who were heterozygous for a variant allele. No episodes of bone marrow suppression were observed in those homozygous for the wild-type gene. What remains unclear, however, is whether knowledge of the patients' genotype would avoid the need for any future hematological monitoring.

Naughton et al. (67) found in a cohort of 135 patients, mostly with systemic lupus erythematosus, that although the single patient homozygous for mutant alleles experienced bone marrow toxicity, only one of the eleven others with drug-induced neutropenia had a polymorphism detected. Clearly, additional unknown polymorphisms may account for some of these patients. Therefore, genotyping may detect the small number of patients who are homozygous for TPMT polymorphisms who are clearly at risk of significant toxicity. In this group, an alternative agent can be used. In heterozygous patients, avoidance of the drug may not be necessary, although a lower dose may be needed to avoid bone marrow or GI toxicity. Taking all the current data into consideration, it appears that genotyping alone is insufficient to identify all patients who are at risk of developing AZA toxicity, and, therefore, regular monitoring is still necessary even when no TPMT polymorphisms are detected.

LEFLUNOMIDE

Pharmacology

Leflunomide is an isoxazole derivative first isolated and described nearly 20 years ago. Leflunomide is a prodrug that is converted nonenzymatically, primarily in the intestinal mucosa and plasma, but also by the liver, to the active metabolite malononitrilamide, termed A77 1726 (68). A77 1726 has a long half-life of approximately two weeks. Treatment with oral leflunomide is initiated with a loading dose of 100 mg once daily for three days and continued at a dose of 10–20 mg once daily. In placebo-controlled trials, leflunomide is superior to placebo in improving signs and symptoms of RA and is comparable with sulfasalazine and MTX in terms of clinical response rate (9,11,69). It is also comparable to MTX (9) and sulfasalazine (11) for reducing the rate of radiographic progression of RA. The overall withdrawal rates in clinical trials are approximately 28%, and these are mostly due to adverse effects including diarrhea, nausea, rash, elevated liver transaminases, and alopecia (9,11,69). To date, there are no studies looking at the pharmacogenetics of this agent in humans. There are however, several potential pathways in which genetic variability may exert an influence.

Mechanism and Site of Action

A77 1726 inhibits cell proliferation in activated lymphocytes in patients with active RA. In vitro data indicate that the drug inhibits the enzyme dihydro-orotate dehydrogenase (DHODH), which is the fourth enzyme utilized in the de novo purine synthesis pathway (70). By inhibiting uridine 5′-monophosphate (UMP) production, the levels of ribonucleotides and deoxyribonucleotides necessary for DNA and RNA synthesis are reduced. The interruption to DNA synthesis results in lymphocyte cell arrest (Fig. 4). The induction of arrest of activated autoimmune lymphocytes by leflunomide thereby reduces the autoimmune response in RA patients. When antirheumatic activity of leflunomide was observed, it was unclear as to whether it inhibited DHODH (71) or tyrosine kinases, which transfer ATPs terminal phosphate to a tyrosine residue on another protein. Davis et al. (71) established that leflunomide had no inhibitory effects on DHODH or tyrosine kinases but noted that A77 1726 had a concentration-dependent inhibitory effect on DHODH, with DHODH requiring both substrate and an electron acceptor. Although it was found that A77 1726 inhibits the activity of tyrosine kinases, the concentrations needed were much greater than the usual therapeutic concentrations seen in RA. DHODase inhibition is therefore potentially the main mechanism of action of this novel

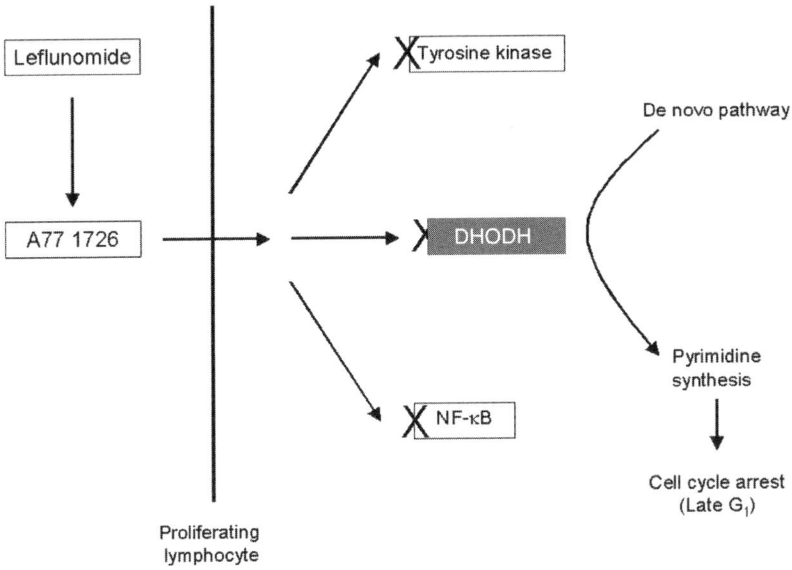

Figure 4 Proposed inflammatory pathways for the active moiety of leflunomide, A77 1726, in rheumatoid arthritis. At pharmacological concentrations, inhibition of DHODH (*gray box*) appears to be the most important mechanism leading to a reduction in pyrimidine synthesis in proliferating lymphocytes and cell cycle. *Abbreviations*: NF-κB, nuclear factor-κB. DHODH, dihydroorotate synthase.

immunosuppressive agent. DHODH has two redox sites, oxidation of dihydro-orotate to orotate, and the oxidation by ubiquinone of dihydroflavin mononucleotide ($FMNH_2$) to flavin mononucleotide (FMN). The long *N*-terminal extension forms a helical membrane-associated motif. This forms the mouth of a hydrophobic tunnel leading into the $FMNH_2$-ubiquinone redox site. A77 1726 binds to a narrow region of the tunnel. The DHODH sites resemble one another as they all carry out the same reaction. However, regions near the active sites can differ. The residues that interact with the inhibitors differ markedly from one organism to another, and a single residue change can lead to resistance (72). A77 1726 is also reported to possess other activities, such as concentration-dependent inhibition of nuclear factor kappa-B activation and nuclear factor kappa-B-dependent reporter gene expression (73). It also has inhibitory effects on oxygen radical, immunoglobulin (Ig)G, and IgM production (74) and interleukin (IL)-1b and IL-2 levels (75). Genetic variability of these pathways, especially of the DHODH enzyme, may therefore account for some of the variability in response to leflunomide observed in clinical practice.

ANTIMALARIAL DRUGS

Antimalarials, such as chloroquine and hydroxychloroquine, are commonly used in the treatment of RA. Although considered to be weaker agents than MTX and sulfasalazine, they are often used in mild disease or in combination with other agents (13). It is known that these drugs accumulate in the acid lysosomes of lymphocytes, macrophages, and polymorphonuclear cells (37,76), where they alter protease function and protein glycosylation. To date there are no studies on genetic polymorphisms and response to antimalarials.

BIOLOGICAL THERAPIES

A treatment may be termed as biological if it is derived from a living organism, unlike traditional drugs, which are chemically synthesized. Within RA, particular interest has focused on two proinflammatory cytokines that have been demonstrated to be critical in the pathophysiology of RA, IL-1, and TNF-α.

TNF-α Blockade

TNF-α is a pro-inflammatory cytokine that mediates both inflammatory synovitis and breakdown of articular cartilage. It also induces the production of other cytokines and matrix metalloproteinases that are important within the rheumatoid joint (77). TNF-α binds to either of the two cellular receptors, p55 or p75, which also exist in soluble shortened forms in different body fluids. These receptors are thought to be involved in the regulation of TNF-α activity (78). Currently three TNF blockers, infliximab, etanercept, and adalimumab are available for use in clinical practice.

Pharmacology and Mechanism of Action

Infliximab

Infliximab is a chimeric anti-TNF-α antibody that consists of a murine antigen-binding region bound to a human IgG1 constant region. It has a high affinity for TNF-α and has a serum half-life (once in steady-state) of 10 days (78). It is administered as a continuous infusion and has been licensed for use in RA and Crohn's disease. It binds to both soluble and cell-bound TNF-α and prevents binding at the TNF receptor (6). It is highly efficacious in the treatment of RA, both in terms of improvement in joint counts and in preventing radiographic damage. Clinical trials have shown it to be superior to MTX (the current "gold standard" DMARD) in terms of both clinical and radiological outcomes (4,79). Immunogenicity is a potential problem with infliximab, with studies showing that up to 25% of the patients develop human antichimeric antibodies (HACA) (80). Within the use of infliximab for Crohn's disease, there is some evidence to suggest that patients who produce antibodies to infliximab have a lower serum concentration of infliximab and shorter duration of response (81). Within RA, infliximab is usually coadministered with MTX to avoid this potential problem, and currently it does not appear that antibodies to infliximab are important in response to treatment.

Etanercept

Etanercept is a recombinant human TNF receptor (p75)–Fc fusion protein. It binds to soluble TNF-α and is administered subcutaneously in a dose of 25 mg twice weekly. It has a half-life of 115 hours (6). Several controlled trials have demonstrated that etanercept has significant benefit in RA, both as monotherapy or in combination with MTX (5,82). It is also licensed for use in juvenile idiopathic arthritis. As etanercept is fully humanized, immunogenicity is not clinically relevant.

Adalimumab (D2E7)

Adalimumab is the first fully human monoclonal antibody that blocks TNF-α. In controlled clinical trials, adalimumab has been shown to be efficacious in treating RA both with and without MTX (83,84).

Genetics of TNF-α

The TNF-α gene is mapped to the MHC Class III region on the short arm of chromosome 6, between the *HLA-B* and *HLA-DR* genes, and is highly polymorphic. Studies suggest that approximately 60% of the variation in TNF-α production is genetically determined (85), and these genes are potential candidates for both susceptibility and severity in RA. At least 14 SNPs have been identified within the TNF-α gene, and functional data exist for some of these polymorphisms (85). Two of the polymorphisms, the −238GA genotype and the +489GA genotype, may be associated with less erosive disease independent of the shared epitope (85,86). Fabris et al. (87) studied 163 RA patients and divided them into severe disease (active RA despite combination DMARD therapy) and moderate disease (responders to MTX). The −238AG genotype was absent in the severe RA group, and they concluded that the −238GG genotype might be associated with a poorer outcome. There was, however, a high proportion of controls with the −238GG genotype, and so its overall significance remains to be confirmed. Cvetkovic et al. (88) investigated TNF polymorphisms via restriction fragment length polymorphisms (RFLPs) and found that patients with the A1A2 genotype (equivalent to −308GA genotype) had more severe disease in terms of both disease activity and functional class, although there was no difference between the groups in terms of the number of DMARDs used. Other workers have failed to find an association between disease severity and the presence of this polymorphism (89). One small study aimed to examine the effects of TNF-α polymorphisms on responses to infliximab in Crohn's disease, but the results were contradictory between the cohorts studied (90).

To date, two other studies have examined the effect of polymorphisms in the TNF-α gene on the outcome of infliximab treatment. Mugnier et al. (91) genotyped 59 patients with established RA treated with infliximab and found that patients with the TNFα −308G/G genotype had a better response to infliximab at 22 weeks than patients carrying at least one copy of the TNFα −308A/G polymorphism. A second study (92) found a similar association, between the TNFα −308G/G genotype and a good clinical response to etanercept. In addition a combination of alleles influencing the production of IL-1 receptor antagonist (IL-1Ra) and TGFβ1 (*A2* allele of the IL-1 receptor antagonist and TGFβ1 +915 GSBC) were also associated with a poor response to etanercept. To date, there are no published studies evaluating pharmacogenetic markers on outcome of adalimumab treatment.

IL-1Ra (Anakinra)

Pharmacology and Mechanism of Action

IL-1 is another key proinflammatory cytokine in the pathogenesis of RA. It is produced by a variety of cells including monocytes, macrophages, and synoviocytes. There are several forms of IL-1, membrane-associated IL-1α and soluble IL-1β. Unlike TNF, activation of the IL-1 pathway also leads to release of its endogenous inhibitor IL-1Ra. Although levels of IL-1Ra are increased in RA patients compared with the healthy controls, the relative increase in IL-1Ra is insufficient to prevent signalling of IL-1 (6,93). Anakinra is a recombinant human IL-1Ra and binds IL-1R, thereby preventing binding of native IL-1. IL-1Ra has a short half-life and is therefore administered daily by a subcutaneous injection. In clinical trials, it has been shown to be efficacious for both clinical improvement and reducing radiological progression of RA (93,94).

Genetics of IL-1

No studies to date have evaluated genetic predictors of response to treatment with IL-1Ra. The genes for IL-1 and IL-1Ra are found on the long arm of chromosome 2. In one study, a polymorphism within the IL-1β promoter sequence (at position 511) was overrepresented in an RA population who had required joint surgery, compared with both patients who had not required surgery and healthy controls (95). This polymorphism may therefore be a marker of RA severity. However, Huang et al. (96) looked at the same polymorphism in a Taiwanese population and did not find an increased allele frequency in the RA group compared with the controls. These and other gene polymorphisms in the IL-1 family may be hypothesized to influence responses to IL-1Ra therapy and clearly require further evaluation.

SUMMARY AND FUTURE DIRECTIONS

Rheumatology is currently in an exciting era of unprecedented new drug development. In addition, the old paradigm of sequential monotherapy with DMARDs is being superseded by the use of DMARD combinations and the introduction of biologic drugs. The use of drugs is still, however, limited by adverse events and limited efficacy and also, in the case of biologics, by the high unit costs of these agents. The study of pharmacogenetics in rheumatology is, as can be seen, at an early stage. In most cases, polymorphisms in a single gene have been studied in isolation. Even using this approach with its inherent limitations, several genes of interest have been identified that may predict efficacy and/or adverse events and need confirmation. There is also clearly a need to extend this work to study drug pathways and gene–gene interactions of relevance more completely. With regard to the biologic agents, pharmacogenetics offers the opportunity to examine predictors of response and nonresponse that may allow better targeting of these expensive therapies to the right patient groups. In the next few years, substantial progress will be made in delineating the genetic contribution to the kinetics and mode of action of the drugs employed in rheumatology.

REFERENCES

1. Fries JF, Williams CA, Morfeld D, Singh G, Sibley J. Reduction in long-term disability in patients with rheumatoid arthritis by disease-modifying antirheumatic drug-based treatment strategies. Arthritis Rheum 1996; 39(4):616–622.
2. Kirwan JR. The effect of glucocorticoids on joint destruction in rheumatoid arthritis. The Arthritis and Rheumatism Council Low-Dose Glucocorticoid Study Group. N Engl J Med 1995; 333(3):142–146.
3. Boers M, Verhoeven AC, Markusse HM, van de Laar MA, Westhovens R, van Denderen JC, van Zeben D, Dijkmans BA, Peeters AJ, Jacobs P, van den Brink HR, Schouten HJ, van der Heijde DM, Boonen A, van Der LS. Randomised comparison of combined step-down prednisolone, methotrexate and sulphasalazine with sulphasalazine alone in early rheumatoid arthritis. Lancet 1997; 350(9074):309–318.

4. Maini R, St Clair EW, Breedveld F, Furst D, Kalden J, Weisman M, Smolen J, Emery P, Harriman G, Feldmann M, Lipsky P. Infliximab (chimeric anti-tumour necrosis factor alpha monoclonal antibody) versus placebo in rheumatoid arthritis patients receiving concomitant methotrexate: a randomised phase III trial. ATTRACT Study Group. Lancet 1999; 354(9194):1932–1939.
5. Moreland LW, Cohen SB, Baumgartner SW, Tindall EA, Bulpitt K, Martin R, Weinblatt M, Taborn J, Weaver A, Burge DJ, Schiff MH. Long-term safety and efficacy of etanercept in patients with rheumatoid arthritis. J Rheumatol 2001; 28(6):1238–1244.
6. Jenkins JK, Hardy KJ. Biological modifier therapy for the treatment of rheumatoid arthritis. Am J Med Sci 2002; 323(4):197–205.
7. Felson DT, Anderson JJ, Meenan RF. The comparative efficacy and toxicity of second-line drugs in rheumatoid arthritis. Results of two metaanalyses. Arthritis Rheum 1990; 33(10):1449–1461.
8. Felson DT, Anderson JJ, Boers M, Bombardier C, Chernoff M, Fried B, Furst D, Goldsmith C, Kieszak S, Lightfoot R. The American College of Rheumatology preliminary core set of disease activity measures for rheumatoid arthritis clinical trials. The Committee on Outcome Measures in Rheumatoid Arthritis Clinical Trials. Arthritis Rheum 1993; 36(6):729–740.
9. Strand V, Cohen S, Schiff M, Weaver A, Fleischmann R, Cannon G, Fox R, Moreland L, Olsen N, Furst D, Caldwell J, Kaine J, Sharp J, Hurley F, Loew-Friedrich I. Treatment of active rheumatoid arthritis with leflunomide compared with placebo and methotrexate. Leflunomide Rheumatoid Arthritis Investigators Group. Arch Intern Med 1999; 159(21):2542–2550.
10. Dougados M, Combe B, Cantagrel A, Goupille P, Olive P, Schattenkirchner M, Meusser S, Paimela L, Rau R, Zeidler H, Leirisalo-Repo M, Peldan K. Combination therapy in early rheumatoid arthritis: a randomised, controlled, double blind 52 week clinical trial of sulphasalazine and methotrexate compared with the single components. Ann Rheum Dis 1999; 58(4):220–225.
11. Smolen JS, Kalden JR, Scott DL, Rozman B, Kvien T, Larsen A, Loew-Friedrich I, Oed C, Rosenberg R. Efficacy and safety of leflunomide compared with placebo and sulphasalazine in active rheumatoid arthritis: A double-blind, randomised, multicentre trial. Lancet 1999; 353(9149):259–266.
12. O'Dell JR, Haire CE, Erikson N, Drymalski W, Palmer W, Eckhoff PJ, Garwood V, Maloley P, Klassen LW, Wees S, Klein H, Moore GF. Treatment of rheumatoid arthritis with methotrexate alone, sulfasalazine and hydroxychloroquine, or a combination of all three medications. N Engl J Med 1996; 334(20):1287–1291.
13. Mottonen T, Hannonen P, Leirisalo-Repo M, Nissila M, Kautiainen H, Korpela M, Laasonen L, Julkunen H, Luukkainen R, Vuori K, Paimela L, Blafield H, Hakala M, Ilva K, Yli-Kerttula U, Puolakka K, Jarvinen P, Hakola M, Piirainen H, Ahonen J, Palvimaki I, Forsberg S, Koota K, Friman C. Comparison of combination therapy with single-drug therapy in early rheumatoid arthritis: a randomised trial. FIN-RACo trial group. Lancet 1999; 353(9164):1568–1573.
14. Dayer JM, Bresnihan B. Targeting Interleukin-1 in the Treatment of Rheumatoid Arthritis. Arthritis Rheum 2002; 46(3):574–578.
15. Pincus T, Marcum SB, Callahan LF. Longterm drug therapy for rheumatoid arthritis in seven rheumatology private practices: II. Second line drugs and prednisone. J Rheumatol 1992; 19(12):1885–1894.
16. Morgan C, Lunt M, Brightwell H, Bradburn P, Fallow W, Lay M, Silman A, Bruce IN. Contribution of patient related differences to multidrug resistance in rheumatoid arthritis. Ann Rheum Dis 2003; 62(1):15–19.
17. Klippel JH, Dieppe PA, Arnett FC. Rheumatology. Vol. 1. In: John H, ed. Klippel, Paul A, Dieppe (section editors), Frank C Arnett. et al., ed. London: Mosby, 1998.
18. Bombardier C, Laine L, Reicin A, Shapiro D, Burgos-Vargas R, Davis B, Day R, Ferraz MB, Hawkey CJ, Hochberg MC, Kvien TK, Schnitzer TJ. Comparison of upper gastrointestinal toxicity of rofecoxib and naproxen in patients with rheumatoid arthritis. VIGOR Study Group. N Engl J Med 2000; 343(21):1520–1528.

19. Deeks JJ, Smith LA, Bradley MD. Efficacy, tolerability, and upper gastrointestinal safety of celecoxib for treatment of osteoarthritis and rheumatoid arthritis: systematic review of randomised controlled trials. BMJ 2002; 325(7365):619–626.
20. Kirchheiner J, Meineke I, Freytag G, Meisel C, Roots I, Brockmoller J. Enantiospecific effects of cytochrome P450 2C9 amino acid variants on ibuprofen pharmacokinetics and on the inhibition of cyclooxygenases 1 and 2. Clin Pharmacol Ther 2002; 72(1):62–75.
21. Brenner SS, Herrlinger C, Dilger K, Murdter TE, Hofmann U, Marx C, Klotz U. Influence of age and cytochrome P450 2C9 genotype on the steady-state disposition of diclofenac and celecoxib. Clin Pharmacokinet 2003; 42(3):283–292.
22. Knox AJ. How prevalent is aspirin induced asthma? Thorax 2002; 57(7):565–566.
23. Jawien J. A new insight into aspirin-induced asthma. Eur J Clin Invest 2002; 32(2):134–138.
24. Sokka T. Contemporary Disease Modifying Antirheumatic Drugs (DMARD) in Patients with Recent Onset Rheumatoid Arthritis in a US Private Practice: Methotrexate as the Anchor Drug in 90% and New DMARD in 30% of Patients. J Rheumatol 2002; 29(12):2521–2524.
25. Hillson JL, Furst DE. Pharmacology and pharmacokinetics of methotrexate in rheumatic disease. Practical issues in treatment and design. Rheum Dis Clin North Am 1997; 23(4):757–778.
26. Chan ESL, Cronstein BN. Molecular action of methotrexate in inflammatory diseases. Arthritis Research 2002; 4(4):266–273.
27. Cronstein BN. The mechanism of action of methotrexate. Rheum Dis Clin North Am 1997; 23(4):739–755.
28. Cutolo M, Sulli A, Pizzorni C, Seriolo B, Straub RH. Anti-inflammatory mechanisms of methotrexate in rheumatoid arthritis. Ann Rheum Dis 2001; 60(8):729–735.
29. Weisberg I, Tran P, Christensen B, Sibani S, Rozen R. A second genetic polymorphism in methylenetetrahydrofolate reductase (MTHFR) associated with decreased enzyme activity. Mol Genet Metab 1998; 64(3):169–172.
30. Montesinos MC, Desai A, Delano D, Chen JF, Fink JS, Jacobson MA, Cronstein BN. Adenosine A2A or A3 receptors are required for inhibition of inflammation by methotrexate and its analog MX-68. Arthritis Rheum 2003; 48(1):240–247.
31. Pisetsky DS, St Clair EW. Progress in the treatment of rheumatoid arthritis. J Am Med Assoc 2001; 286(22):2787–2790.
32. Bathon JM, Martin RW, Fleischmann RM, Tesser JR, Schiff MH, Keystone EC, Genovese MC, Wasko MC, Moreland LW, Weaver AL, Markenson J, Finck BK. A comparison of etanercept and methotrexate in patients with early rheumatoid arthritis. N Engl J Med 2000; 343(22):1586–1593.
33. Wolfe F, Hawley DJ, Cathey MA. Termination of slow acting antirheumatic therapy in rheumatoid arthritis: a 14-year prospective evaluation of 1017 consecutive starts. J Rheumatol 1990; 17(8):994–1002.
34. van Ede AE, Laan RF, Blom HJ, Huizinga TW, Haagsma CJ, Giesendorf BA, de Boo TM, van de Putte LB. The C677T mutation in the methylenetetrahydrofolate reductase gene: a genetic risk factor for methotrexate-related elevation of liver enzymes in rheumatoid arthritis patients. Arthritis Rheum 2001; 44(11):2525–2530.
35. Urano W, Taniguchi A, Yamanaka H, Tanaka E, Nakajima H, Matsuda Y, Akama H, Kitamura Y, Kamatani N. Polymorphisms in the methylenetetrahydrofolate reductase gene were associated with both the efficacy and the toxicity of methotrexate used for the treatment of rheumatoid arthritis, as evidenced by single locus and haplotype analyses. Pharmacogenetics 2002; 12(3):183–190.
36. Kumagai K, Hiyama K, Oyama T, Maeda H, Kohno N. Polymorphisms in the thymidylate synthase and methylenetetrahydrofolate reductase genes and sensitivity to the low-dose methotrexate therapy in patients with rheumatoid arthritis. Int J Mol Med 2003; 11(5):593–600.
37. Choy E, Panayi G. Mechanisms of action of second-line agents and choice of drugs in combination therapy. Clin Exp Rheumatol 1999; 17(6 suppl 18):S20–S28.
38. Box SA, Pullar T. Sulphasalazine in the treatment of rheumatoid arthritis. Brit J Rheumatol 1997; 36(3):382–386.

39. Kitas GD, Farr M, Waterhouse L, Bacon PA. Influence of acetylator status on sulphasalazine efficacy and toxicity in patients with rheumatoid arthritis. Scand J Rheumatol 1992; 21(5):220–225.
40. Pullar T, Hunter JA, Capell HA. Effect of acetylator phenotype on efficacy and toxicity of sulphasalazine in rheumatoid arthritis. Ann Rheum Dis 1985; 44(12):831–837.
41. Hein DW. Arylamine N-acetyltransferase (NAT) nomenclature. www.louisville.edu/medschool/pharmacology/NAT2.html. 2004.
42. Tanaka E, Taniguchi A, Urano W, Nakajima H, Matsuda Y, Kitamura Y, Saito M, Yamanaka H, Saito T, Kamatani N. Adverse effects of sulfasalazine in patients with rheumatoid arthritis are associated with diplotype configuration at the N-acetyltransferase 2 gene. J Rheumatol 2002; 29(12):2492–2499.
43. Sabbagh N, Delaporte E, Marez D, Lo-Guidice JM, Piette F, Broly F. NAT2 genotyping and efficacy of sulfasalazine in patients with chronic discoid lupus erythematosus. Pharmacogenetics 1997; 7(2):131–135.
44. Ricart E, Taylor WR, Loftus EV, O'Kane D, Weinshilboum RM, Tremaine WJ, Harmsen WS, Zinsmeister AR, Sandborn WJ. N-Acetyltransferase 1 and 2 genotypes do not predict response or toxicity to treatment with mesalamine and sulfasalazine in patients with ulcerative colitis. Am J Gastroenterol 2002; 97(7):1763–1768.
45. Munro R, Capell HA. Penicillamine. Brit J Rheumatol 1997; 36(1):104–109.
46. Emery P, Panayi GS, Huston G, Welsh KI, Mitchell SC, Shah RR, Idle JR, Smith RL, Waring RH. D-Penicillamine induced toxicity in rheumatoid arthritis: the role of sulphoxidation status and HLA-DR3. J Rheumatol 1984; 11(5):626–632.
47. Madhok R, Zoma A, Torley HI, Capell HA, Waring R, Hunter JA. The relationship of sulfoxidation status to efficacy and toxicity of penicillamine in the treatment of rheumatoid arthritis. Arthritis Rheum 1990; 33(4):574–577.
48. Layton MA, Jones PW, Alldersea JE, Strange RC, Fryer AA, Dawes PT, Mattey DL. The therapeutic response to D-penicillamine in rheumatoid arthritis: influence of glutathione *S*-transferase polymorphisms. Rheumatology 1999; 38(1):43–47.
49. Maetzel A, Wong A, Strand V, Tugwell P, Wells G, Bombardier C. Meta-analysis of treatment termination rates among rheumatoid arthritis patients receiving disease-modifying anti-rheumatic drugs. Rheumatology 2000; 39(9):975–981.
50. Singal DP, Reid B, Green D, D'Souza M, Bensen WG, Buchanan WW. Polymorphism of major histocompatibility complex extended haplotypes bearing HLA-DR3 in patients with rheumatoid arthritis with gold induced thrombocytopenia or proteinuria. Ann Rheum Dis 1990; 49(8):582–586.
51. ten Wolde S, Dijkmans BA, van Rood JJ, Claas FH, de Vries RR, Hazes JM, van Riel PL, van Gestel A, Breedveld FC. Human leucocyte antigen phenotypes and gold-induced remissions in patients with rheumatoid arthritis. Brit J Rheumatol 1995; 34(4):343–346.
52. Alarcon GS, Barger BO, Acton RT, Koopman WJ. HLA antigens and gold toxicity in American blacks with rheumatoid arthritis. Rheumatol Int 1986; 6(1):13–17.
53. Hakala M, van Assendelft AH, Ilonen J, Jalava S, Tiilikainen A. Association of different HLA antigens with various toxic effects of gold salts in rheumatoid arthritis. Ann Rheum Dis 1986; 45(3):177–182.
54. Stockman A, Zilko PJ, Major GA, Tait BD, Property DN, Mathews JD, Hannah MC, McCluskey J, Muirden KD. Genetic markers in rheumatoid arthritis relationship to toxicity from D-penicillamine. J Rheumatol 1986; 13(2):269–273.
55. Clarkson RW, Sanders PA, Grennan DM. Complement C4 null alleles as a marker of gold or D-penicillamine toxicity in the treatment of rheumatoid arthritis. Brit J Rheumatol 1992; 31(1):53–54.
56. Evans TI, Small RE, Redford TW, Han J, Moxley G. Tumor necrosis factor microsatellite markers TNFa5b5 and TNFa6b5 influence adverse reactions to parenteral gold in Caucasians. J Rheumatol 1999; 26(11):2303–2309.
57. Suarez-Almazor ME, Spooner C, Belseck E, Dr Maria Suarez-Almazor HSRVAMC. Azathioprine for rheumatoid arthritis. The Cochrane Library (Oxford) 2001 issue 2 (10 p) (3 ref 16 bib) (Update Software, online or CD ROM, updated quarterly) (Oxford). 2000.

58. Lennard L, Van Loon JA, Weinshilboum RM. Pharmacogenetics of acute azathioprine toxicity: relationship to thiopurine methyltransferase genetic polymorphism. Clin Pharmacol Ther 1989; 46(2):149–154.
59. Jeurissen ME, Boerbooms AM, van de Putte LB. Pancytopenia related to azathioprine in rheumatoid arthritis. Ann Rheum Dis 1988; 47(6):503–505.
60. Yates CR, Krynetski EY, Loennechen T, Fessing MY, Tai HL, Pui C-H, Relling MV, Evans WE. Molecular diagnosis of thiopurine *S*-methyltransferase deficiency: genetic basis for azathioprine and mercaptopurine intolerance. Ann Intern Med 1997; 126(8):608–614.
61. Ameyaw MM, Collie-Duguid ES, Powrie RH, Ofori-Adjei D, McLeod H-L. Thiopurine methyltransferase alleles in British and Ghanaian populations. Hum Mol Genet 1999; 8(2):367–370.
62. McLeod HL, Pritchard SC, Githang'a J, Indalo A, Ameyaw MM, Powrie RH, Booth L, Collie-Duguid ES. Ethnic differences in thiopurine methyltransferase pharmacogenetics: evidence for allele specificity in Caucasian and Kenyan individuals. Pharmacogenetics 1999; 9(6):773–776.
63. Weinshilboum RM, Raymond FA, Pazmino PA. Human erythrocyte thiopurine methyltransferase: radiochemical microassay and biochemical properties. Clin Chim Acta 1978; 85(3):323–333.
64. Stolk JN, Boerbooms AM, de Abreu RA, de Koning DG, van Beusekom HJ, Muller WH, van de Putte LB. Reduced thiopurine methyltransferase activity and development of side effects of azathioprine treatment in patients with rheumatoid arthritis. Arthritis Rheum 1998; 41(10):1858–1866.
65. McLeod HL, Lin JS, Scott EP, Pui CH, Evans WE. Thiopurine methyltransferase activity in American white subjects and black subjects. Clin Pharmacol Ther 1994; 55(1):15–20.
66. Black AJ, McLeod HL, Capell HA, Powrie RH, Matowe LK, Pritchard SC, Collie-Duguid ES, Reid DM. Thiopurine methyltransferase genotype predicts therapy-limiting severe toxicity from azathioprine. Ann Intern Med 1998; 129(9):716–718.
67. Naughton MA, Battaglia E, O'Brien S, Walport MJ, Botto M. Identification of thiopurine methyltransferase (TPMT) polymorphisms cannot predict myelosuppression in systemic lupus erythematosus patients taking azathioprine. Rheumatology (Oxford) 1999; 38(7):640–644.
68. Fox RI, Herrmann ML, Frangou CG, Wahl GM, Morris RE, Strand V, Kirschbaum BJ. Mechanism of action for leflunomide in rheumatoid arthritis. Clin Immunol 1999; 93(3):198–208.
69. Emery P, Breedveld C, Lemmel EM, Kaltwasser JP, Dawes PT, Gomoe B, Van der Bosch F, Nordstrom D, Bjorneboe O, Dahl R, et al., the Multinational Leflunomide Study Group. A comparison of the efficacy and safety of leflunomide and methotrexate for the treatment of rheumatoid arthritis. Rheumatology 2000; 39:655–665.
70. Ruckemann K, Fairbanks LD, Carrey EA, Hawrylowicz CM, Richards DF, Kirschbaum B, Simmonds HA. Leflunomide inhibits pyrimidine de novo synthesis in mitogen-stimulated T-lymphocytes from healthy humans. J Biol Chem 1998; 273(34):21682–21691.
71. Davis JP, Cain GA, Pitts WJ, Magolda RL, Copeland RA. The immunosuppressive metabolite of leflunomide is a potent inhibitor of human dihydroorotate dehydrogenase. Biochemistry 1996; 35(4):1270–1273.
72. Liu S, Neidhardt EA, Grossman TH, Ocain T, Clardy J. Structures of human dihydroorotate dehydrogenase in complex with antiproliferative agents. Structure 2000; 8(1):25–33.
73. Manna SK, Aggarwal BB. Immunosuppressive leflunomide metabolite (A77 1726) blocks TNF-dependent nuclear factor-kappa B activation and gene expression. J Immunol 1999; 162(4):2095–2102.
74. Siemasko K, Chong AS, Jack HM, Gong H, Williams JW, Finnegan A. Inhibition of JAK3 and STAT6 tyrosine phosphorylation by the immunosuppressive drug leflunomide leads to a block in IgG1 production. J Immunol 1998; 160(4):1581–1588.
75. Cao WW, Kao PN, Aoki Y, Xu JC, Shorthouse RA, Morris RE. A novel mechanism of action of the immunomodulatory drug, leflunomide: Augmentation of the immunosuppressive

cytokine, TGF-beta 1, and suppression of the immunostimulatory cytokine, IL-2. Transplantation Proceedings 1996; 28(6):3079–3080.

76. Munster T, Furst DE. Pharmacotherapeutic strategies for disease-modifying antirheumatic drug (DMARD) combinations to treat rheumatoid arthritis (RA). Clin Exp Rheumatol 1999; 17(6 suppl 18):Suppl-36.
77. Choy EH, Panayi GS. Cytokine pathways and joint inflammation in rheumatoid arthritis. N Engl J Med 2001; 344(12):907–916.
78. Case JP. Old and new drugs used in rheumatoid arthritis: a historical perspective. Part 2: the newer drugs and drug strategies. Am J Ther 2001; 8(3):163–179.
79. Lipsky PE, van der Heijde DM, St Clair EW, Furst DE, Breedveld FC, Kalden JR, Smolen JS, Weisman M, Emery P, Feldmann M, Harriman GR, Maini RN. Infliximab and methotrexate in the treatment of rheumatoid arthritis. Anti-Tumor Necrosis Factor Trial in Rheumatoid Arthritis with Concomitant Therapy Study Group. N Engl J Med 2000; 343(22):1594–1602.
80. Feldmann M, Elliott MJ, Woody JN, Maini RN. Anti-tumor necrosis factor-alpha therapy of rheumatoid arthritis. Adv Immunol 1997; 64:283–350.
81. Baert F, Noman M, Vermeire S, Van Assche G, D'Haens G, Carbonez A, Rutgeerts P. Influence of immunogenicity on the long-term efficacy of infliximab in Crohn's disease. N Engl J Med 2003; 348(7):601–608.
82. Weinblatt ME, Kremer JM, Bankhurst AD, Bulpitt KJ, Fleischmann RM, Fox RI, Jackson CG, Lange M, Burge DJ. A trial of etanercept, a recombinant tumor necrosis factor receptor: Fc fusion protein, in patients with rheumatoid arthritis receiving methotrexate. N Engl J Med 1999; 340(4):253–259.
83. Kempeni J. Update on D2E7: a fully human anti-tumour necrosis factor alpha monoclonal antibody. Ann Rheum Dis 2000; 59(suppl 1):i44–i45.
84. Weinblatt ME, Keystone EC, Furst DE, Moreland LW, Weisman MH, Birbara CA, Teoh LA, Fischkoff SA, Chartash EK. Adalimumab, a fully human anti-tumor necrosis factor alpha monoclonal antibody, for the treatment of rheumatoid arthritis in patients taking concomitant methotrexate: the ARMADA trial. Arthritis Rheum 2003; 48(1):35–45.
85. Verweij CL. Tumour necrosis factor gene polymorphisms as severity markers in rheumatoid arthritis. Ann Rheum Dis 1999; 58:Suppl-6.
86. van Krugten MV, Huizinga TW, Kaijzel EL, Zanelli E, Drossaers-Bakker KW, van de LP, Hazes JM, Zwinderman AH, Breedveld FC, Verweij CL. Association of the TNF +489 polymorphism with susceptibility and radiographic damage in rheumatoid arthritis. Genes Immun 1999; 1(2):91–96.
87. Fabris M, Di PE, D'Elia A, Damante G, Sinigaglia L, Ferraccioli G. Tumor necrosis factor-alpha gene polymorphism in severe and mild-moderate rheumatoid arthritis. J Rheumatol 2002; 29(1):29–33.
88. Cvetkovic JT, Wallberg-Jonsson S, Stegmayr B, Rantapaa-Dahlqvist S, Lefvert AK. Susceptibility for and clinical manifestations of rheumatoid arthritis are associated with polymorphisms of the TNF-alpha, IL-1beta, and IL-1Ra genes. J Rheumatol 2002; 29(2):212–219.
89. Brinkman BM, Huizinga TW, Kurban SS, van der Velde EA, Schreuder GM, Hazes JM, Breedveld FC, Verweij CL. Tumour necrosis factor alpha gene polymorphisms in rheumatoid arthritis: association with susceptibility to, or severity of, disease? Brit J Rheumatol 1997; 36(5):516–521.
90. Mascheretti S, Hampe J, Kuhbacher T, Herfarth H, Krawczak M, Folsch UR, Schreiber S. Pharmacogenetic investigation of the TNF/TNF-receptor system in patients with chronic active Crohn's disease treated with infliximab. Pharmacogenomics J 2002; 2(2):127–136.
91. Mugnier B, Balandraud N, Darque A, Roudier C, Roudier J, Reviron D. Polymorphism at position −308 of the tumor necrosis factor alpha gene influences outcome of infliximab therapy in rheumatoid arthritis. Arthritis Rheum 2003; 48(7):1849–1852.
92. Padyukov L, Lampa J, Heimburger M, Ernestam S, Cederholm T, Lundkvist I, Andersson P, Hermansson Y, Harju A, Klareskog L, Bratt J. Genetic markers for the efficacy of tumour necrosis factor blocking therapy in rheumatoid arthritis. Ann Rheum Dis 2003; 62(6):526–529.

93. Nuki G, Bresnihan B, Bear MB, McCabe D, European Group Of Clinical Investigators. Long-term safety and maintenance of clinical improvement following treatment with anakinra (recombinant human interleukin-1 receptor antagonist) in patients with rheumatoid arthritis: extension phase of a randomized, double-blind, placebo-controlled trial. Arthritis Rheum 2002; 46(11):2838–2846.
94. Bresnihan B. Effects of anakinra on clinical and radiological outcomes in rheumatoid arthritis. Ann Rheum Dis 2002; 61(suppl 2):ii74–ii77.
95. Crilly A, Maiden N, Capell HA, Madhok R. Predictive value of interleukin 1 gene polymorphisms for surgery. Ann Rheum Dis 2000; 59(9):695–699.
96. Huang CM, Tsai FJ, Wu JY, Wu MC. Interleukin-1beta and interleukin-1 receptor antagonist gene polymorphisms in rheumatoid arthritis. Scand J Rheumatol 2001; 30(4):225–228.

11
Polymorphisms in Cardiovascular Medicine: The Role of Genetic Variants in Disease Diagnosis and Drug Response

Yasmin
Clinical Pharmacology Unit, University of Cambridge, Cambridge, U.K.

David N. Cooper
Institute of Medical Genetics, Cardiff University, Cardiff, U.K.

John R. Cockcroft
Wales Heart Research Institute, Cardiff University, Cardiff, U.K.

INTRODUCTION

Cardiovascular disease (CVD), including stroke, is the leading cause of illness and death worldwide, and is eminently preventable. Genetic studies have demonstrated that in most cardiovascular conditions, specific inherited polymorphisms can influence the therapeutic response. Moreover, it is apparent that there is considerable interindividual variation in the effectiveness of cardiovascular system drugs. These differences are due to both environmental factors (e.g., salt intake, smoking) and genetic variation. Ultimately, they result in abnormalities in gene expression (over-, under-, zero-, or defective production of an enzyme) that yield phenotypic changes that are of pathological significance in such disorders as hypertension, atherosclerosis, coronary heart disease, myocardial infarction, and arterial stiffness. Molecular genetic studies have also identified defects in ion channels, contractile or structural proteins, and signaling molecules that play a role in disease pathogenesis.

Inherited differences in drug metabolizing enzymes are usually monogenic codominant traits. However, the overall clinical effect of most drugs is influenced by multiple genes involved in the mechanistic pathways of drug absorption, metabolism, disposition, and interaction with the target receptor (1). Therefore, for any given drug, one gene may determine the extent of drug activation, a second may affect drug excretion, and still a third may determine receptor sensitivity. The overall effect of a given drug may thus be influenced by polymorphism in a number of different genes and therefore potentially by individual-specific combinations and permutations of polymorphic alleles.

In the following sections, we review polymorphisms that are thought to play an important role in the treatment of CVD.

POLYMORPHISM IN THE HUMAN GENOME

> Even at birth the whole individual is destined to die, and perhaps his organic disposition may already contain the indication of what he is to die from.
>
> —Sigmund Freud, *The Dissolution of the Oedipus Complex* (1924)

Most polymorphisms are expected to be neutral with respect to fitness. However, those polymorphisms that occur either within gene coding or promoter regions may affect either the structure/function of the gene product (2) or the expression of the gene (3) and may therefore have the potential to be of phenotypic or even of pathological significance. It should be noted that although most polymorphisms are of the single nucleotide (SNP) variety, there are some gene-associated polymorphisms in the human genome of other types, for example, triplet repeat copy number, gene deletion, gene duplication, intragenic duplication, microinsertion, inversion, gene fusion, and gene copy number (4).

The mechanisms by which polymorphisms are maintained in human populations are likely to be varied. The neutralist theory assumes no selection on the alleles of a polymorphic locus, and the frequency of an allele may therefore increase simply by *genetic drift* (the change of allele frequency due to random sampling). Such "transient polymorphisms" often remain at a low frequency in the population before being lost or may instead increase in frequency under the influence of either genetic drift or positive selection until one allele reaches fixation. Most known polymorphisms are probably of this type. However, if the alternative alleles are not neutral with respect to fitness, the DNA polymorphisms may be maintained by selection pressure, possibly overdominant selection (also known as "heterozygote advantage" or "balanced polymorphisms").

In practice, the relationship between a polymorphism and a disease susceptibility should usually be interpreted in terms of *linkage disequilibrium*. Linkage disequilibrium is said to be present when certain alleles at one locus occur with certain alleles of another locus on the same chromosome at frequencies greater than can be attributed to chance alone. For our purposes, it can be considered to be due to a mutation occurring in a gene a number of generations ago. This mutant gene has then increased in frequency within the population, affected individuals of succeeding generations inheriting not only the mutant gene but also the particular alleles of neighboring polymorphisms. Gradually, the relationship between the marker alleles and the mutant gene will decay due to recombination. As a consequence, marker/disease associations from different populations can be extremely difficult to interpret, although both polymorphic allele frequency and linkage phase can be established in any one population. Also either or both can differ dramatically between populations.

Association studies employing polymorphisms located within or in close proximity to potential candidate genes can be a powerful approach to the epidemiological analysis of complex disorders (5). However, the results of such studies are notoriously difficult to replicate (6). One of the problems we face both in interpreting and comparing the results of disease association studies is that these studies will often vary with respect to the polymorphism(s) used, the population examined, the exact definition of disease phenotype employed, and the statistical methodology adopted. The possibility of confounding factors (e.g., population stratification, life style, nutritional status) is omnipresent, as is the use of poorly selected and inappropriate controls. Another caveat is reporting bias; there will be a tendency to only report significant associations whereas negative findings will either not be published or published only in more obscure lower-impact journals.

In some cardiovascular conditions, disease associations are evident in polymorphic *haplotypes* rather than with individual SNPs (7). Haplotypes are specific combinations of alleles of closely linked polymorphisms. Disease–haplotype associations are also explicable in terms of linkage disequilibrium and probably reflect the nonadditive effects of individual SNPs on gene function/expression. Interactions between polymorphic alleles at different loci are also possible. Studies that seek combinatorial effects of polymorphisms at multiple loci may however be at risk of failing to allow for multiple testing in their significance assessment. Indeed, some disease associations may be found only in a given age or ethnic group or in one sex but not the other. Such findings may simply allow one to conclude that if one looks hard enough for an association, one will find another sooner or later. It should therefore be no surprise that significant associations are sometimes found with alternative alleles in different studies focusing on different clinical phenotypes or on different ethnic groups. Also, unsurprising is the fact that "disconfirmation" of previously published positive findings is a common occurrence in this research area (5).

As discussed below, less common types of gene-associated polymorphisms relevant to cardiovascular medicine include an indel (combined micro-insertion/micro-deletion) polymorphism in the apolipoprotein E (*APOE*) gene (8), a gross insertion polymorphism involving an *Alu* sequence introduced into the angiotensin I-converting enzyme (*ACE*) gene (9), and a microinsertion/deletion polymorphism in the plasminogen activator inhibitor-1 (*PAI1*) gene (10). This *PAI1* polymorphism is due to the insertion or deletion of a single G residue within the promoter sequence (10); the *ins* allele contains an interleukin 1-responsive element, which is absent in the *del* allele, suggesting that individuals homozygous for the *del* allele could exhibit an altered PAI1 response during the acute phase reaction (10).

POLYMORPHISM IN CARDIOVASCULAR DISEASE

The list of genes, implicated as playing a significant role in the regulation of cardiovascular signaling pathways, is certainly large. Table 1 summarizes some of these genes and their polymorphisms associated with altered cardiovascular function. In this chapter, we focus on: (*i*) the major pathways with their "well-established" proteins and polymorphisms, (*ii*) the emerging proteins and polymorphisms of the cardiovascular matrix and arterial stiffening, which are recognized as independent predictors of increased cardiovascular risk, (*iii*) the lipid, inflammation and coagulation system polymorphisms that are important in predicting increased cardiovascular risk, (*iv*) genetic polymorphism of cardiovascular drug metabolism (e.g., cytochrome P450 system), (*v*) evidence for genetic polymorphisms affecting responses to drugs with adverse reactions, and (*vi*) a perspective on pharmacogenetics in cardiovascular medicine.

Renin–Angiotensin–Aldosterone System (RAAS)

The Renin–angiotensin–aldosterone system (RAAS) plays a crucial role in the development and progression of CVD by promoting sodium absorption, cardiac remodeling and norepinephrine release, and other potentially detrimental effects (Fig. 1). It also plays a significant role in controlling several elements of the extracellular matrix components; manipulating this system can however reverse experimental cardiac fibrosis (11). Drugs that interfere with this system have proved to be among the most successful therapeutic agents for a variety of CVDs.

Table 1 Examples of Gene Polymorphisms Associated with Cardiovascular Function and Their Frequencies[a]

Gene	Chromosome location	Polymorphism	Allele frequency (%)[a]		Disease/cardiovascular function	References
			Caucasians	African Americans		
Angiotensinogen (*AGT*)	1q41-q45	Met235**Thr**	42.2	77	Angiotensinogen levels	(185)[a]
					Coronary artery disease	(12)
					Blood pressure	(18)
						(154)
Angiotensin (*ACE*)	17q23	I/**D**	56.2	60.3	Angiotensin-converting enzyme levels	(185)[a]
						(20)
					Carotid wall thickness	(26)
					Heart failure	(31)
					Pulse pressure	(27)
Angiotensin II type1 receptor (*ATR1*)	3q21-q25	A1166**C**	29	9	Blood pressure	(185)[a]
					Arterial stiffness	(159)
						(156,157)
Aldosterone synthase (*CYP11B2*)	8q21-q22	T-344**C**	50.3	79	Left ventricle size and mass	(186)[a]
					Aldosterone levels	(35)
					Arterial stiffness	(33)
						(34)
β-2 adrenergic receptor (*ADRB2*)	5q31-q32	Arg16**Gly**	43	49	Coronary artery disease	(187)[a]
		Gln27**Glu**	35	18	Heart failure	(45)
						(41)
						(46)

Nitric oxide synthase (*NOS3*)	7q35-q36	Glu298**Asp**	39.6	—	Coronary artery disease	(55)[a]
					Myocardial infarction	(56)
					Essential hypertension	(54)
Elastin (*ELN*)	7q11.2	**Ser**425Gly	36	—	Large artery stiffness	(68)[a]
					Distensibility	(66)
						(67)
Fibrillin (*FBN1*)	15q21.1	**2–3**	9.4	—	Large artery stiffness	(95)
					Pulse pressure	(94)
Apolipoprotein E (*APOE*)	19q13.2	**E4**	13.4	19.6	Coronary heart disease/ myocardial infaction	(105) (123)
					Cholesterol level	(99)
					Aortic wall thickness	(188)
Choslesteryl ester transfer protein (*CETP*)	16q13	*Taq*I B1**B2**	0.42	—	Cholesteryl ester transfer protein levels	(68) (105) (181)[a]
C-reactive protein (*CRP*)	1q21-q23	1444C>**T**	26	—	C-reactive protein levels	(120)[a]
					Coronary heart disease risk	(123)
					Arterial stiffness	(119)
Interleukin-6 (*IL6*)	7p21	−174G>**C**	37	—	Interleukin-6 levels	(124)[a]
					Coronary heart disease mortality	(123)

[a]Frequency of the allele in bold type.

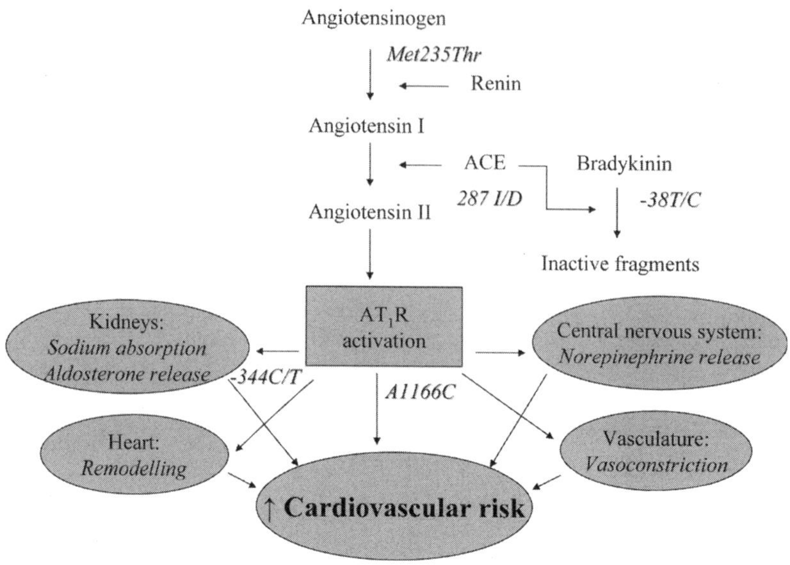

Figure 1 Components and effects of renin–angiotensin–aldosterone system and polymorphisms.

Angiotensinogen

Angiotensinogen (AGT) is the most extensively studied of the candidate genes in CVD and sits at the head of the RAAS pathway. A number of studies have linked the *AGT* locus on chromosome 1 to essential hypertension. The Met235Thr polymorphism in the *AGT* gene is associated with an increase in plasma AGT levels (12). The relationship of *AGT* gene variants to human CVD/myocardial infarction is less certain, with several studies reporting a positive association (13,14) but others reporting no association (15,16). In coronary artery disease patients, AGT concentrations were found to be higher in 235Thr (TT) homozygotes (14). A recent meta-analysis of 45,267 subjects also confirmed that TT homozygotes and MT heterozygotes for the Met235Thr polymorphism exhibited increased AGT levels (17). Tiret et al. (16) also showed that the number of antihypertensive medications being taken by 235Thr carriers was greater than in controls. Further, in untreated essential hypertensives, the *AGT* gene was found to be an independent predictor of the blood pressure response to ACE inhibitor therapy (18); the best response occurred in carriers of the 235 Thr allele.

Angiotensin-Converting Enzyme

Another gene in this pathway that has been studied extensively is the *ACE* gene, on account of the variable clinical efficacy of drugs that interfere with this pathway, inhibition of which leads to a decrease in both blood pressure and cardiovascular mortality (19). *ACE* not only plays a central role in the renin-angiotensin system but also in the kallikrein-kinin pathways, thereby promoting the formation of angiotensin II and inactivating bradykinin. The insertion (I)/deletion (D) polymorphism in intron 16 of the *ACE* gene located on chromosome 17 (due to the presence/absence of a 287-bp *Alu* repeat sequence) has received particular attention because of its influence on circulating *ACE* activity (9). In fact, some 50% of the genetic variance in serum *ACE* levels has been attributed to polymorphic variation in the *ACE* gene. Individuals homozygous for the deletion allele (DD) have been shown to have twice the serum levels compared with those homozygous for the insertion allele (II), with heterozygous individuals (ID) having intermediate levels (20). The morbidity associated with the *ACE* DD genotype (21) and the D allele (22) in left ventricular hypertrophy (23), myocardial infarction (24), cerebral ischemic stroke (25), and increasing carotid wall thickness (26) suggests that polymorphic variation in *ACE* gene exerts an important influence on a variety of different aspects of the heart and vascular tree. The I/D polymorphism also appears to exert an influence on pulse pressure with age and hence may increase cardiovascular risk (27). Although the D allele has been associated with an increased risk of various cardiovascular conditions, the situation in hypertension is controversial. The inconsistent results are exemplified by the fact that the I allele has tended to track with high blood pressure in some studies, albeit below the level of statistical significance (18,28).

In summary, the homozygous DD genotype of the insertional *ACE* gene polymorphism may be an independent risk factor for coronary heart disease, especially in individuals who lack other conventional risk factors, such as hypertension or hypercholesterolemia. If confirmed, this suggests the possibility of using drugs that act on the renin-angiotensin system (such as ACE inhibitors) in individuals genetically defined as being at high risk of heart disease.

The human I/D polymorphism may also play a role in pharmacogenetics (see section "Renin-Angiotensin System Drugs"). Thus, although some studies have failed to demonstrate a difference in blood pressure response to ACE inhibitors or other drugs (18,29,30), recent data indicate that knowledge of *ACE* genotype may help in the partitioning of patients into potential responders and nonresponders and also in helping to determine the overall prognosis (31).

Aldosterone Synthase

Aldosterone is a mineralocorticoid hormone that controls sodium balance and intravascular volume, thereby helping to regulate blood pressure. It is synthesized in the adrenal cortex from deoxycorticosterone by a mitochondrial CYP450 enzyme, aldosterone synthase (known as *CYP11B2*). The *CYP11B2* gene encoding this enzyme is located on chromosome 8 and several polymorphisms have been identified in its upstream regulatory region. The polymorphism at −344 C/T in the promoter region has been associated with elevated plasma aldosterone levels (32) and also left ventricular diameter and mass in young adults free of clinically overt disease. In these studies, individuals with a CC genotype exhibited increased aldosterone levels (33), increased arterial stiffness (34), and increased left ventricular size and mass. The left ventricular size, mass, and to some extent, diastolic function have also been associated with the −344CC genotype (35). By contrast, the −344 C/T polymorphism was not found to influence the risk of myocardial infarction either directly or via interaction with other drugs.

β_2 Adrenergic Receptor (β_2AR)

The human β_2AR is a member of the G-protein-linked seven-transmembrane domain receptor family. β_2ARs are of particular interest because the sequence of the human β_2AR gene (*ADRB2*) is highly variable, giving rise to a coding region with numerous polymorphisms (36,37). The human β_2AR is encoded by an intronless gene located on chromosome 5. Four amino acid polymorphisms have been reported within the *ADRB2* gene; all are single-base substitutions. The two common polymorphisms in the extracellular domain of the *ADRB2* gene, Arg16Gly and Gln27Glu, appear to have functional significance when exposed to exogenously administered β_2AR agonists. For example, in transfected Chinese hamster fibroblasts and in primary cultured smooth muscle cells expressing these variants, the Gly16 version of the receptor undergoes enhanced agonist-promoted downregulation of receptor number, as compared with the Arg16 form of the receptor. By contrast, Glu27

β_2AR is relatively resistant to such downregulation as compared with the Gln27 form of the receptor, but only when co-expressed with Arg16 (37,38). The third polymorphism in the intercellular domain, Thr164Ile, also has several functional effects, which include lower binding affinities for agonists and deficient coupling of the receptor to adenylate cyclase. Transgenic mice expressing Thr164Ile variant receptor targeted to the heart manifested impaired myocardial signaling and function (39).

β_2AR polymorphisms have been implicated in the pathogenesis of essential hypertension, both on the basis of evidence suggesting altered β_2-mediated vasodilatation (40–42) and on the basis of linkage studies (43). Some studies (44), but not all (45), have demonstrated the relationship between certain β_2AR polymorphic alleles and hypertension, presumably because the expression of these receptor forms exerts a vasodilatory influence on vascular smooth muscle. The risk appears to be greater for those possessing Gly16 and Glu27 alleles, the latter (Glu27 allele) having an odds ratio for occurrence of hypertension of 1.80 (44). Given the massive heterogeneity of hypertension, it is not surprising to find that β_2AR polymorphisms are responsible only for exerting a relatively small effect. Several studies have associated the Ile164 allele with heart failure (46). Indeed, individuals with the Ile164 receptor experienced an increased risk of either death or transplant compared with the Thr164 homozygotes. A subsequent study measured exercise capacity and showed substantially reduced exercise capacity in Ile164 allele carriers (47). Importantly, several studies have also demonstrated a relationship between *ADRB2* genotype and some measure of vascular relaxation in response to agonist infusion (41,42,48,49). In a study by Brodde et al. (50) of healthy subjects, the Ile164 allele carriers showed decreased responsiveness (heart rate and systolic time interval) to β_2AR agonist infusions as compared with Thr164 homozygotes. This suggests that the alternative alleles of the Ile/Thr164 polymorphism have physiologic effects even in the absence of a disease phenotype, such as heart failure. The clinical implications are that, in patients carrying the Thr164Ile β_2AR polymorphism (Ile164 allele), the therapeutic efficacy of such treatment with β_2AR agonists might initially be lower than in patients with the wild-type genotype (Thr/Thr). However, with ongoing treatment (and thus β_2AR desensitization), this disadvantage might disappear because desensitization in these patients is likely to be less than in wild-type β_2AR patients.

These polymorphisms have also been extensively evaluated in respiratory disease: these effects are discussed in detail in the relevant chapter 6 in this book.

Nitric Oxide Synthases

Nitric oxide (NO) is an important regulatory molecule involved in cardiovascular homeostasis, neuronal transmission, and immune defence. NO is synthesized from L-arginine by a family of three enzymes [nitric oxide synthases (NOS)] (51). NO is produced by the vascular endothelium under basal conditions, and its production is stimulated by a variety of receptor agonists and also by shear stress. It also acts locally to prevent platelet and leucocyte adhesion (52). NO dilates all types of blood vessels studied by stimulating soluble guanylyl cyclase and by increasing cyclic guanosine mono phosphate (GMP) in smooth muscle cells. NO released by endothelial cells acts as a major endogenous vasodilator, counterbalancing the vasoconstriction produced by the sympathetic nervous system, the renin-angiotensin system, and endothelin. Further, blockade of NO synthesis with inhibitory L-arginine analogs leads to significant peripheral vasoconstriction and, depending on the species studied, increases blood pressure (53).

Abnormal endothelial NOS activity could result from mutations in the coding sequence of the 26 exon endothelial cell eNOS (*NOS3*) gene located on chromosome 7.

The human *NOS3* gene exhibits significant interindividual variation. Studies have reported an association between the Glu298 allele of the Glu298Asp *NOS3* polymorphism and hypertension (54), coronary artery disease (55), myocardial infarction (56,57), and coronary spasm (58). However, further studies are required to determine how this amino acid substitution exerts its effects. The only study performed on the effect of variation in the *NOS3* gene on aortic stiffness failed to find any association between aortic stiffness and the Glu298Asp polymorphism, although it did confirm the higher frequency of the 298G allele in hypertensives, as compared with the controls (59). In this study, small differences in pulse wave velocity (PWV) were noted between different groups (GG and GT homozygotes had a higher PWV than the TT homozygotes), but these failed to reach statistical significance. Such small differences could be important, as a 4% difference in PWV would equate to an ~8% difference in aortic distensibility, which would be equivalent to aging ~10 years (60). This suggests that either larger numbers of subjects are required or a less variable measure of arterial stiffness may be needed. Indeed, it is possible that *NOS3* could modulate arterial phenotypes other than aortic PWV, such as wave reflection and stiffness in muscular arteries.

Recently, clinical and experimental studies have identified other proteins associated with the arterial stiffening process. The following paragraphs describe some of these matrix proteins and their associated polymorphisms that are involved in the arterial stiffening process and may thus be associated with increased cardiovascular risk.

ECM Proteins

Premature arterial stiffening has emerged as a key determinant of cardiovascular risk. The stiffness of the large arteries depends on a number of factors, including structural elements within the arterial wall (such as elastin and collagen), smooth muscle tone, and distending (mean arterial) pressure and also a variety of genetic influences. Elastin and collagen are the main extracellular matrix (ECM) proteins of the arterial wall. The breakdown of elastin, collagen, and other components of the cardiovascular matrix (e.g., gelatin) is mediated by enzymes, such as the elastases and matrix metalloproteinases (MMPs). In recent years, the focus has shifted to the genetic variation in these matrix proteins and enzymes owing to their involvement in atherogenesis and arterial wall remodeling.

Elastin (ELN)

Elastin is a critical autocrine factor that maintains vascular homeostasis through a combination of biomechanical support and biologic signaling. The structure and function of this protein may be altered either by defective synthesis or in response to physiological and pathological changes in the vessel wall. *ELN* is encoded by a single gene on human chromosome 7, whose transcription is influenced by a number of factors, such as insulin-like growth factor I.

Several lines of evidence support the view that disruption of arterial elastic fibres and intimal proliferation in the large elastic arteries results in a quantitative and/or qualitative modification of elastin during vascular development that is of pathogenetic importance (61,62). Molecular genetic studies on knockout mice (61,62), human genetic disorders (Supravalvular aortic stenosis, Williams syndrome, Marfan syndrome), and normotensive adults led to the identification of deletions, more subtle mutations, and several polymorphisms in the *ELN* gene (e.g., *Bgl*I, Ser422Gly), which disrupt the elastic fibers, leading to a narrowed lumen, which in turn affects the biomechanical properties of the arterial wall (63–68). Hanon *et al.*(68) examined the association between the Ser422Gly polymorphism and carotid arterial distensibility in 320 subjects without evidence of CVD and who had never been treated pharmacologically. The Ser422 allele (AA and AG genotypes) was found to be associated significantly with decreased distensibility of the carotid artery, as compared with the individuals with the GG genotype. Moreover, this relationship was evident even after adjustment for age and mean pressure, and it was more prominent in patients over 50 years of age. By contrast, no association was observed between these genotypes and arterial parameters at the radial artery. This may be because the carotid artery is an elastic artery with high amounts of elastin and collagen fibres, whereas the radial artery is a muscular artery composed principally of arterial smooth muscles.

Although several enzymes, such as serum elastase activity (SEA) and lysyl oxidase are involved in the degradation of elastin fibres and increased cardiovascular risk, to our knowledge there are no data to suggest that *ELN* gene polymorphisms influence levels of elastase activity or evidence for *ELN* variants that can be modulated by drugs.

Matrix Metalloproteinases

Matrix metalloproteinases (MMPs) are a family of enzymes involved in the process of normal development and growth and play a fundamental role in the degradation of the arterial wall (69). Under normal physiological conditions, the proteolytic activities of MMPs are precisely regulated at a variety of levels, including transcription, activation of the precursor zymogens, interaction with specific ECM components, and inhibition by endogenous inhibitors in the vascular wall, involving tissue inhibitors of metalloproteinases (TIMPs). Various cytokines, hormones, and growth factors, as well as shear stress and oxidative stress, are known to modulate these enzymes. Recent observations suggest that genetic diversity of expression of various members of the MMP family may contribute to the progression of CVDs (70). Increased expression of MMPs, as assessed by mRNA and protein levels, gelatinolytic activity, and decreased TIMP levels have been demonstrated in aneurysmal aortae (71). A 10-fold higher level of MMP9 expression is observed in aneurysm tissues than in normal aorta.

A total of 15 MMP genes have been identified (70). The polymorphisms that influence MMP gene expression and that are associated with susceptibility to coronary heart disease, aortic aneurysm, and age-related arterial stiffening are summarized in Table 2. These polymorphisms have an effect on transcription and may, consequently, play a role in the regulation of ECM proteolysis. Of all the MMPs, the *MMP9* (also known as gelatinase B) gene located on chromosome 20 (72) may be particularly important in arterial wall remodeling as it has been associated with adverse cardiovascular outcomes. Moreover, a recent study of the *MMP9* locus identified 10 sequence variants, four of which were in the promoter region, five in the coding region, and one in the 3′ untranslated sequence. The promoter polymorphisms are thought to be functional because they exhibit different transcriptional activities and they may consequently play a role in the regulation of ECM proteolysis. Interestingly, MMP9 concentration is also predictive of cardiovascular mortality in patients with coronary artery disease (73,74). Indeed, Blankenberg et al. (73) reported significantly higher circulating MMP9 levels in patients who had had a fatal cardiovascular event than in those who did not. Increased levels of MMPs have also been observed during the development and progression of atherosclerosis (75). However, the possible role of MMPs in hypertension remains confusing because both increased and decreased MMP levels have been reported (76–78). Nevertheless, recent in vivo studies demonstrated that MMP inhibitors could be used to prevent the degradation of elastic fibers following vascular injury and reduce the development of neointima formation.

Table 2 Matrix Metalloproteinase Gene Polymorphisms in Cardiovascular Conditions

Gene	Chromosome location	Polymorphism[a]	Frequency (%) in Caucasians	Disease studied	References
MMP2	16q21	C-1306**T**	17	Aneurysmal coronary artery disease	(189)[a]
MMP3	11q23.3	−1171/5A/**6A**	19	Aneurysmal coronary artery disease	(189)[a]
		−1612del/ins		Intracranial aneurysm	(190)
				Myocardial infarction	(191)
				Abdominal aortic aneurysm	(79)
				Common carotid geometry	(80)
				Age-related aortic stiffening	(82)
				Coronary atherosclerosis	(85)
				Coronary heart disease	(84)
					(87)
MMP9	20q11.2-q13.1	C-1562**T**	19	Coronary atherosclerosis	(72)[a]
				Intracranial aneurysm	(191)
				Aneurysmal coronary artery disease	(189)
		R-279**Q**	35	Coronary artery disease	(73)
				Intracranial aneurysm	(192)
				Abdominal aortic aneurysm	(193)
					(80)
MMP12	11q22.2-22.3	A-82**G**	10	Aneurysmal coronary artery disease	(189)[a]
				Coronary atherosclerosis	(194)

[a]Frequency of the allele in bold type.

A functional 5A/6A polymorphism has also been described in the promoter of the *MMP3* (Stromelysin-1) gene located on chromosome 11. MMP3 levels degrade ECM and are associated with atherogenesis and plaque rupture. Interestingly, at the clinical level, both alleles have been associated with coronary events and aortic aneurysms (79,80). By contrast, the 6A allele has been claimed to be associated with increased carotid intima media thickness, progression of coronary artery disease in post-bypass patients, and elastic properties of large arteries (81–85). Individuals homozygous for the 6A allele exhibited greater progression of angiographically evident disease than those with a 5A5A genotype (84). In the study by Medley et al. (85) the 5A6A heterozygous genotype was found to be associated with large artery stiffness in older but not in younger individuals at low cardiovascular risk. Moreover, individuals homozygous for the 5A allele exhibited a fourfold higher level of *MMP3* gene expression in dermal biopsies, as compared with subjects who were heterozygous. Because large artery stiffness is the primary cause of isolated systolic hypertension, the clinical implications of this study includes a predisposition to this condition in individuals homozygous for the *MMP3* promoter polymorphism.

In older populations, where isolated systolic hypertension is more common, treatment with long-term ACE inhibitors and calcium antagonists results in some pressure-independent decreases in arterial stiffness [review by Dart et al. in Ref. (86)]. In the REGRESS study (87), patients with 5A6A and 6A6A genotypes on medication (statins) experienced fewer clinical events than the placebo group. The LOCAT study also presented similar findings (88). These results suggest that stromelysin gene promoter polymorphisms confer a genotype-specific response to medication.

Although statins decrease the secretion of MMPs in experimental models, their role in reducing MMPs in vivo is unclear. The only data from aneurysm patients, indicated a reduction in both the total and active MMP levels with statin treatment (89). MMP inhibitors, such as marimastat, reduced MMP2 activity in an in vitro model (90), but the role of other MMP inhibitors and antihypertensive therapy in reducing MMP levels is controversial. However, antihypertensive treatment with calcium channel blockers significantly increased plasma concentrations of active MMP9 (76) and collagen metabolism (92,91).

Fibrillin1

Fibrillin1 (*FBN1*) (encoded by the *FBN1* gene on chromosome 15 and known to be involved in Marfan syndrome) is the major component of 10–12-nm microfibrils. *FBN1* plays a role in tropoelastin deposition and elastic fiber formation, in addition to possessing both load-bearing and anchoring functions within the arterial wall. There is some evidence that subtle and relatively frequent abnormalities of *FBN1* function might contribute to arterial disease, albeit to a lesser exent than the rarer pathological mutations do in Marfan syndrome. Recently, a tandem nucleotide repeat polymorphism has been identified in the *FBN1* gene. Some alleles have been found to be associated with systemic sclerosis (93) with pulse pressure in healthy subjects (94) and most recently with increased arterial stiffness in coronary artery disease patients (95). Medley et al. (95) showed that patients with the 2-3 genotype of the TAAAA repeat tended to have stiffer arteries, higher pulse pressure, and more severe coronary artery disease than patients with other genotypes (2-2 or 2-4). This suggests that the 2-3 genotype in the *FBN1* gene may be an important factor contributing to risk associated with pulse pressure and large artery stiffening.

Genetic variations in the proteins constituting the aortic wall and regulating the turnover of the ECM are likely to influence elastic properties and therefore are good candidates for involvement in determining large artery stiffness. Subjects in future studies, not just in

Marfan syndrome but also in other groups, such as coronary artery disease, should be genotyped to investigate whether the variable response to beta blockade observed in Marfan syndrome can be predicted by genotype and whether alternative drugs should be used to protect the aorta in some patients.

Lipid Pathway

Elevated cholesterol and other dyslipidemias are major risk factors for atherosclerotic diseases and CVDs. Several polymorphisms in lipid pathways (Fig. 2), involving apolipoproteins A-I and IV, B, E, C-II and III, cholesteryl ester transfer protein (CETP), and others have been associated with cardiovascular conditions. The following section describes apolipoprotein E (ApoE) and CETP polymorphisms.

Apolipoprotein E (ApoE)

The gene that is most comprehensively studied in this pathway is that encoding ApoE on chromosome 19. ApoE is synthesized in the liver and intestine and is found in association with triglyceride-rich lipoproteins. Polymorphism in the *APOE* gene determines the greatest fraction (around 5%) of the population variance in low-density lipoprotein (LDL) cholesterol of the known gene variants related to lipoprotein metabolism. In humans, there are three common alleles, designated *E2*, *E3*, *E4*, that give rise to three homozygous—22,33,44—and three heterozygous genotypes—32,42,34. Corbo et al. (96) found that the *E3* allele was the most frequent in all human populations tested and that its frequency was always negatively correlated with that of *E4*. The *E4* allele is also one of the few polymorphisms that has repeatedly been shown to be a good predictor of CVD/myocardial infarction (97–99) and is thus potentially an important genetic marker for risk stratification. The most likely explanation for the increased risk associated with the *E4* allele is that these individuals have a preponderance of small dense LDLs, which are prone to oxidation.

The *APOE* gene variants also differ with respect to response to statin therapy: Individuals with an *E4* allele tend to have a lesser response, and those with the *E2* allele a

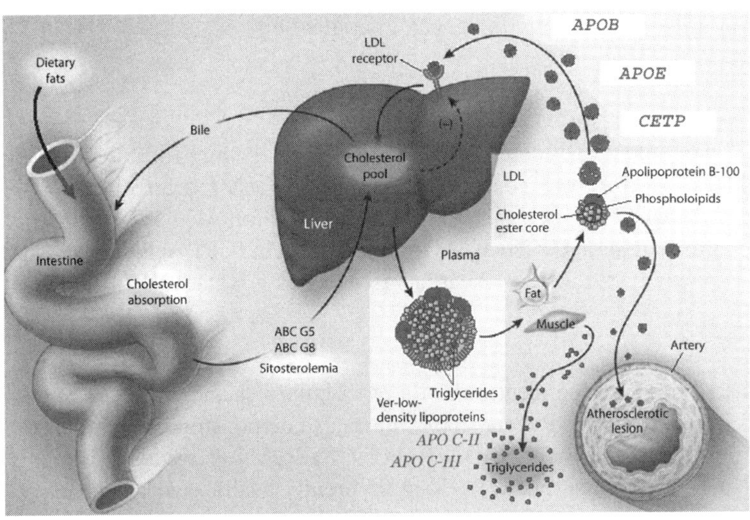

Figure 2 Genetic polymorphisms in the lipid pathway.

greater response to statins. Importantly, in the 4S study, the risk of death or a major coronary event in survivors of myocardial infarction was related to the APOE genotype. The *E4* allele carriers had nearly a twofold increased risk of dying in the follow-up period, compared with other patients. Also, *E4* allele-bearing patients on statins benefited more than those without the *E4* allele (100). APOE genotypes that have been shown to influence plasma cholesterol level had, however, no effect on the hypolipidemic efficacy of colestipol (101). Reports of response to fibrates in relation to the *APOE* gene variation are conflicting (102,103). With regard to HMG Co-A reductase, there have been no reports of variants of the gene itself that influence the efficacy of the treatment.

Cholesterol Ester Transfer Protein (CETP)

CETP is involved in reverse cholesterol transport, and several polymorphisms with a functional impact on plasma high-density lipoprotein (HDL) cholesterol and triglycerides have been identified (104). CETP mediates the transfer of neutral lipids between lipoproteins and plays a central role in HDL metabolism. The *B2* allele of the *Taq*IB polymorphism of the *CETP* gene located on chromosome 16, a silent base change in the nucleotide 277 of the first intron, is associated with decreased CETP activity and increased HDL concentration (105,106). Kuivenhoven et al. (105) reported a significant genotype-dependent association of the *CETP Taq*IB polymorphism with the progression of coronary atherosclerosis in the placebo group, as compared with the treatment group: carriers of the B1B1 genotype had the highest CETP and the lowest HDL concentrations and the fastest progression of atherosclerosis. Ordovas et al. (106) found the CETP activity to be decreased in *B2* allele carriers. In addition to the *Taq*IB polymorphism, several other *CETP* SNPs have also been associated with interindividual variation in CETP plasma and HDL cholesterol levels and the risk of CVD (107–109).

Interestingly, polymorphisms in the *CETP* gene have been shown to influence the effectiveness of hypolipidemic drugs and dietary intervention. In the REGRESS study, statin therapy slowed the progression of coronary atherosclerosis in the B1B1 *CETP Taq*IB carriers but not in the B2B2 carriers (105). However, in the WOSCOPS trial this association was not observed. Nevertheless, the B1B1 *CETP Taq*IB homozygotes have also been shown to serve as a marker of lipoprotein response to dietary intervention (110,111). These results suggest that polymorphisms in the *CETP* gene could influence the effects of therapy (diet or statins) in the general population.

Inflammation

Inflammation is a key component of atherosclerosis, and genes coding for inflammatory proteins and cytokines are therefore good candidates for coronary heart disease risk. Inflammation is characterized by a local reaction, which may be followed by activation of systemic acute phase reactant proteins [such as C-reactive protein (CRP) and interleukin6 (IL6)], which are associated with increased cardiovascular risk.

C-Reactive Protein (CRP)

CRP has emerged as a strong, independent predictor of vascular risk and is associated with endothelial dysfunction (112–116). Recent studies have also demonstrated a relationship between increased pulse pressure, PWV, and CRP (117,118). Recently, we demonstrated a link between CRP and pulse pressure and PWV in apparently healthy individuals (119). Some common polymorphisms (−717G>A and +1441C>T) have been identified in the chromosome 1-located *CRP* gene. In the Brull et al. (120) study, the +1444T allele was associated significantly with the elevated CRP levels, even after adjustments for other confounding factors. In healthy subjects, the +1444TT homozygotes had higher CRP levels than +1444C allele carriers, both at baseline and after exercise. In coronary artery bypass graft (CABG) patients, genotype did not influence the baseline CRP, although +1444TT homozygotes had raised CRP levels compared with the +1444C allele carriers. This result is in keeping with the hypothesis that this variant increases susceptibility to vascular disease. However, if the CRP level is a marker for, rather than a mediator of, atherosclerosis, then future studies of this polymorphisms will be required to establish the genotype-specific risk thresholds for CRP in the prediction of CHD risk.

Interleukin6 (IL6)

IL6 is a pleiotropic cytokine involved in the regulation of the acute phase response. Elevated levels of IL6 are associated with the development and severity of coronary disease (121,122). Two common polymorphisms (−174 G>C and −572 G>C) have been identified in the promoter region of the *IL6* gene located on chromosome 22. The role of IL6 in determining the pathogenesis of aneurysmal disease is evidenced by the finding that −174 C allele carriers have increased IL6 levels and display increased mortality with a relative risk of 2.95 over a 5-year follow-up period (123). In patients with CABG, 6 hours after the procedure, peak IL6 levels rose to a significantly higher level in patients with the −572C allele (CC and CG genotypes) than in those with the −572GG genotype (124). In the same cohort, the −174CC homozygotes had significantly elevated IL6 levels, when compared with −174G allele carriers. These effects were significant even after adjustment for other variables. Two other studies also demonstrated the link between the −174C allele and higher CHD mortality (125,126). In the WOSCOPS study, subjects with the −174CC genotype and on medication exhibited a reduced risk of coronary heart diseases with pravastatin treatment (127). These results strongly support the role of the genotype not just with plasma IL6 levels in an acute inflammatory situation but also with mortality.

Coagulation Factors VII and V

The blood clotting system requires precise control of factors within and outside the coagulation cascade to prevent fatal bleeding or unwanted thrombosis. One common coding sequence polymorphism (Arg/Gln353) has been found in the coagulation factor VII (*F7*) gene. Plasma levels of factor VII vary significantly in the general population, are associated with cardiovascular risk, and are known to be influenced by a number of different environmental factors, including sex, age, and cholesterol and triglyceride levels. The Gln variant, which occurs at a frequency of ~10% in various populations, is associated with a 20% to 25% reduction in the level of plasma factor VII activity as a result of impaired secretion (128). This relatively high frequency is suggestive of a balanced polymorphism and could indicate that the Gln variant confers some benefit, for example, protection against thrombosis, myocardial infarction, or arterial disease (129).

Another missense polymorphism of hemostatic significance is factor V Leiden. Factor V (*F5*) Leiden increases the risk of myocardial infarction, stroke, and venous thrombosis in men (130), and in a subgroup of patients, thrombosis is associated with coinheritance of gene mutations that modify the factor V Leiden phenotype (131). The variant, which underlies the phenomenon of activated protein C resistance, results from the substitution of Arg506 by Gln in coagulation factor V (*F5*). Factor Va serves as a cofactor in the activation of prothrombin by factor Xa, and the factor V Leiden variant is relatively resistant to activated protein C-mediated inactivation. Between 1% and 7% of the Caucasian population possess the factor V Leiden mutation (132), which may therefore be regarded as a fairly frequent polymorphism with phenotypic effect. Because the factor V Leiden mutation is also associated with a relative risk of ~6.0 for venous thrombosis, this also represents a polymorphism with clinical effect. Why is this factor V variant so common? Its high frequency in the general population suggests that it confers, or has conferred, some selective advantage on its bearers. Dahlbäck (132) speculated that a slight hypercoagulable state associated with possession of the factor V Leiden variant might have been advantageous in certain situations, such as traumatic injury and childbirth. Consistent with this postulate, carriers of the factor V Leiden variant have a significantly reduced risk of bleeding during surgery (133) and childbirth (134), despite a higher than normal risk of fetal loss (135).

CYP450 System

The cytochromes are a family of proteins (enzymes) that play a key role in the oxidative metabolism of drugs (e.g., β-blockers, antihypertensives, antiarrhythmics, monoamine oxidase inhibitors, and so on). Approximately 70% of the human liver CYPs are accounted for by CYP1A2, CYP2A6, CYP2B6, CYP2C, CYP2D6, CYP2E1, and CYP3A (136). CYP2D6 is of particular clinical importance both because a number of commonly prescribed drugs are substrates of this enzyme and also due to interindividual and ethnic differences in its ability to perform its role in drug metabolism. In addition, *CYP2D6* polymorphism has been extensively studied and associated with metabolism of debrisoquine and sparteine. The *CYP2D6* gene on chromosome 22 that encodes this enzyme is highly polymorphic and more than 50 allelic variants have been identified, although many of these occur in a very small number of individuals. Although most of these variants are polymorphic, these do not have any direct effect on the expression or activity of the enzyme they encode. Nonetheless, these variants partition the population into three phenotypes in terms of their ability to metabolize drugs to either active or inactive metabolites: extensive metabolizers (EM), poor metabolizers (PM), and ultrarapid metabolizers (URM), as shown in Figure 3. Individuals capable of efficient drug metabolism are termed EM, whereas individuals with a deficiency in metabolism, typically resulting from the mutation or deletion of both alleles of the gene, are termed PM. Conversely, over-expression due to *CYP2D6* gene amplification results in URM. The prevalence of genetic variants and their clinical impact varies substantially in the three groups across all racial and population groups. For example, approximately 5% to 10% of the Caucasians and 2% to 3% of the black Americans, and 1% of the Asians are PMs of CYP2D6 (137,138).

From the alleles identified, *CYP2D6*4* is the most common allele among PMs. This allele is associated with a splice site mutation and as a consequence does not produce a functional enzyme (139). In addition, the *CYP2D6*3* allele, which contains a frameshift mutation, also produces a PM phenotype. The *CYP2D*5* allele, which is a complete gene mutation, also produces this PM phenotype. The earliest evidence for polymorphic expression of *CYP2D6* was observed in the clinical trials of antihypertensive treatment debrisoquine. Liver biopsy studies established that those patients who were PMs of debrisoquine had a deficiency in CYP450 mono-oxygenase activity resulting from ineffective binding of substrate to the enzyme (140). Because the *CYP2D6* polymorphisms are recessive traits, the heterozygous individuals with one active and one mutant allele manifest metabolism of the substrate, which does not differ overtly from a person of normal phenotype. However, these heterozygous individuals may display a slightly increased metabolic rate that points to a deficiency of, or a reduction in, metabolic capacity. These

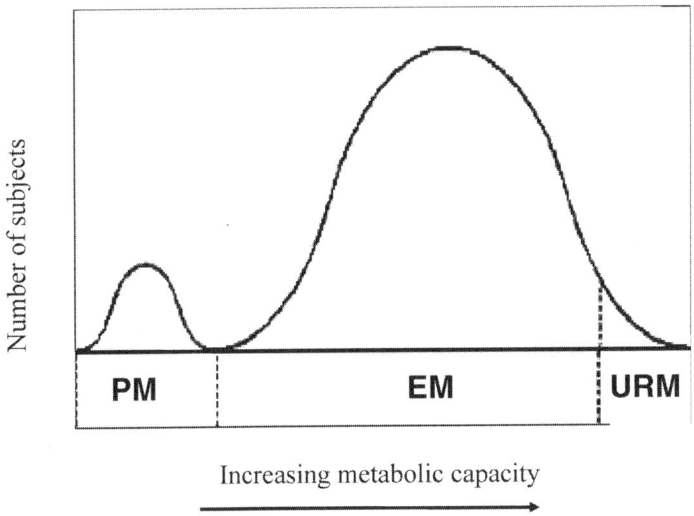

Figure 3 Cytochrome P450 enzyme showing polymorphic distribution. *Abbreviations*: PM, poor metabolizers; EM, extensive metabolizers; URM, ultra rapid metabolizers.

individuals are the EMs and represent the great majority of the population. URMs, on the other hand, occur as a result of the duplication of the *CYP2D6*2* allele. The enzyme produced by the *CYP2D6*2* allele is similar to that produced by the *CYP2D6*1* allele. However, certain individuals may inherit 2, 3, 4, 5, or as many as 13 gene copies arranged in tandem and thus produce proportionally higher amounts of the enzyme (141). The other SNPs detected are numbered as indicated in the standardized *CYP2D6* nomenclature (142).

As mentioned previously, a number of drugs are metabolized by these enzymes, and it is possible that the *CYP2D6*-related genotype interacts with target polymorphisms (e.g., beta-adrenergic receptor polymorphisms) and polymorphisms in genes involved in cardiovascular pathophysiology (e.g., *ACE* I/D polymorphism) to influence overall response to beta-blockers. One study found that the clearance of the R(+) enantiomer of carvedilol was 66% lower, and the area under the concentration-versus-time curve was 156% higher among PMs than EMs (143). *CYP2D6* allelic variants also associated with adverse drug reactions through various mechanisms (see the chapter on adverse drug reactions) (144,145). *CYP2D6* PMs manifest reduced clearance of the antianginal drug perhexilene, which accumulates in such organs as liver and nerves, causing hepatotoxicity and peripheral neuropathy (146). Although tremendous progress has been made in elucidating the molecular basis of variation in P450 enzyme expression and activity, the adverse effect in PMs probably represents the greatest impact of *CYP2D6* polymorphic variant observed in clinical practice.

GENETIC POLYMORPHISMS AND RESPONSE TO DRUGS

It is now commonly accepted that individual drug response is determined by both genetic and nongenetic factors. Polymorphisms may influence drug response in three ways, through (*i*) pharmacokinetic interactions (e.g., caused by the polymorphisms in the CYP450 system), (*ii*) pharmacodynamic gene–drug interactions (e.g., that involve gene products expressed as receptors, which are relevant to the pharmacodynamics of drugs such as β-adrenergic receptor antagonists), and (*iii*) genes that are in the causal pathway of disease and are able to modify the effect of drugs, such as APOE (147). Therefore, identifying genetic variants that discriminate between responders and nonresponders and using these to ascertain which patients are likely to be susceptible to adverse drug reactions promises to revolutionalize drug therapy. In the following section, we discuss some polymorphisms that influence individual responses to various cardiovascular drugs.

Renin–Angiotensin System Drugs (ACE Inhibitors)

The renin–angiotensin system (RAS) has an important role in cardiovascular health and disease, and polymorphisms of the ACE, AGT, angiotensin-II type 1 receptor (*AGTR1*), and *CYP11B2* genes have been targeted for pharmacological research owing to the genetic variation they manifest (refer to previous section). The possibility that variation in these genes may alter drug response is therefore of considerable interest. ACE inhibitors and AT_1R blockers have proved efficacious in managing CVDs, such as heart failure, myocardial infarction, hypertension, vascular disease, and nephropathy.

As mentioned earlier, the ACE *D* allele has been associated with higher circulating and tissue-activity levels and greater AGTR1 expression than the I allele (9,148–150). Similarly, hypertensive patients on ACE inhibitors and carrying the DD genotype showed significant reductions in blood pressure and plasma angiotensin II levels (151,152). Left ventricular hypertrophy and endothelial function also improved in individuals bearing the DD genotype, in comparison with those with the II genotype (29,153). By contrast, other reports showing the pharmacogenetic basis of ACE inhibitors and *ACE* genotypes were inconsistent (18,150). This suggests that genetic mechanisms are not always disease-specific. Disparities in results may be due to differences in the therapeutic agents used, the duration of drug exposure, or the dose administered. In addition, differences in the study populations may also have influenced the results, particularly because the RAS polymorphisms are known to differ in frequency between racial groups. The other possible explanation for these conflicting data is that other genetic variants in the RAS, including *AGT* and *AGTR1* polymorphisms, interact with the *ACE* I/D polymorphism to influence drug response (Fig. 1).

The *AGT* gene Met235Thr polymorphism also affects RAS activity and drug responses. The 235Thr allele has been found to be associated with higher AGT levels and enhanced blood pressure response to ACE inhibitors (14,18,154). In the Schunkert et al. (154) study, the systolic and diastolic blood pressures were higher, and the likelihood of using two or more antihypertensive medications was 2.1 times higher, with the 235Thr allele.

The vascular AGTR1 mediates many detrimental effects of angiotensin II, including vasoconstriction, cardiac remodeling, and aldosterone secretion. The 1166C allele of the gene encoding *AGTR1* A1166C polymorphism has also been associated with increased arterial responsiveness to angiotensin II in ischemic heart disease and increased arterial stiffness in hypertensives (155–158). Benetos et al. (157) showed that the 1166C allele was associated with a greater response to ACE inhibitor therapy. The carriers of the C allele manifested a threefold reduction in carotid to femoral PWV (a measure of aortic stiffness) when given perindopril as compared with the AA homozygotes. The *AGTR1* gene was also found to be predictive of the blood pressure response to a single dose of losartan, with significantly greater reductions in mean arterial pressure in the 1166C allele carriers than in the 1166A homozygotes (159). However, a study of hypertensives did not reveal any association between this polymorphism and blood pressure responses to ACE inhibition (18).

The aldosterone synthase (*CYP11B2*) gene polymorphism C-344T has also been associated with responsiveness to ACE inhibition (160). Following treatment, the left ventricular ejection fraction improved in patients who harbored the 344C allele to a greater extent than those with the 344T allele.

RAS polymorphisms associated with adverse reactions to ACE inhibitors: In general, ACE inhibitors are well tolerated in young and older adults and improve a variety of cardiovascular functions. However, the RAS polymorphisms have been associated with adverse reactions, such as the "ACE inhibitor-related cough" and other effects (e.g., angioedema). The II genotype has been associated with increased susceptibility to the development of cough during the treatment period (161). After 4 weeks of therapy, the threshold of cough was significantly reduced for individuals bearing the II genotype but not in individuals bearing the DD genotype. The reported incidence of dry cough is variable, and the reason why ACE inhibitors cause coughing in only certain individuals is still unclear. However, the appearance of this cough in association with ACE inhibitors is thought to be related to the activity of the bradykinin B2 (*BDKRB2*) receptor gene (162), because treatment with these agents increases the concentration of bradykinin. This in turn may lead to the activation of proinflammatory peptides (e.g., prostaglandins) and to the local release of histamine in airways, which is responsible for the adverse reaction, such as cough, in some patients. It has also been speculated that these adverse effects are genetically predetermined: in particular, involving variants of the genes encoding *ACE*, *chymase* and bradykinin B2 receptor (*BDKRB2*). Interestingly, a recent study supports this view; a significant association has been observed between the TT genotype and T allele of the -38C/T polymorphism in the bradykinin B2 (*BDKRB2*) gene and ACE inhibitor-related cough in patients with a history of cough, compared with cough-free subjects receiving ACE inhibitors.

Much of the data on RAS polymorphisms and drug response indicates that a genotypic test may predict the therapeutic efficacy of ACE inhibitors. However, inconsistencies in the reported data means that the situation remains unclear at present. These discordant results are not surprising in view of the complex signaling pathway of RAS as shown in Figure 1.

β-Adrenoreceptor Blocking Drugs (β-Blockers)

β-Blockers are extensively used in cardiovascular conditions, such as heart failure and hypertension. Polymorphisms in the RAS genes, and the α and β-ARs have been assessed for their impact on β-blocker response. The best example of the pharmacogenetic interaction between β-blockers and the *ACE* I/D polymorphism is provided by patients with heart failure. McNamara et al. (31) studied the influence of *ACE* I/D polymorphism in heart failure and showed reduced survival in patients carrying the *D* allele. The *D* allele has previously been suggested to be deleterious in conditions, such as myocardial infarction, left ventricular hypertrophy, and hypertrophic cardiomyopathy (22,163). β-Blocker treatment abolished the deleterious effects on heart-failure prognosis associated with the *D* allele, whereas the adverse impact was increased in patients who were not on β-blockers at the time of entry into the trial (31). This suggested a possible pharmacogenetic interaction between *ACE* I/D polymorphism and β-blocker therapy. However, the mechanisms underlying this remain unclear, and these findings have not, as yet, been replicated in other studies. It nevertheless appears that increased angiotensin II concentrations associated with the D allele may cause increased activation of the sympathetic nervous system and that patients with the D allele may thus derive greater benefit from pharmacological intervention to decrease sympathetic nervous system activity (e.g., β-blocker therapy).

The response to β-agonists has also been reported to be influenced by the β_1- and β_2AR gene polymorphisms. Homozygosity for the Arg389 genotype of the β_1-adrenergic receptor (*ADRB1*) gene was shown to be associated with hypertension and a higher double product (blood pressure × heart rate) than patients with at least one 389Gly allele (148,164). However, whether the antihypertensive effect of β-blocker therapy is influenced by these polymorphisms is less certain. The one study of Arg389Gly polymorphism and its possible effect on response to β-blockade (atenolol and bisoprolol) in hypertensive patients reported that both heart rate and blood pressure fell by a similar amount irrespective of genotype after four weeks of β-blocker treatment (165). The other well-studied drug receptor is the β_2AR, and three polymorphisms (Arg16Gly, Gln27Glu, Thr164Ile) in the *ADRB2* gene have been associated with hypertension, heart failure, and also asthma and other respiratory phenotypes. The Gly16 allele imparts attenuated vasodilatory responses to catecholamines (42) and is also a major determinant of β_2-agonist bronchodilator response (166,167). As discussed previously, the 164Ile allele of the β_2AR has been shown to affect the clinical outcome in heart failure patients (46). The increased risk of death and/or cardiac transplant was estimated to be almost fivefold in patients with the 164Ile allele. β-Blocker treatment did not influence the risk associated with this polymorphism. The other two polymorphisms, Arg16Gly and Gln27Glu, did not influence the clinical outcome in these patients.

Polymorphisms in the gene coding for the CYP2D6 enzyme, which catalyzes the metabolism of β-blockers, such as metoprolol, carvedilol, timolol, and propanolol, may also affect β-blocker response. It is possible that the *CYP2D6*-related genotype interacts with drug target polymorphisms (e.g., β-AR polymorphisms) and polymorphisms in genes involved in cardiovascular pathophysiology (e.g., *ACE* I/D polymorphism) to influence the overall response to β-blockers.

β-AR polymorphisms associated with adverse reactions to β-blockers: Although β-blockers are very effective agents in the treatment of heart failure and hypertension, they are also associated with several adverse effects, particularly fatigue, slow heart rate, coldness of the extremities, sleep disturbances, shortness of breath, dizziness, and so on. It is not known whether any polymorphic alleles or a particular genotype of the β-AR (*ADRB*) gene influence these adverse effects. As mentioned previously, however, the *CYP2D6* genotype might be involved because the P450 enzyme metabolizes these agents.

Lipid-Lowering Drugs (Statins, Fibrates)

Hydroxymethylglutaryl coenzyme-A (HMGCoA) reductase inhibitors, better known as "statins," are the most potent lipid-lowering agents, consistently documented to prevent or reduce cardiovascular events in primary and secondary prevention (168–170). The therapeutic potential of this type of drug is probably far greater than previously anticipated (171). Many of the nonlipid lowering effects of statins could be of major relevance to a variety of disease processes. For example, statins enhance nitric oxide production and improve endothelial function, display anti-inflammatory potency, inhibit integrins, and lower circulating adhesion molecules (172,173). As with statins, fibrates have also been shown to reduce coronary risk (LOCAT study); the beneficial nonlipid effects with respect to atherosclerotic prevention include antithrombotic effects (decrease in fibrinogen and PAI1), anti-inflammatory activity (inhibition of TNF-α-induced endothelial expression of VCAM-1 and IL6), and decrease in plasma uric acid (174).

A number of studies of candidate genes involved in the lipid pathway have identified genetic polymorphisms influencing the clinical response to statins, not only on LDL plasma levels but also in terms of lipid-lowering outcomes and/or clinical events (Table 3).

Table 3 Examples of Genetic Polymorphisms Affecting Responses to Therapeutic Agents

Gene/gene product	Medication	Drug effect associated with polymorphism	References
Angiotensin-converting enzyme (*ACE*)	ACE inhibitors	Left ventricular mass reduction	(150)
		Blood pressure reduction	(152,196)
		Endothelial function improvement	(196)
		Arterial stiffness	(153)
		Survival after cardiac transplantation	(29)
		Renal protection	(31)
		ACE inhibitor-related cough	(197)
			(161)
Angiotensinogen (*AGT*)	ACE inhibitors	Blood pressure reduction	(18)
Bradykinin B2 receptor (*BDKRB2*)	ACE inhibitors	ACE inhibitor-induced cough	(198)
β_2-Adrenergic receptor (*ADRB2*)	β_2-Agonists	Cardiovascular effects (increased heart rate, cardiac index, peripheral vasodilation)	(41) (199)
		Susceptibility to agonist-induced desensitization	(48)
		Bronchodilation	(42)
			(200)
			(46)
Angiotensin-converting enzyme (*ACE*)	Statins	Lipid changes (reductions in total cholesterol, LDL cholesterol, increase HDL and APOB concentrations)	(183) (201)
Apolipoprotein E (*APOE*)		Progression/regression of atherosclerotic lesions, decrease in coronary artery diameter, death	(177) (176)
Choslesteryl ester transfer protein (*CETP*)			(105)
			(100)
			(106)
Stromelysin-1 (*MMP3*)	Statins	Cardiovascular events reduction (death, myocardial infarction, stroke, angina)	(87)
		Decreased risk of repeated angioplasty	
Prothrombin (*F2*)	Oral contraceptives	Increased risk of deep vein and cerebral vein thrombosis	(184)
Factor V (*F5*)			

Abbreviations: LDL, low-density lipoproteins; HDL, high-density lipoproteins.

Although a number of variants have been identified, this section deals with polymorphisms (e.g., APOE and CETP) associated with lipid-lowering therapy. In addition, the pharmacogenetic interaction of statins with *ACE I/D* (175) and MMP3 (84) is also discussed.

Despite a majority of publications describing a cholesterol reduction in APO *E4* carriers (105,106,176–178), there are some contradictory reports (100,102) on the effects of APOE polymorphism on the efficacy of hypolipidemic drugs. *APOE* genotype probably plays a key role in the LDL cholesterol-lowering response to statins. As discussed earlier, in the 4S study, the risk of death or coronary event in survivors of myocardial infarction was related to the APOE genotype (100). Among patients who received placebo and who had at least one APO *E4* allele, the relative risk of death from all causes was 1.9. The detrimental impact of the *E4* allele was not evident among patients who received simvastatin. From the literature, it is evident that APO *E4* allele is also associated with an enhanced response (in terms of LDL reduction) to dietary intervention but a reduced response to statin-induced LDL cholesterol-lowering. This modest effect of LDL cholesterol reduction in response to statins seen in APO *E4* individuals may actually be due to the low HMGCo-A reductase activity itself (179).

CETP provides another example of a pharmacogenetic intervention interacting with the genotype to bring about lipid-lowering. CETP plays a key role in distributing cholesteryl esters among HDLs, LDLs, and very low-density lipoproteins (VLDLs). As mentioned previously, one variant in the *CETP* gene is referred to as *B1* and its absence as *B2*. The *B2* allele of the *Taq*IB polymorphism has been shown to be associated with decreased CETP activity, increased HDL cholesterol, and faster progression of coronary atherosclerosis (105). However, there was no difference in plasma lipoprotein response to statins between the genotypes (B1B1, B1B2, B2B2). Moreover, B2B2 carriers with low CETP and high HDL levels did not respond to therapy in terms of disease regression. The pravastatin-treated patients with a B2B2 genotype derived no benefit from the treatment, as measured by changes in mean coronary artery lumen, whereas B1B1 genotype-treated patients had significantly less atherosclerotic progression than the placebo group. The WOSCOPS study also did not find any interaction between *CETP* genotype and statin therapy (180). However, untreated patients with angiographic coronary artery disease who carried the *B2* allele had higher rates of death/nonfatal myocardial infarction over 2.4 years follow-up (181). Statin therapy was associated with greater benefit in these high-risk *B2* carriers than in the B1B1 homozygotes. Although both *APOE* and *CETP* variants are promising as drug targets, additional clarification of risk and pharmacogenetic associations is needed.

From this literature, it is clear that the response to statins is not based on lipid levels but rather upon genotypes. These studies have identified genetic subgroups of placebo-treated patients with ischemic heart disease who had an increased risk of major coronary events. In general, treatment abolished the harmful effects associated with the genetic variant. The evidence is based on clinical outcome data. Therefore, future large-scale population studies are required to complement the results from the clinical trials and small-scale selected population cohorts.

It has also been demonstrated that statins may reduce ACE activity (175). However, the data regarding the influence of the *ACE* I/D polymorphism on the effectiveness of statins are controversial (182,183). In the LCAS study, subjects with the DD genotype displayed the strongest reduction of coronary atherosclerosis with statin therapy, whereas in the REGRESS trial, statins reduced coronary atherosclerosis less strongly in DD than ID or II genotypes. A CARE substudy focused upon whether the glycoprotein IIIa (ITGB3) PI^{A1A2} and *ACE* I/D polymorphisms were associated with fatal coronary events or non-fatal myocardial infarction (183). In this study, the greatest benefit of pravastatin treatment occurred in patients with a glycoprotein IIIa PI^{A1A2} genotype who also carried at least one *D* allele of the *ACE* gene.

A functional polymorphism in the stromelysin-1 (*MMP3*) gene (5A/6A) has been described (84). Evidence suggests that stromelysin activity is important in connective tissue remodeling associated with atherogenesis and plaque rupture. In this study, patients homozygous for the *6A* allele displayed greater progression of angiographic disease than those with other genotypes. de Maat et al. (87) in their REGRESS study, investigated the influence of 5A/6A polymorphism on statins and showed no differences in prognostic baseline characteristics, disease severity, or lipid values among the three genotypic groups (5A5A, 5A6A, 6A6A). But, pravastatin therapy reduced clinical events most effectively among the *6A* allele carriers (5A6A or 6A6A genotypes). Moreover, these beneficial changes were independent of the effects of pravastatin on lipid levels, raising the possibility that this agent exerts a pleiotropic effect not merely on stromelysin expression or activity. Similar findings were observed in the LOCAT study (88). These results indicate that the stromelysin-1 gene promoter polymorphism confers a genotype-specific response to statins.

Although statins decrease the secretion of MMPs in vitro models, their role in reducing MMPs in vivo is unclear. The only data from aneurysm patients demonstrated a reduction in both total and active MMP levels in the tissue with statins (89). To our knowledge, there are no reports of variants in other MMPs, such as *MMP2*, *9*, or *12*, that could be modulated by drugs. Should this be the case, then such treatment may provide new ways to manipulate and target arterial wall remodeling in specific arterial beds in individual patients.

Polymorphisms in the lipid pathway associated with adverse reactions to statins: In general, HMGCo-A reductase inhibitors are well tolerated, although in a minority of patients severe adverse effects, such as myopathy or rhabdomyolysis, may develop. The incidence of these potentially life-threatening side effects increases with (*i*) coadministration of drugs that are metabolized via the same pharmacokinetic pathways and (*ii*) high-dose statin therapy (e.g., dementia).

Other Drugs

Antiplatelet (e.g., aspirin) and anticoagulant (e.g., warfarin) agents are commonly used to prevent and treat cardiovascular thrombolic events. Several genetic polymorphisms have been identified in the coagulation *F5* and *F7* genes. The G1691A variant in the *F5* gene and the G20210A variant in the prothrombin (*F2*) gene are established risk factors for venous thrombosis. In women who carried the prothrombin variant and were on oral contraceptives, the OR rose from 10.2 to 149. The relative risk was sixfold higher for prothrombin A20210 variant and ninefold higher for *F5* A1691 carriers (184) in deep vein thrombosis patients. There is also evidence that the *F5* genotype is directly correlated with prothrombotic phenotype and anticoagulant/antiplatelet treatment. However, the treatment that is currently available is not ideal, in that warfarin requires regular monitoring and lowers natural anticoagulant levels and also procoagulant factors. This is likely to change soon with the introduction of orally active direct thrombin inhibitors, such as ximelagatran. The effects of the anticoagulant "warfarin" are discussed in detail in the relevant chapter on hematological aspects of pharmacogenetics.

A PERSPECTIVE ON PHARMACOGENETICS IN CARDIOVASCULAR MEDICINE

It is clear from the numerous examples reviewed here that genetic polymorphisms can be an important determinant of predicting cardiovascular risk. It is equally clear that these genetic variants determine drug disposition and response in humans. The outcome data with HMGCo-A reductase inhibitors (statins) are particularly interesting in this respect. These studies, conducted in fairly large populations and with specific clinical endpoints (beyond lipid-lowering), focused on the polymorphic genes encoding the proteins, such as *APOE*, *CETP*, and *stromelysin-1*, and showed how the genotype might be associated with worse prognosis.

REFERENCES

1. Evans WE, Johnson JA. Pharmacogenomics: the inherited basis for inter-individual differences in drug response. Ann Rev Genomics Hum Genet 2001; 2:9–39.
2. Ng PC, Henikoff S. Accounting for human polymorphisms predicted to affect protein function. Genome Res 2002; 12:436–446.
3. Hoogendoorn B, Coleman SL, Guy CA, et al. Functional analysis of human promoter polymorphisms. Hum Mol Genet 2003; 12:2249–2254.
4. Cooper DN. Human Gene Evolution. Oxford: BIOS Scientific, 1999.
5. Hirschhorn JN, Lohmueller K, Byrne E, Hirschhorn K. A comprehensive review of genetic association studies. Genet Med 2002; 4:45–61.
6. Ioannidis JPA, Trikalinos TA, Ntzani EE, et al. Genetic associations in large versus small studies: an empirical assessment. Lancet 2003; 361:567–571.
7. Ozaki K, Ohnishi Y, Iida A, et al. Functional SNPs in the lymphotoxin-alpha gene that are associated with susceptibility to myocardial infarction. Nat Genet 2002; 32:650–654.
8. Fullerton SM, Clark AG, Weiss KM, et al. Apolipoprotein E variation at the sequence haplotype level: implications for the origin and maintenance of a major human polymorphism. Am J Hum Genet 2000; 67:881–900.
9. Rigat B, Hubert C, Alhenc-Gelas F. et al. An insertion/deletion polymorphism in the angiotensin I-converting enzyme gene accounting for half the variance of serum enzyme levels. J Clin Invest 1990; 86:1343–1346.
10. Dawson SJ, Wiman B, Hamsten A, et al. The two allele sequences of a common polymorphism in the promoter of the plasminogen activator inhibitor-1 (PAI-1) gene respond differently to interleukin-1 in HepG2 cells. J Biol Chem 1993; 268:10739–10745.
11. Varo N, Iraburu MJ, Varela M, Lopez B, Etayo JC, Diez J. Chronic AT (1) blockade stimulates extracellular collagen type I degradation and reverses myocardial fibrosis in spontaneously hypertensive rats. Hypertension 2000; 35:1197–1202.
12. Jeunemaitre X, Sourbrier F, Kotelevstev YV, et al. Molecular basis of human hypertension: role of angiotensnogen. Cell 1992; 72:169–180.
13. Katsuya T, Koike G, Yee TW, et al. Association of angiotensinogen gene T235 variant with increased coronary heart disease. Lancet 1995; 355:434–442.
14. Winkelmann BR, Russ AP, Nauck M, et al. Angiotensinogen M235T polymorphism is associated with plasma angiotensinogen and cardiovascular disease. Am Heart J 1999; 137:698–705.
15. Ludwig EH, Borecki IB, Ellison RC, et al. Associations between candidate loci angiotensin-converting enzyme and angiotensinogen with coronary heart disease and myocardial infarction: the NHLBI Family Heart Study. Ann Epidemiol 1997; 7:3–12.
16. Tiret L, Ricard S, Poirier O, et al. Genetic variation at the angiotensiogen locus in relation to high blood pressure and myocardial infarction: the ECTM study. J Hypertens 1995; 13:311–317.

17. Sethi AA, Nordestgaard BG, Tybjaerg-Hansen A. Angiotensinogen gene polymorphism, plasma angiotensinogen, and risk of hypertension and ischaemic heart disease: a meta-analysis. Arterioscler Thromb Vasc Biol 2003; 23:1269–1275.
18. Hingorani AD, Jia H, Stevens PA, Hopper R, Dickerson JE, Brown MJ. Renin-angiotensin system gene polymorphisms influence blood pressure and the response to angiotensin converting enzyme inhibition. J Hypertension 1995; 13:1602–1609.
19. Yusuf S, Sleight P, Pogue J, et al. Effects of an angiotensin-converting-ezyme inhibitor, ramipril, on cardiovascular events in high risk patients. The Heart Outcomes Prevention Evaluation Study investigators (see comments). New Engl J Med 2000; 342:145–153.
20. Rioux PP. Clinical trials in pharmacogenetics and pharmacogenomics: methods and applications. Am J Health Syst Pharm 2000; 57:887–898.
21. Evans AE, Poirer O, Kee F, Lecerf L, et al. Polymorphisms of the angiotensin-converting-enzyme gene in subjects who die from coronary heart disease. QJM 1994; 87:211–214.
22. Schunkert H, Hense S, Holmer SR, Stender M, Perz S, et al. Association between deletion polymorphism of the angiotensin-converting enzyme gene and left ventricular hypertrophy. New Engl J Med 1994; 330:345–348.
23. Montgomery HE, Should the contribution of ACE gene polymorphism to left ventricular hypertrophy be reconsidered? Heart 1997; 77:489–490.
24. Samani NJ, Thompson JR, O'Toole L, Channer K, Woods KL. A meta-analysis of the association of the deletion allele of the angiotensin-converting enzyme gene with myocardial infarctions. Circulation 1996; 94:708–712.
25. Sharma P. Meta-analysis of the *ACE* gene in ischaemic stroke. J Neurol Neurosurg Psych 1998; 64:227–230.
26. Sayed-Tabatabaei FA, Houwing-Duistermaat JJ, van Duijn CM, Witteman JCM. Angiotensin-converting enzyme gene polymorphism and carotid artery wall thickness. A meta-analysis. Stroke 2003; 34:1634–1639.
27. Safar ME, Lajemi M, Rudnichi A, Asmar R, Benetos A. Angiotensin-converting enzyme D/I gene polymorphism and age-related changes in pulse pressure in subjects with hypertension. Arterioscl Thromb Vasc Biol 2004; 24:1–5.
28. Zee RYL, Lou Y, Griffiths LR, Morris BJ, et al. Association of a polymorphism of the angiotensin I converting enzyme gene with essential hypertension. Biochem Biophys Res Commun 1992; 184:9–15.
29. Sasaki M, Oki T, Luchi A, et al. Relationship between the angiotensin converting enzyme gene polymorphism and the effects of enalapril on left ventricular hypertrophy and impaired diastolic filling in essential hypertension: M-mode and pulsed Doppler echocardiographic studies. J Hypertens 1996; 14:1403–1408.
30. Dudley C, Keavney B, Casadei B et al. Prediction of patient responses to antihypertensive drugs using genetic polymorphisms: investigation of rennin-angiotensin system genes. J Hypertens 1996; 14:259–262.
31. McNamara DM, Holubkov R, Janosko, et al. Pharmacogenetic interactions between beta-blocker therapy and the angiotensin-converting enzyme deletion polymorphism in patients with congestive heart failure. Circulation 2001; 103:1644–1648.
32. Paillard F, Chansel D, Brand E, Benetos A, Thomas F, et al. Genotype-phenotype relationships for the renin-angiotensin-aldosterone system in normal population. Hypertension 1999; 34:423–429.
33. Pojoga L, Gautier S, Blanc H, Guyene TT, et al. Genetic determination of plasma aldosterone levels in essential hypertension. Am J Hypertens 1998; 11:856–860.
34. Hautanena A, Lankien L, Kupari M, et al. Associations between aldosterone synthase gene polymorphism and adrenocortical function in males. J Int Med 1998; 244:11–18.
35. Kupari M, Hautanen A, Lankinen L, Koskinen P, Virolainen J, et al. Associations between human aldosterone synthase (CYP11B2) gene polymorphisms and left ventricular size, mass and function. Circulation 1998; 97:569–575.
36. Reihauss E, Innis M, Macintyre N, Liggett SB. Mutations in the gene encoding for the beta 2-adrenergic receptor in normal and asthmatic subjects. Am J Respir Cell Mol Biol 1993; 8:334–339.

37. Green SA, Turki J, Innis M, Liggett SB. Influence of beta 2-adrenergic receptor impart distinct agonist-promoted regulatory properties. Biochemistry 1994; 33:9414–9419.
38. Green SA, Turki J, Bejarno P, Hall IP, Liggett SB. Influence of β_2-adrenergic receptor genotypes on signal transduction in human airway smooth muscle cells. Am J Respir Cell Mol Biol 1995; 13:25–33.
39. Turki J, Lorenz JN, Green SA, Donnelly ET, et al. Myocardial signalling defects and impaired cardiac function of a human beta 2-adrenergic receptor polymorphism expressed in transgenic mice. Proc Natl Acad Sci USA 1996; 93:10483–10488.
40. Skrabal F, Kotano P, Luft FC. Mini review: inverse regulation of α-2 and β-2 adrenergic receptors in salt sensitive hypertension: an hypothesis. Life Sci 1989; 45:2061–2076.
41. Cockcroft JR, Gazis AG, Cross DJ, Wheatley A, et al. β-2 adrenoceptor polymorphism determines vascular reactivity in humans. Hypertension 2000; 36:371–375.
42. Hoit BD, Suresh DP, Craft L, Walsh RA, Liggett SB. β_2-adrenergic receptor polymorphisms at amino acid 16 differentially influence agonist-stimulated blood pressure and peripheral blood flow in normal individuals. Am Heart J 2000; 139:537–542.
43. Svetkey LP, Chen Y-T, McKeown S-P, Preis L, et al. Preliminary evidence of linkage of salt sensitivity in black Americans at the β-2 adrenoceptor locus. Hypertension 1997; 29:918–922.
44. Bray MS, Kruskall J, Li L, Ferrell R, Kardia S, et al. Positional genomic analysis identifies β_2-adrenergic receptor gene as a susceptibility locus for human hypertension. Circulation 2000; 101:2877–2882.
45. Jia H, Sharma P, Hopper R Dickerson C, et al. β_2-Adrenoceptor gene polymorphisms and blood pressure in East Anglian Caucasians. J Hypertens 2000; 18:687–693.
46. Liggett SB, Wagoner LE, Craft LL, Hornung RW, et al. The Ile164 β2-adrenergic receptor polymorphism adversely affects the outcome of congestive heart failure. J Clin Invest 1998; 102:1534–1539.
47. Wagoner LE, Craft LL, Singh LL, Suresh DP, Zengel PW, et al. Polymorphisms of the the β_2-adrenergic receptor determine exercise capacity in patients with heart failure. Circ Res 2000; 86:834–840.
48. Gratze G, Fortin J, Labugger R, Binder A, Kotano P, et al. β_2-Adrenergic receptor variants affect resting blood pressure and agonist-induced vasodilation in young adult Caucasians. Hypertension 1999; 33:1425–1430.
49. Perregaux D, Chaudhuri A, Rao S, Airen A, et al. Brachial vascular reactivity in blacks. Hypertension 2000; 36:866–871.
50. Brodde OE, Buscher R, Tellkamp R, Radke J, Dhein S, Insel PA. Blunted cardiac responses to receptor activation in subjects with Thr164Ile beta(2)-adrenoceptors. Circulation 2001; 103:1048–1050.
51. Wang Y, Marsden PA. Nitric oxide synthases: biochemical and molecular regulation. Curr Opin Nephrol Hypertens 1995; 4:12–22.
52. Moncada S, Higgs A. The L-Arginine nitric oxide pathway. New Engl J Med 1993; 329:2002–2012.
53. Haynes WG, Noon JP, Walker BR, Webb DJ. L-NMMA increases blood pressure in man. Lancet 1993; 342:931–932.
54. Miyamoto Y, Saito Y, Kajiyama N, Yoshimura M, et al. Endothelial nitric oxide synthase gene is positively associated with essential hypertension. Hypertension 1998; 32: 3–8.
55. Hingorani A, Liang CF, Fatibene J, Lyon A, et al. A common variant of the endothelial nitric oxide synthase ($Glu^{298} \rightarrow Asp$) is a major risk factor for coronary artery disease in the UK. Circulation 1999; 100:1515–1520.
56. Hibi K, Ishigami T, Tamura K, Mizushima S, et al. Endothelial nitric oxide synthase gene polymorphism and acute myocardial infarction. Hypertension 1998; 32:521–526.
57. Shimasaki Y, Yasue H, Yoshimura M, Nakayama M, et al. Association of the missense mutation Glu298Asp variant of the endothelial nitric oxide synthase gene with myocardial infarction. J Am Coll Cardiol 1998; 31:1506–1510.

58. Yoshimura M,Yasue H, Nayakama M, Shimsaki Y, et al. A missense Glu298Asp variant in the endothelial nitric oxide synthase gene is associated with coronary spasm in the Japanese. Hum Genet 1998; 103:65–69.
59. Lacolley P, Gautier S, Poirier O, Pannier B, et al. Nitric oxide synthase gene polymorphisms, blood pressure and aortic stiffness in normotensive and hypertensive subjects. J Hypertens 1998; 16:31–35.
60. Avolio AP, Deng FQ, Li WQ, Luo YF, et al. Effects of aging on arterial distensibility in populations with high and low prevalence of hypertension: Comparision between urban and rural communities in China. Circulation 1985; 71:202–210.
61. Li DY, Brooke B, Davis EC, Mecham RP, et al. Elastin is an essential determinant of arterial morphogenesis. Nature 1998; 393:276–280.
62. Li DY, Faury G, Taylor DG, Boyle WA, et al. Novel arterial pathology in mice and humans hemizygous for elastin. J Clin Invest 1998; 102:1783–1787.
63. Ewart AK, Morris AC, Atkinson D, Weishan J, et al. Hemizygosity at the elastin locus in a developmental disorder. Nat Genet 1993; 5:11–15.
64. Tassabehji M, Metcalfe K, Donnai D, Hurst J, et al. Elastin: genomic structure and point mutations in patients with supravalvular aortic stenosis. Hum Mol Genet 1997; 6:1029–1036.
65. Ewart AK, Morris CA, Ensing GJ, Loker J, et al. Human vascular disorder, supravalvular aortic stenosis, maps to chromosome 7. Proc Natl Acad Sci USA1993; 90: 3226–3230.
66. Tromp G, Christiano A, Goldstein N, Indik Z, et al. A to G polymorphism in the *ELN* gene. Nucleic Acids Res 1991; 19:4314.
67. Raybouldd MC, Birley AJ, Hulten M. A *Bgl* I polymorphism in the human elastin gene (*ELN*). Clin Genet 1994; 46:212–213.
68. Hanon O, Luong V, Mourard JJ, Bortolotto LA, Jeunemaitre X, Girerd X. Aging, carotid artery distensibility, and the Ser422Gly elastin gene polymorphisms in humans. Hypertension 2001; 38:1185–1189.
69. Wossner JF. Matrix metalloproteinases and their inhibitors in connective tissue remodelling. FASEB 1991; 5:2145–2154.
70. Henney AM, Ye S, Zhang B, Jormsjo S, Whatling C, Eriksson P, Hamsten A. Genetic diversity in the matrix metalloproteinase family. Effects on function and disease progression. Ann NY Acad Sci 2000; 902:27–37.
71. Thompson RW, Holmes DR, Mertens RA, Liao S, Botney MD, Mencham RP, Welgus HG, Parks WC. Production and localization of 92-kilodalton gelatinase in abdominal aortic aneurysms. An elastolytic metalloproteinase expressed by aneurysm-infiltrating macrophages. J Clin Invest 1995; 96:318–326.
72. Zhang B, Ye S, Herrmann SM, et al. Functional polymorphism in the regulatory region of gelatinase B gene in relation to severity of coronary atherosclerosis. Circulation 1999; 99:1788–1794.
73. Blankenberg S, Rupprecht HJ, Poirier O, Bickel C, Smieja M, Haffner G, Meyer J, Cambien F, Tiret L, for the AtheroGene investigators. Plasma concentrations and genetic variation of matrix metalloproteinase 9 and prognosis of patients with cardiovascular disease. Circulation 2003; 107:1579–1585.
74. Montaner J, Molina CA, Monasterio J, Abilleira S, Arenillas JF, Ribo M, Quintana M, Alvarez-Sabin J. Matrix metalloproteinase-9 pretreatment level predicts intracranial hemorrhagic complications after thrombolysis in human stroke. Circulation 2003; 107: 598–603.
75. Galis SZ, Khatri JJ. Matrix metalloproteinases in vascular remodelling and atherogenesis. The good, the bad, and the ugly. Cir Res 2002; 90:251–262.
76. Zervoudaki A, Economou E, Stefanadis C, Pitsqvos C, Tsioufis K, Aggeli C, et al. Plasma levels of extracellular matrix metalloproteinases 2 and 9 in patients with essential hypertension before and after antihypertensive treatment. J Hum Hypertens 2003; 17:119–124.
77. Li-Saw-Hee FL, Edmunds E, Blann AD, Beevers DG, Lip GH. Matrix metalloproteinase-9 tissue inhibitor mettaloproteinase-1 levels in essential hypertension. Relationship to left ventricular mass and anti-hypertensive therapy. Int J Cardiol 2000; 75:43–47.

78. Laviades C, Varo N, Fernandez J, Mayor G, Gil MJ, Monreal I, Diez J. Abnormalities of the extracellular degradation of collagen type I in essential hypertension. Circulation 1998; 98:535–540.
79. Terashima M, Akita H, Kanazawa K, Inoue N, et al. Stromelysin promoter 5A/6A polymorphism is associated with acute myocardial infarction. Circulation 1999; 99: 2717–2719.
80. Yoon S, Tromp G, Vongpunsawad S, Ronkainen A, et al. Genetic analysis of MMP3, MMP9 and PAI-1 in Finnish patients with abdominal aortic or intracranial aneurysms. Biochem Biophys Res Commun 1999; 265:563–568.
81. Rauramaa R, Vaisanen SB, Luong LA, Schmidt-Trucksass A, et al. Stromelysin-1 and interleukin-6 gene promoter polymorphisms are determinants of asymptomatic carotid artery atherosclerosis. Arterioscler Thromb Vasc Biol 2000; 20:2657–2662.
82. Gnasso A, Motti C, Irace C, Carallo C, Liberatoscioli L, Bernardini S, Massoud R, Mattioli PL, Federici G, Cortese C. Genetic variation in human stromelysin gene promoter and common carotid geometry in healthy male subjects. Arteriosclers Thromb Vasc Biol 2000; 20:1600–1605.
83. Ghilardi G, Biondi MA, DeMonti M, Turri O, et al. Matrix metalloproteinase-1 and matrix metalloproteinase-3 gene promoter polymorphisms are associated with carotid artery stenosis. Stroke 2002; 33:2408–2412.
84. Ye S, Watts GF, Mandalia S, Humphries SE, Henney AM. Preliminary report: genetic variation in the human stromelysin promoter is associated with progression of coronary atherosclerosis. Br Heart J 1995; 73:209–215.
85. Medley TL, Kingwell B, Gatza CD, Pillay P, Cole TJ. Matrix metalloproteinase-3 genotype contributes to age-related aortic stiffening through modulation of gene and protein expression. Circ Res 2003; 92:1–8.
86. Dart AM, Kingwell BA. Pulse pressure—a review of mechanisms and clinical relevance. J Am Coll Cardiol. 2001; 37:975–984.
87. de Maat MP, Jukema JW, Ye S, et al. Effect of stromelysin-1 promoter on efficacy of pravastatin in coronary atherosclerosis and restonosis. Am J Cardiol 1999; 83:852–856.
88. Humphries SE, Luong LA, Talmud PJ, et al. The 5A/6A polymorphism in the promoter of the stromelysin-1 (MMP3) gene predicts progression of angiographically determined coronary artery disease in men in the LOCAT gemfibrozil study. Lipid coronary angiography trial. Atherosclersosis 1998; 139:49–56.
89. Nagashima H, Aoka Y Sakomura Y, Sakuta A, Aomi S, Ishizuka N, Hagiwara N, Kawana M, Kasanuki H. A 3-hydroxy-3-methylglutaryl coenzyme A reductase inhibitor, cerivastatin, suppress production of matrix metalloproteinase-9 in human abdominal aortic aneurysm wall. J Vasc Surg 2002; 36:158–163.
90. Laufs U, La Fatta V, Plutzky J, Liao JK. Upregulation of endothelial nitric oxide synthase by HMG CoA reductase inhibitors. Circulation 1998; 97:1129–1135.
91. Kitakaze M, Karasawa A, Kobayashi H, Tanaka H, Kuzuya T, Hori M. Benidipine: a new Ca^{2+} channel blocker with a cardioprotective effect. Cardiovas Drug Review 1999; 17:1–15.
92. Hirono O, Fatema K, Nitobe J, Takeishi Y, Kaneko K, Shiga R, Kubota I. Long term effects of benidipine hydrochloride on severe left ventricular hypertrophy and collagen metabolism in patients with essential hypertension. J Cardiol 2002; 39:195–204.
93. Tan FK, Wang N, Kuwana M, et al. Association of fibrillin-1 single nucleotide polymorphism haplotypes with systemic sclerosis in Choctaw and Japanese populations. Arthritis Rheumatism 2001; 44:893–901.
94. Powell J, Turner R, Henney A, et al. An association between arterial pulse pressure and variation in the fibrillin-1 gene. Heart 1997; 78:396–398.
95. Medley TL, Cole TJ, Gatza CD, Wang WYS, Dart AM, Kingwell BA. Fibrillin-1 genotype is associated with aortic stiffness and disease severity in patients with coronary artery disease. Circulation 2002; 105:810–815.
96. Corbo RM, Scacchi R. Apoliporotein E (*APOE*) allele distribution in the world. Is *APOE**4 a 'thrifty' allele? Ann Hum Genet 1999; 63:310–310.

97. Boerwinkle E, Ellsworth DL, Hallman DM, Biddinger A. Genetic analysis of atherosclerosis: a research paradigm for the common chronic diseases. Hum Mol Genet 1996; 5:1405–1410.
98. Winkelmann BR, Hager J. Genetic variation in coronary heart disease and myocardial infarction: methodological overview and clinical evidence. Pharmacogenomics 2000; 1: 73–94.
99. Wilson PW, Myers RH, Larson MG, Ordovas JM, et al. Apolipoprotein E alleles, dyslipidemia, and coronary heart disease: the Framingham offspring study. J Am Med Assoc 1994; 272:1666–1671.
100. Gerdes LU, Gerdes C, Kervinen K, et al. The apolipoprotein epsilon4 allele determines prognosis and the effect on prognosis of simvastatin in survivors of myocardial infarction: a substudy of the Scandinavian simvastatin survival study. Circulation 2000; 101:1366–1371.
101. Korhonen T, Hannuksela ML, Seppanen S, Kervinen K, Kesaniemi YA, Savolainen MJ. The effect of the apolipoprotein E phenotype on cholesteryl ester transfer protein activity, plasma lipids and apolipoprotein A I levels in hypercholesterolaemic patients on colestipol and lovastatin treatment. Eur J Clin Pharmacol 1999; 54:903–910.
102. Sanllehy C, Casals E, Rodriuez-Villar C, et al. Lack of interaction of apolipoprotein E phenotype with the lipoprotein response to lovastatin or gemfibrozil in patients with primary hypercholesterolaemia. Metabolism 1998; 47:560–565.
103. Yamada M. Influence of apolipoprotein E polymorphism on bezafibrate treatment response in dyslipidemic patients. J Atheroscler Thromb 1997; 4:40–44.
104. Yamashita S, Maruyama T, Hirano KL, et al. Molecular biology and pathophysiological aspects of plasma cholesteryl ester transfer protein. Biochem Biophys Acta 2000; 1529:257–275.
105. Kuivenhoven JA, Jukema JW, Zwindermann AH, et al. The role of common variant of the cholesteryl ester transfer protein gene in the progression of coronary atherosclerosis. New Engl J Med 1998; 338:86–93.
106. Ordovas JM, Cupples LA, Corella D, et al. Association of cholesteryl ester transfer protein-TaqIB polymorphism with variations in lipoprotein subclasses and coronary heart disease risk: the Framingham study. Arterioscler Thromb Vasc Biol 2000; 20:1323–1329.
107. Agellon LB, Quinet EM, Gillette TG, et al. Organisation of the human *CETP* gene. Biochemistry 1990; 29:1372–1376.
108. Agerholm-Larsen B, Nordesgaard BG, Steffensen R, et al. Elevated high density lipoprotein cholesterol is a risk factor for ischaemic heart disease in white women when caused by a mutation in the *CETP* gene. Circulation 2000; 101:1907–1912.
109. Agerholm-Larsen B, Tybjaerg-Hansen A, Schnohr P, et al. Common *CETP* mutations, decreased high density lipoprotein cholesterol and possible decreased risk of ischaemic heart disease. The Copenhagen City Heart study. Circulation 2000; 102:2197–2203.
110. Dullaart KP, Hoogenberg K, Riemenes SS, et al. *CETP* gene polymorphism is a determinant of HDL cholesterol and of the lipoprotein response to a lipid lowering diet in type 1 diabetes. Diabetes 1997; 46:2082–2087.
111. Wallace AJ, Humphries SE, Fisher RM, et al. Genetic factors associated with resposnse to low density lipoprotein subfractions to change in the nature of dietary fat. Atherosclerosis 2000; 149:387–394.
112. Koenig W, Froehlich M, Sund M, Doering A, Fischer H, Loewel H, Hutchinson W, Pepys M. C-reactive protein (CRP) predicts risk of coronary heart disease (CHD) in healthy middle-aged men: results from the MONICA-Augburg cohort study, 1984–85-1992 [abstr]. Circulation 1997; 96(suppl I):I–99.
113. Wu DM, Chu NF, Shen MH, Chang JB. Plasma C-reactive protein levels and their relationship to anthropometric and lipid characteristics among children. J Clin Epidemiol 2003; 56:94–100.
114. Fichtlscherer S, Rosenberger G, Walter DH, Breuer S, Dimmeler S, Zeiher AM. Elevated C-reactive protein levels and impaired endothelial vasoreactivity in patients with coronary artery disease. Circulation 2000; 102:1000–1006.
115. Abramson JL, Weintraub WS, Vaccarino V. Association between pulse pressure and C-reactive protein among apparently healthy US adults. Hypertension 2002; 39:197–202.

116. Cleland SJ, Sattar N, Petrie JR, Forouhi NG, Elliott HL, Connell JM. Endothelial dysfunction as a possible link between C-reactive protein levels and cardiovascular disease. Clin Sci 2000; 98:531–535.
117. London GM, Marchias SJ, Guerin AP, Metivier F, Adda H, Pannier B. Inflammation, arteriosclerosis, and cardiovascular therapy in hemodialysis patients. Kidney Int 2003; 84:S88–S93.
118. Preston GA, Barrett CV, Alcorta DA, Hogan SL, Dinwiddle L, Jennette JC, Falk RJ. Serum matrix metalloproteinases MMP-2 and MMP3 levels in dialysis patients vary independently of CRP and IL 6 levels. Nephron 2002; 92:817–823.
119. Yasmin, McEniery CM, Wallace S, Mackenzie IS, Cockcroft JR, Wilkinson IB. C-reactive protein is associated with arterial stiffness in apparently healthy individuals. Arterioscler Thromb Vasc Biol 2004; 24:969–974.
120. Brull DJ, Serrano N, Zito F, Jones L, et al. Human *CRP* gene polymorphism influences *CRP* levels. Implications for the prediction and pathogenesis of coronary heart disease. Arterioscler Thromb Vasc Biol 2003; 23:2063–2069.
121. Ridker PM, Rafia N, Stampfer MJ, Hennekens CH. Plasma concentration of interleukin-6 and risk of future myocardial infarction among apparently healthy men. Circulation 2000; 101:1767–1772.
122. Gabriel AS, Ahnve S, Wretlind B, Martinsson A. Il-6 and IL-1 receptor antagonist in stable angina pectoris and relation of IL-6 to clinical findings in acute myocardial infarction. J Intern Med 2000; 248:61–66.
123. Humphries SE, Talmud PJ, Hawe E, Bolla M, Day INM, Miller GJ. Apolipprotein E4 and coronary heart disease in middle-aged men who smoke: a prospective study. Lancet 2001; 358:115–119.
124. Brull DJ, Montgomery J, Sanders J, Dhamrait S, et al. Interleukin-6 gene −174G>C and −572G>C promoter polymorphisms are strong predictors of plasma interleukin-6 levels after coronary artery bypass surgery. Arterioscler Thromb Vasc Biol 2001; 21: 1458–1463.
125. Jones KG, Brull DJ, Sian M, Brown LC, et al. Interleukin-6 and the prognosis of abdominal aortic aneurysm. Circulation 2001; 103:2260–2265.
126. Georges JL, Loukaci V, Poirer O, Evans A, et al. Interleukin-6 gene polymorphisms and susceptibility to myocardial infarction. J Mol Med 2001; 79:300–305.
127. Basso F, Lowe GDO, Rumley A, McMahon AD, et al. Interleukin-6 −174G>C polymorphism and risk of coronary heart disease in West of Scotland Coronary Prevention Study (WOSCOPS). Arterioscler Thromb Vasc Biol 2002; 22:599–604.
128. Feng D, Tofler GH, Larson MG, et al. Factor VII gene polymorphism, factor VII levels, and prevalent cardiovascular disease: the Framingham Heart Study. Arterioscler Thromb Vasc Biol 2000; 20:593–600.
129. Girelli D, Russo C, Ferraresi P, et al. Polymorphisms in the factor VII gene and the risk of myocardial infarction in patients with coronary artery disease. New Engl J Med 2000; 343:774–780.
130. Ridker PM, Hennekens CH, Lindpainter K, Stampfer MJ, et al. Mutation in gene coding for coagulation factor V and the risk of myocardial infarction, stroke, and venous thrombosis in apparently healthy men. New Engl J Med 1995; 85:1504–1508.
131. DeStefano V, Martinelli I, Mannucci PM, et al. The risk of recurrent venous thromboembolism among heterozygous carriers of the G202010A proThrombin gene mutation. Br J Haematol 2001; 113:630–635.
132. Dahlbäck B. Physiological anticoagulation. Resistance to activated protein protein C and venous thromboembolism. J Clin Invest 1994; 94: 923–927.
133. Donahue BS, Gailani D, Higgins MS, et al. Factor V Leiden protects against blood loss and transfusion after cardiac surgery. Circulation 2003; 107:1003–1008.
134. Lindqvist PG, Svensson PJ, Dahlback B, Marsal K. Factor V Q506 mutation (activated protein C resistance) associated with reduced intrapartum blood loss—a possible evolutionary selection mechanism. Thromb Haemost 1998; 79:69–73.
135. Rey E, Kahn SR, David M, Shrier I. Thrombophilic disorders and fetal loss: a meta-analysis. Lancet 2003; 361:901–908.

136. Lin JH, Lu AYH. Inhibition and induction of cytochrome P450 and the clinical implication. Clin Pharmacokinet 1998; 35:361–391.
137. Relling MV, Cherrie J, Schell MJ, et al. Lower prevalence of the debrisoquin oxidative poor metabolizer phenotype in American black versus white subjects. Clin Pharmacol Ther 1991; 50:308–313.
138. Nakamura K, Goto F, Ray WA, et al. Inter-ethnic differences in genetic polymorphism of debrisoquin and mephenytoin hydroxylation between Japanese and Caucasian populations. Clin Pharmacol Ther 1985; 38:402–408.
139. Kagimoto M, Heim M, Kagimoto K, et al. Multiple mutations of the human cytochrome P450IID6 gene (*CYP2D6*) in poor metabolizers of debrisoquine. Study of the functional significance on individual mutations by expression of chimeric genes. J Biol Chem 1990; 265:17209–17214.
140. Mahgoub A, Idle JR, Dring LG, et al. Polymorphic hydroxylation of desbrisoquine in man. Lancet 1977; 2:584–586.
141. Johansson I, Lundqvist E, Bertilsson L, et al. Inherited amplification of an active gene in the cytochrome P450 *CYP2D* locus as a cause of ultrarapid metabolism of debrisoquine. Proc Natl Acad Sci USA 1993; 90:11825–11829.
142. http://www.imm.ki.se/CYPalleles.
143. Zhou HH, Wood AJ. Stereoselective disposition of carvedilol is determined by *CYP2D6*. Clin Pharmacol Ther 1995; 57:518–524.
144. Eichelbaum M, Gross AS. The genetic polymorphism of debrisoquine/sparteine metabolism-clinical aspects. Pharmacol Ther 1990; 46:377–394.
145. PirMohamed M, Park BK. Cytochrome 450 enzyme polymorphism and adverse drug reactions. Toxicology 2003; 192:23–32.
146. PirMohamed M, Park BK. Genetic susceptibility to adverse drug reactions. Trends Pharmacol Sci 2001; 22:298–305.
147. Maitland-van der Zee AH, de Boer A, Leufkens HGM. The interface between pharmacoepidemiology and pharmacogenetics. Eur J Pharmacol 2000; 410:13–22.
148. Johnnson JA, Humma A. Pharmacogenetics of cardiovascular drugs. Briefings in Fundamental Genomics and Proteomics 2002; 1:1–14.
149. Tiret L, Rigat B, Visvikis S, et al. Evidence from combined segregation and linkage analysis, that a variant of the angiotensin I converting enzyme (ACE) gene controls plasma ACE levels. Am J Hum Genet 1992; 51:197–205.
150. Kohno M, Yokokawa K, Minami M, Kano H, Yasunari K, et al. Association between angiotensin-converting enzyme gene polymorphisms and regression of left ventricular hypertrophy in patients treated with angiotensin-converting enzyme inhibitors. Am J Med 1999; 106:544–549.
151. Diegeuz-Lucena JL, Aranda-Lara P, Ruiz-Galdon M, et al. Angiotensin I converting enzyme genotypes and angiotensin II receptors. Response to therapy. Hypertension 1996; 28: 98–103.
152. Stavroulakis GA, Makris TK, Krespi PG, Hatzizacharias AN, et al. Predicting response to chronic antihypertensive treatment with fosinopril: the role of angiotensin-converting enzyme gene polymorphism. Cardiovas Drugs Ther 2000; 14:427–432.
153. Prasad A, Narayanan S, Husain S, et al. Insertion-deletion polymorphism of the *ACE* gene modulates reversibility of endothelial dysfunction with ACE inhibition. Circulation 2000; 14:427–432.
154. Schunkert H, Hense HW, Gimenez-Roqueplo AP, Steiber J, et al. The angiotensinogen T235 variant and the use of antihypertensive drugs in a population based cohort. Hypertension 1997; 29:628–633.
155. Van Geel PP, Pinto PP, Voors AA, et al. Angiotensin II type I receptor A1166C gene polymorphism is associated with an increased response to angiotensin II in human arteries. Hypertension 2000; 35:717–721.
156. Benetos A, Gautier S, Ricard S, et al. Influence of angiotensin-converting enzyme and angiotensin-II type I receptor gene polymorphisms in aortic stiffness in normotensive and hypertensive patients. Circulation 1996; 94:698–703.

157. Benetos A, Cambien F, Gautier S, et al. Influence of angiotensin II type I receptor gene polymorphism on the effects of perindopril and nitrendipine on arterial stiffness in hypentensive individuals. Hypertension 1996; 28:1081–1084.
158. Lajemi M, Labat C, Gautier S, Lacolley P, et al. Angiotensin II type 1 receptor −153A/G and 1166A/C gene polymorphisms and increase in aortic stiffness with age in hypertensive subjects. J Hypertens 2001; 19:407–413.
159. Miller JA, Thai K, Sholey JW. Angiotensin II type 1 receptor gene polymorphism predicts response to losartan and angiotensin II. Kidney Int 1999; 56:2173–2180.
160. Tiago AD, Badenhorst D, Skudicky D, Woodiwiss AJ, Candy GP, Brooksbank R, et al. An aldosterone synthase gene variant is associated with improvement in left ventricular fraction in dilated cardiomyopathy. Cardiovasc Res 2002; 54:584–589.
161. Takahashi T, Yamaguchi E, Furuya K, Kawakami Y. The ACE gene polymorphism and cough threshold for capaicin after cilazapril usage. Respir Med 2001; 95:130–135.
162. Mukae S, Itoh S, Aoki S, Iwata T, Nishio K, Sato R, Katagiri T. Association of polymorphisms of the renin angiotensin system and bradykinin B2 receptor with angiotensin converting enzyme inhibitor-related cough. J Hum Hypertens 2002; 16:857–863.
163. Cambien F, Poirier O, Lecerf L, Evans A, Cambou JP, et al. Deletion polymorphism in the gene for angiotensin-converting enzyme is a potent risk factor for myocardial infarction. Nature 1992; 359:641–644.
164. Humma LM, Puckett BJ, Richardson HE, et al. Effect of beta1-adrenoceptor genetic polymorphisms on resting hemodynamics in patients undergoing diagnostic testing for ischaemia. Am J Cardiol 2001; 88:1034–1037.
165. O'Shaughnessy KM, Fu B, Dickerson C, Thurston D, Brown MJ. The gain-of-function G389R variant of the beta1-adrenoceptor does not influence blood pressure or heart rate response to beta blockade in hypertensive subjects. Clin Sci 2000; 99:233–238.
166. Liggett SB. The pharmacogenetics of $\beta 2$ adrenergic receptors: relevance to asthma. J Allergy Clin Immun 2000; 105:487–492.
167. Liggett SB. Pharmacogenetics of beta-1- and beta-2-adrenergic receptors. Pharmacology 2000; 61:167–173.
168. LaRosa JC, He J, Vupputuri S. Effect of statins on risk of coronary disease a meta-analysis of randomized controlled trials. J Am Med Assoc 1999; 282:2340–2346.
169. Serruys PW, de Feyter P, Macaya C, et al. Fluvastatin for prevention of cardiac events following successful first percutaneous coronary intervention: a randomized controlled trial. J Am Med Assoc 2002; 287:3215–3222.
170. Shepherd J, Blauw GJ, Murphy MB, et al. Pravastatin in elderly at risk of vascular disease (PROSPER): a randomized controlled trial. Lancet 2002; 360:1623–1630.
171. Ichihara K, Satoh K. Disparity between angiographic regression and clinical event rates with hydrophobic statins. Lancet 2002; 359:2195–2198.
172. Frenette PS. Locking a leucocyte integrin with statins. New Engl J Med 2001; 345:1419–1421.
173. Marz W, Winkelmann BR. HMG CoA reductase inhibition in the treatment of atherosclerosis: effects beyond lipid lowering. J Kardiol 2002; 9:284–294.
174. Dela Serna G, Cadarso C. Fenojibrate decreases plasma fibrinogen, improves lipid profile and reduces uricemia. Clin Pharmacol Ther 1999; 66:166–172.
175. Faggiotto A, Paoletti R. State-of-the-Art lecture. Statins and blockers of the renin-angiotensin system: vascular protection beyond their primary mode of action. Hypertension 1999; 34:987–996.
176. Ballantyne CM, Herd JA, Stein EA, et al. Apolipopotein E genotypes and response of plasma lipds and progression-regression of coronary atherosclerosis to lipid lowering drug therapy. J Am Coll Cardiol 2000; 36:1572–1578.
177. Pedro-Botet J, Schaefer EJ, Bakker-Arkema RG, Black DM, et al. Apolipoprotein E genotypes affects plasma lipid response to atorvastatin in a gender specific manner. Atherosclerosis 2001; 158:183–193.
178. Marques-Vidal P, Bongard V, Ruidavets JB, Fauvel J, et al. Effect of apolipoprotein E alleles and angiotensin converting enzyme insertion/deletion polymorphisms on lipid and

lipoprotein markers in middle-aged men and in patients with stable angina pectoris or healed myocardial infarction. Am J Cardiol 2003; 92:1102–1105.

179. Hagberg JM, Wilund KR, Ferrell RE. Apo E gene and gene-environment effects on plasma lipoprotein-lipid levels. Physiol Genomics 2000; 4:101–108.
180. Freeman DJ, Wilson V, McMahon AD, et al. A polymorphism of the cholesteryl ester transfer protein (*CETP*) gene predicts cardiovascular events in the West of Scotland Coronary Prevention Study (WOSCOPS). Atherosclerosis 2000; 151:91.
181. Carlquist JF, Muhlestein JB, Horne BD, Hart NI, et al. The cholesterol ester transfer protein *Taq*IB gene polymorphism predicts clinical benefit to statin therapy in patients with significant coronary artery disease. Am Heart J 2003; 146(6):1007–1014.
182. Van Geel PP, Pinto YM, Zwinderman AH, et al. The angiotensin-converting enzyme deletion type gene is associated with ischaemic events and a blunted effect of lipid lowering treatment on angiographically defined coronary atherosclerosis [abstr]. Eur Heart J 1997; IS:1.
183. Bray PF, Cannon CP, Goldschimdt-Clermont P, Moye LA, et al. The platelet PI (AZ) and angiotensin-converting enzymel (PCE) D allele polymorphisms and the risk of recurrent events after acute myocardial infarction. Am J Cardial 2001; 88:347–352.
184. Martinelli I, Taioli E, Bucciarelli P, et al. Interaction between the G20210A mutation of the proThrombin gene aand oral contraceptive use in deep vein Thrombosis. Arterioscler Thromb Vasc Biol 1999; 19:700–703.
185. Wang JG, Staessen JA. Genetic polymorphisms in the renin-angiotensin system: relevance for susceptibility to cardiovascular disease. Eur J Pharmacol 2000; 410:289–302.
186. Zhu H, Sagnella GA, Dong Y, Miller MA, Onipinla A, Markandu ND, MacGregor GA. Contrasting associations between aldosterone synthase gene polymorphisms and essential hypertension in blacks and in whites. J Hypertens 2003; 21:87–95.
187. Xie HG, Stein CM, Kim RB, Gainer JV, Sofowora G, Dishy V, et al. Human beta2-adrenergic receptor polymorphisms: no association with essential hypertension in black or white Americans. Clin Pharmacol Ther 2000; 67:670–675.
188. Lee JH, Tang MX, Schupf N, Stern Y, Jacobs DM, Tycko B, Mayeux R. Mortality and apolipoprotein E in Hispanic, African-American, and Caucasian elders. Am J Med Genet 2001; 103:121–127.
189. Lamblin N, Bauters C, Hermant X, Lablanche JM, Helbecque N, Amouyel P. Polymorphisms in the promoter regions of MMP-2, MMP3, MMP-9, MMP-12 genes as determinants of anueursymal coronary artery disease. J Am Coll Cardiol 2002; 40:43–48.
190. Humphries SE, Martin S, Cooper J, Miller G. Interaction between smoking and the stromelysin-1 (*MMP3*) gene 5A/6A promoter polymorphism and risk of coronary heart disease in healthy men. Ann Hum Genet 2002; 66:343–352.
191. Zhang B, Dhillon S, Geary I, Howell WM, Iannotti F, Day INM, Ye S. Polymorphisms in matrix metalloproteinase-1, 3, 9 and 12 genes in relation to subarachnoid hemorrhage. Stroke 2001; 32:2198–2202.
192. Shimajiri S, Arima N, Tanimoto A, et al. Shortened microsatellite d(CA)21 sequence down-regulates promoter activity of matrix metalloproteinase 9. FEBS 1999; 455:70–74.
193. Peters DG, Kassam A, St Jean PL, et al. Functional polymorphism in the matrix metalloproteinase-9 promoter as a potential risk factor for intracranial aneurysm. Stroke 1999; 30:2612–2616.
194. Jormsjo S, Ye S, Moritz J, Walter DH, Dimmeler S, Zeiher AM, Henney A, Hamsten A, Eriksson P. Allele-specific regulation of matrix metalloproteinase-12 gene activity is associated with coronary artery luminal dimensions in diabetic patients with manifest coronary artery disease. Circ Res 2000; 86:998–1003.
195. O'Toole L, Stewart M, Padfield P, Channer K. Effect of insertion/deletion polymorphism of the angiotensin-converting enzyme gene on responses to angiotensin-converting enzyme inhibitors in patients with heart failure. J Cardiovasc Pharmacol 1998; 32:988–994.
196. Ohmichi N, Iwai N, Uchida Y, Schichini G, et al. Relationship between the response to the angiotensin converting enzyme (inhibiton) imidapril and the angiotensin converting enzyme genotype. Am J Hypertens 1997; 10:951–955.

197. Perna A, Ruggenenti P, Testa A, et al. ACE genotype and ACE inhibitors induced renoprotection in chronic proteinuric nephropathies. Kidney Int 2000; 57:274–281.
198. Mukae S, Aoki S, Itoh S, Iwata T, Ueda H, Katagiri T. Bradykinin B2 receptor gene polymorphism is associated with angiotensin converting enzyme inhibitor-related cough. Hypertension 2000; 118:1091–1094.
199. Drysdale CM, McGraw DW, Stack CB, et al. Complex promoter and coding region beta 2-adrenergic receptor haplotypes alter receptor expression and predict in vivo responsiveness. Proc Natl Acad Sci USA 2000; 97:483–488.
200. Martinez FD, Graves PE, Baldini M, Solomons S, et al. Association between genetic polymorphisms of the beta 2 adrenoreceptor and response to albuterol in children with and without a history of wheezing. J Clin Invest 1997; 100:3184–3188.
201. Marian AJ, Sofavi F, Ferlic L, Dunn JK, et al. Interactions between angiotensin-I converting enzyme insertion/deletion polymorphism and response of plasma lipids and coronary autherosclerosis to treatment with fluvastatin: the lipoprotein and coronary atherosclerosis study. J Am Coll Cardiol 2000; 35:89–95.

12
Pharmacogenetics and Metabolic Disease

Simon Constable and Munir Pirmohamed
Department of Pharmacology and Therapeutics, University of Liverpool, Liverpool, U.K.

INTRODUCTION

Diabetes mellitus (DM), hyperlipidemia, and osteoporosis are common diseases, responsible, directly and indirectly, for significant morbidity and mortality worldwide. Each condition presents a variety of very specific management problems, but they are unified by a common theme—they are frequently asymptomatic and often manifest through their complications. This chapter focuses on the current level of understanding and the role of pharmacogenetics in the management of these three metabolic diseases. The influence of genes on the pharmacokinetics of the currently available drugs is discussed, and the interaction between genes and the environment in pathophysiology, including the response to drug therapy, is also considered.

DIABETES MELLITUS

DM is an increasing global health burden affecting more than 150 million people worldwide, with an ever increasing incidence and a prevalence that varies from population to population (1). The vast majority of patients suffering from DM have type 2 DM, a multifaceted and heterogeneous metabolic syndrome characterized by fasting and postprandial hyperglycemia–due to peripheral insulin resistance—resulting in a decreased insulin-mediated glucose disposal, increased endogenous glucose production (mainly from the liver), and impaired pancreatic insulin secretion (2–4). Insulin resistance, or reduced responsiveness to circulating concentrations of insulin, is an early defect in type 2 DM and is often present years before the onset of hyperglycemia and the clinical diagnosis of diabetes (5). Therapeutic strategies with single or combination therapy have targeted the metabolic defects seen in type 2 DM either individually or in concert.

Diabetes as a Genetic Disease

Heredity plays a significant, but variable, role in the etiology of DM—both type 1 and type 2 diabetes show a familial predisposition, indicating the involvement of genetic factors in determining individual susceptibility to the disease. The etiology and pathophysiology of each type of DM, however, is very different, suggesting that different genes are likely to be involved in this predisposition. The genetic basis of type 1 DM is complex and likely to be due to genes of both large and small effect. Population-based twin studies have confirmed an increased concordance in monozygotic (MZ) pairs, with a concordance of 30% to 40% compared with a concordance rate in dizygotic (DZ) pairs of 5% to 10% (6,7). Based on the results of these twin studies, it is clear that susceptibility to type 1 DM is determined, in part, by genetic risk factors but that probably <50% of the total risk can be attributed to the effects of shared genes. Similarly, in type 2 DM, twin studies have shown higher concordance rates in MZ than DZ twins, but there is a substantial amount of variability in concordance rates between different populations (6,8,9). It appears that the genetic model for type 2 DM is more complex, with multiple genes located on different chromosomes being associated with this condition (10). These findings are similar to those obtained for other common human disorders that exhibit familial aggregation but not simple Mendelian patterns of transmission of risk and is further complicated by numerous environmental factors that also contribute to the clinical manifestation of the disorder.

In type 2 DM there is evidence for a genetically programmed β-cell dysfunction that is unmasked by the failure to compensate for increasing insulin resistance (11). The work of Morris et al. (12) illustrates the synergism between genetic predisposition and the environmental pressure represented by obesity. Furthermore, in the case of maturity-onset diabetes of the young (MODY), the genetic cause of diabetes is an important determinant of the response to oral hypoglycemic drugs. This has implications for the wider management of diabetes in the future. The hope is that identification of the genes involved in β-cell dysfunction in MODY will lead to the uncovering of genes for the more common non-MODY forms of type 2 DM.

Diabetes largely exerts its effects on morbidity and mortality via its long-term macrovascular and microvascular complications (summarized in Table 1). There is now increasing evidence to show that genetic factors, together with elevated blood glucose, play an important role in the susceptibility to these complications. Polymorphisms of

Table 1 The Complications of Diabetes

Organ system/disease	Clinical manifestations
Eye disease	Retinopathy
	Cataracts
Neuropathy	Autonomic
	Diffuse symmetrical polyneuropathy
	Mononeuropathies
Nephropathy	
Hypertension	
Dyslipidemia	
Macrovascular disease (atherosclerosis)	Cerebrovascular disease
	Coronary artery disease (angina, acute coronary syndromes, heart failure)
	Peripheral vascular disease
Diabetic foot disease	Foot ulceration
Miscellaneous	Charcot's arthropathy
	Cheiroarthropathy
	Necrobiosis lipoidica diabeticorum
	Dermopathy
	Osteopenia

different genes, mainly from the renin–angiotensin system, have been studied extensively, and some of them have been suggested to contribute to the development of complications, especially nephropathy. This clearly has potential implications in management. However, very little is understood about the specific interaction between drugs and genes in this area, and therefore this review will focus on the role of pharmacogenetics in the management of type 2 DM per se. This is the field that has attracted the most research attention thus far.

Antidiabetic Drugs and Genetic Polymorphisms of CYP450 Enzymes

Cytochrome P450 (CYP) 2C9 hydroxylates a wide array of drugs in a diverse range of therapeutic categories—about 16% of the drugs in current clinical use, including drugs used for DM. The sulfonylureas, tolbutamide, glibenclamide, glimepiride, and glipizide are all CYP2C9 substrates (13–15). Nateglinide, an amino acid (δ-phenylalanine) derivative that improves early-phase insulin secretion and reduces mealtime glucose excursions, is also predominantly metabolized by CYP2C9 (and to a lesser extent by CYP3A4) (16–21).

Polymorphisms in *CYP2C9* (especially **2* and **3* variants) are known to reduce enzyme activity to 5% to 12% of the wild-type (*CYP2C9*1*) activity. Thus, polymorphisms in *CYP2C9*, especially in the rare individuals who are homozygous for the *CYP2C9*3* alleles, are likely to lead to a reduced dosage requirement and predisposition to severe toxicity—specifically the risk of life-threatening hypoglycemia.

The archetypal antidiabetic drug most widely studied with respect to *CYP2C9* polymorphisms is tolbutamide (22). It is metabolized almost exclusively by methylhydroxylation process that accounts for 85% of the tolbutamide clearance; this is the initial and rate-limiting step in metabolism (23,24). In vitro and in vivo evidence suggests that *CYP2C9* solely mediates the hydroxylation of tolbutamide. This drug is therefore widely accepted as a prototypic substrate for the assessment of hepatic *CYP2C9* activity and indeed has been used a probe substrate in many pharmacokinetic studies (25,26). An early study of tolbutamide metabolism suggested that approximately 30% of the subjects were poor metabolizers (PMs) (27). The pharmacokinetics of tolbutamide in 50 nondiabetic subjects, including twins, showed an almost ninefold variation in the elimination rate constant, with half-lives varying from 2.9 hours to 25.0 hours. However, at the time of those studies, the genetic basis of interindividual variability had not been defined. Although many subsequent studies failed to find a single individual who could be classified as a PM (28), later studies incorporating genotyping have shown that prolonged half-life is a consequence of the possession of allelic variants of the *CYP2C9* isoform (29–31). In accordance with this, expressed recombinant *CYP2C9*3* has been shown to exhibit lower intrinsic clearance (V_{max}/K_m) for tolbutamide methylhydroxylation than the wild type, caused by a higher K_m value without a change of the V_{max} values. In a further study, the relationship between *CYP2C9* genotype and tolbutamide plasma clearance (CL/F) in 23 healthy subjects expressing all six *CYP2C9* allele combinations has been evaluated and is summarized in Table 2 (32). According to this study, intermediate and slow metabolizers may be predicted to comprise approximately 12% and 1% of the population, respectively. These results are consistent with other work in this field (33,34). Most of these studies have been performed in Caucasians, and it is therefore important to remember that interethnic differences in the frequencies of the allelic variants may lead to varying prevalences of adverse effects associated with sulfonylureas.

Pharmacodynamic monitoring remains the rational option for monitoring tolbutamide treatment (35). To evaluate the pharmacokinetic–pharmacodynamic relationship, nondiabetic healthy subjects were monitored for blood/serum glucose (and plasma insulin)

Table 2 The Relationship Between *CYP2C9* Genotype and Phenotype

Tolbutamide clearance (Lhr^{-1})	Genotype	Metabolizer phenotype
0.97	**1/*1*	Extensive
0.88	**1/*2*	Extensive
0.75	**2/*2*	Extensive
0.56	**1/*3*	Intermediate
0.45	**2/*3*	Intermediate
0.16	**3/*3*	Slow

Abbreviations: **1*, Wild-type allele; *2, Arg144Cys; *3, Ile359Leu.
Source: From Ref. 14.

following tolbutamide administration (500 mg administered orally) with or without a glucose/dextrose challenge in three prospective studies (32–34). No relationship between glucose or insulin concentrations and *CYP2C9* genotype was reported by Lee et al. (34) and Kirchheiner et al (32). Furthermore, hypoglycemia was not observed, even without additional carbohydrate administration after tolbutamide. In contrast, in another study, evaluating Korean subjects, the enhancement in serum glucose increase relative to baseline was significantly lower in *CYP2C9*1/*3* heterozygotes, compared with homozygotes for the wild-type allele (33). The reason for such a difference is not entirely clear, but *CYP2C19* may also contribute to the metabolism of tolbutamide, and there is a relatively high *CYP2C19* PM genotype frequency in Korean and East Asian populations (compared with the Caucasians).

Genetic polymorphisms of *CYP2C9* have also been shown to affect the pharmacokinetics of glibenclamide and glimepiride in healthy volunteers (14,15). Glibenclamide AUC (area under concentration curve) was 280% higher in individuals heterozygous for the *CYP2C9 *3* allele (15). In *CYP2C9*3* homozygotes, the oral clearance was reduced by more than 50% in comparison with the individuals with *CYP2C9*1/*1* genotype (14). Similar results have also been shown for glimepiride, with the AUC in *CYP2C9*3* heterozygotes being increased by 267%, compared with individuals with the **1/*1* genotype (15). In both studies, however, blood glucose responses to glibenclamide and glimepiride were not significantly affected, whereas the insulin secretion after glibenclamide ingestion was higher in subjects with the **3/*3* genotype, compared with the other genotypes (14).

The effect of genetic polymorphisms in another *CYP2C* gene product, *CYP2C8*, on the pharmacokinetics and pharmacodynamics of the new meglitinide analog, repaglinide, has been studied in 28 healthy volunteers (36). There were 19 subjects (68%) with the *CYP2C8*1/*1* genotype (wild-type), six subjects (21%) with the *CYP2C8*1/*3* genotype, and three subjects (11%) with the *CYP2C8*1/*4* genotype. Unexpectedly, the *CYP2C8*3* variant allele was associated with reduced plasma concentrations of repaglinide. The mean AUC of repaglinide was 45% lower, and the peak concentration in plasma was 39% lower in subjects with the *CYP2C8*1/*3* genotype, compared with those with the *CYP2C8*1/*1* genotype. However, no statistically significant differences were found in the blood glucose response to repaglinide between the genotypes.

The clinical consequences of *CYP2C9* polymorphisms for the treatment with oral hypoglycemic agents are largely unclear because the relevant patient studies have not been undertaken. Further data are necessary to evaluate whether dosage adjustment on the basis of genotype is needed in diabetic patients. There appears to be discordance between the pharmacokinetic and pharmacodynamic responses elicted. This is likely to be multifactorial—a reflection of study design, the fact that the studies have been carried out in healthy volunteers rather than diabetic patients, but most importantly this may be attributable to the complex counterregulatory mechanisms that exist in glucose homeostasis. Blood glucose levels in nondiabetics are regulated by several factors, the most important being the counteracting hormones, insulin and glucagon. Decreases in blood glucose caused by oral hypoglycemic-triggered insulin secretion may have been concealed by a counteracting glucagon secretion that keeps the blood glucose levels constant. In diabetic patients, however, the regulation of blood glucose levels and insulin secretion is of course impaired, and thus a greater risk for hypoglycemia cannot be excluded in diabetic people with reduced CYP2C9 activity and higher concentrations of antidiabetic drug. Given the relative ease of pharmacodynamic monitoring and the lack of correlation between the kinetics and dynamics of antidiabetic compounds, it can be argued that monitoring of blood sugar, rather that genotyping, may be more clinical and cost-effective. Whether this is true or false awaits further study. Nevertheless, a clearer understanding of the pharmacokinetic–pharmacodynamic relationship in diabetic patients in the presence of *CYP2C9* polymorphisms is required.

The Chlorpropamide-Alcohol Flush (CPAF)

The CPAF is one of the earliest recognized examples of pharmacogenetics in the management of DM. Many diabetics who take the sulfonylurea, chlorpropamide, experience facial flushing after drinking even small amounts of alcohol. Sulfonylurea-induced alcohol intolerance is seen mainly, but not exclusively, with chlorpropamide and is similar to the interaction between alcohol and disulfiram. The mechanism of the reaction, however, is unclear. The main symptom is facial flushing that occurs more commonly in diabetic than in nondiabetic subjects. It has therefore been proposed that this symptom could be used as a diagnostic test for a certain subset of patients with type 2 DM (37,38). Interestingly, patients who demonstrate CPAF have a noticeably lower prevalence of late complications of diabetes (microangiopathy, macroangiopathy, and neuropathy) than nonflushers. The flush reaction is accompanied by an increase in blood acetaldehyde concentrations, suggesting an inhibition of aldehyde dehydrogenase activity (39,40).

Different prevalences of CPAF have been reported by different authors in type 1 DM, type 2 DM, or healthy subjects. This could be due to different methodological approaches or the different criteria for evaluating CPAF. Bonisolli et al. (41) investigated the association between CPAF and the fast acetylator phenotype (AP) in type 1 and type 2 diabetic patients. An association between fast AP and CPAF was found in type 2 but not in type 1 DM. In addition, a linear relationship was found between the rate of acetylation and the speed of ascent of facial skin temperature after chlorpropamide and alcohol in type 2 diabetics but not in type 1 diabetics. However, many authors do not consider the CPAF test to be sufficiently sensitive and specific, and despite a great deal having been published on the test, its value remains poorly defined (42–45).

Sulfonylurea Sensitivity and MODY

MODY is a relatively rare form of familial diabetes and is part of the differential diagnosis of diabetes presenting in the first three decades of life. MODY is now known to differ fundamentally from type 2 DM in its etiology and is classified separately as type 3A. The key characteristics of this condition are an young age of onset (often before the age of 25 years), noninsulin dependence (absence of features of type 1 DM, with C-peptide positivity and no requirement for insulin within five years of diagnosis), and an autosomal-dominant mode of inheritance (46). At least two consecutive generations are affected with a family member diagnosed (before the age of 25). This is very much a heterogeneous group of disorders with wide variability in the severity of the hyperglycemia and the age at which it becomes clinically manifest. Several genetic subtypes of MODY have now been described, and these are all characterized by mild fasting hyperglycemia in otherwise normal individuals (Table 3) (47). Mutations in six genes have been shown to cause MODY, with two different types of monogenic mutation (48). Glucokinase MODY is caused by mutations in the gene for the glycolytic enzyme glucokinase, and transcription factor MODY is caused by mutations in transcription factors (such as hepatocyte nuclear factor genes *HNF-1*α, *HNF-4*α, and *HNF-1*β and insulin promoter factor-1) (49). There are clear clinical differences between these two different types of MODY, reflecting quantitative and qualitative differences in pancreatic β-cell dysfunction. Glucokinase MODY is relatively mild and characterized by nonprogressive hyperglycemia, which is caused by a stable defect and resetting of the pancreatic glucose sensor. It can be treated with diet alone, and complications are rare. In contrast, MODY caused by mutations in the transcription factors lead to a progressive β-cell defect in insulin secretion, an increasing requirement for treatment, and all the complications usually associated with type 2 DM (50). Diagnostic molecular testing is available for the more common genes involved, although approximately 15% to 20% of the families fitting MODY criteria do not have mutations in any of the known genes (48). A stepwise approach to the etiological investigation of young adults with DM is recommended (51,52). Alternative molecular tests may also be appropriate to identify these patients, with markers downstream of the genetic defect. For example, the haploinsufficiency of the gene coding for *HNF-1*α is associated with reduced serum apolipoprotein M levels, which may be a useful marker for MODY3 patients (53).

Heterozygous mutations in the *HNF-1*α gene are the most common cause of MODY accounting for between 1% and 2% of all cases of DM (57). Isolated case reports have suggested that patients with *HNF-1*α MODY (MODY3) are more sensitive to the hypoglycemic effects of sulfonylureas, compared with the patients with type 2 DM (58–61). Hyperexcitability of the pancreas to sulfonylureas has been described in one healthy glucose-tolerant person with an *HNF-1*α mutation who showed a greater response to intravenous tolbutamide than healthy controls (62). This has subsequently been demonstrated in a randomized cross-over trial comparing the response to a sulfonylurea and metformin in patients with diabetes caused by either *HNF-1*α mutations or type 2 DM (63). Patients

Table 3 Most Common Maturity-Onset Diabetes of the Young Subtypes

Subtype	Mutation	Chromosome	Approximate frequency	End result	References
MODY1	*HNF-4*α	20q	5%	Impaired pancreatic β-cell function	(54)
MODY2	GCK (glucokinase)	7p	10%	Defect in glucose sensing	(55)
MODY3	*HNF-1*α	12q	65%	Impaired pancreatic β-cell function	(56)

with diabetes caused by mutations in the *HNF-1α* gene showed a greater improvement in glycemia in response to treatment with the sulfonylurea gliclazide, in comparison with matched (for body-mass index and degree of glycaemia) patients with type 2 DM. This was not attributable to changes in the hepatic metabolism of the drug but reflects preserved ß-cell function and a preserved insulin secretory response to sulfonylureas in patients with MODY. This has important implications for the management of such patients—the increased sensitivity to sulfonylureas would suggest that this class of drug should be used, alongside an appropriate diet, as initial treatment, instead of a biguanide, or even insulin therapy, and at a reduced dosage to improve glycemic control (63). Hypoglycemia may be more common in these patients, and thus the use of very low doses of sulfonylureas is important. Pearson et al. (63) recommend a starting dose of 20–40 mg gliclazide (or equivalent) in this subgroup of patients. Furthermore, cessation of sulfonylureas should be undertaken cautiously as there may be a marked deterioration in glycemic control.

The effects of sulfonylureas are initiated by the drug binding to ATP-sensitive K^+ (K_{ATP}) channels, inducing membrane depolarization, activation of voltage-gated Ca^{2+} channels, and subsequent degranulation of insulin-containing vesicles (64). Mice lacking the *HNF-1α* gene have a dramatic reduction in insulin secretory response to glucose (65,66) and a good insulin secretory response to glibenclamide. Although this has been demonstrated to be accompanied by impaired hepatic clearance and elevated plasma concentrations of the drug (67), the expression of the glycolytic enzymes, glucokinase and liver pyruvate kinase, is also reduced in the pancreatic islets of *HNF-1α*-deficient mice compared with the wild-type mice (68,69). This suggests that the glucose metabolism pathway is a key site of action on *HNF-1α*, and that in *HNF-1α* deficiency, the genetic ß-cell defect is upstream of the sulfonylurea receptor. Therefore, it is proposed that the good insulin secretory response to sulfonylureas in spite of the poor response to glucose in MODY3 diabetes is the result of a bypass in a severe defect in glucose metabolism and that the signaling pathway downstream of the sulfonylurea receptor is preserved (63). This is illustrated in Figure 1. The challenge for pharmacogenetics in the future is to assist in the identification of a larger group of patients who will respond to specific treatments depending on the predominant underlying pathophysiology.

The PPARγ Gene and Sensitivity to Thiazolidinediones

Thiazolidinediones are a novel class of antidiabetic medication that exert multiple effects beyond glycemic control and may have beneficial effects on cardiovascular risk factors. They decrease insulin resistance and reduce cardiovascular risk by improving various aspects of the cardiovascular dysmetabolic syndrome. They may reduce accelerated atherosclerosis associated with type 2 DM not only by improving glycemia and decreasing plasma insulin levels but also by increasing high-density lipoprotein (HDL) and decreasing triglyceride levels, improving blood pressure, improving fibrinolysis, and reducing vessel wall abnormalities.

Although discovered more than two decades ago, it was not until the mid-1990s that their molecular mechanism of action was elucidated. Thiazolidinediones are synthetic ligands that activate nuclear receptors called peroxisome proliferator-activated receptors (PPARs). Once activated, the PPARs form heterodimers with another nuclear receptor, the 9-cis-retinoic acid receptor (RXR). By binding to specific DNA sequences, these PPAR/RXR heterodimers regulate transcription and translation of proteins involved in glucose and lipid metabolism (70,71). There are three subtypes of PPARs currently identified: PPARα, PPARβ (also known as PPARδ, NUC-1, and FAAR), and PPARγ. The antidiabetic actions of thiazolidinediones correspond to their ability to activate PPARγ receptors found in key target tissues

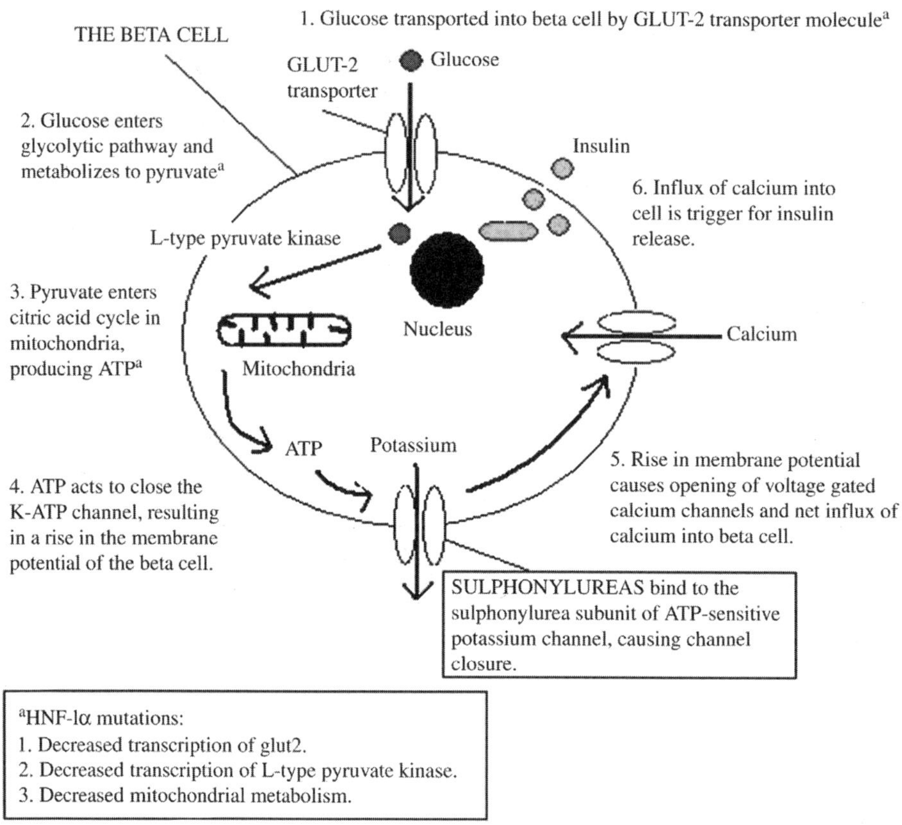

Figure 1 Glucose-induced insulin secretion, sulfonylureas, and the *HNF-1α* mutation. *Abbreviations*: GLUT-2, glucose transporter in hepatocyte and pancreatic β-cell; ATP, adenosine triphosphate; K-ATP, potassium-ATP channel. *Source*: Adapted from Ref. 63.

of insulin action, namely, adipose tissue, skeletal muscle, and liver. Currently, two structurally diverse PPARγ agonists are used in clinical practice: pioglitazone (Actos®) and rosiglitazone (Avandia®). Troglitazone was withdrawn from the market in March 2000 because of its association with idiosyncratic hepatotoxicity, an effect that had been postulated to be influenced by mutations of the glutathione-*S*-transferase genotype (72). In a study by Watanabe et al. (72) genotype analysis was performed on 110 patients who had been prescribed troglitazone, evaluating 68 polymorphic sites in 51 candidate genes relating to drug metabolism, apoptosis, production and elimination of reactive oxygen species, and also the signal transduction pathways of PPARγ2 and insulin. A strong correlation with transaminase elevations was observed only in patients with the combined glutathione-*S*-transferase *GSTT1-GSTM1* null genotype.

The interaction between Thiazolidinediones and the PPAR represents another model of pharmacogenomics. Thiazolidinediones has been shown to decrease plasma glucose concentrations in patients with type 2 DM (73–75), but clinical studies have shown that 10–25% of the patients treated with thiazolidinediones do not achieve a 15% reduction in fasting plasma glucose or do not convert from impaired glucose tolerance to normal glucose tolerance (76). The molecular reasons for the differential responses have not been determined, although it has been postulated that that differences in the PPARγ genotype may modify the response to thiazolidinedione treatment. Different genetic variants of the PPARγ gene have been shown to affect drug action in vitro (77). The most common variant in the PPARγ gene, the Pro12Ala variant, occurs at a frequency of 12% to 15% (78–83), whereas other mutations are very rare (84–86). In a clinical study, the Pro12Ala and the Pro12Pro variants in the PPARγ gene, however, were not associated with a favorable response to pioglitazone in patients with type 2 DM (87). Although these preliminary results would suggest that these variants in the PPARγ gene do not determine the response to pioglitazone, it is unclear whether other variants in the gene, or indeed variants in downstream pathways from this receptor, are important determinants of efficacy or adverse effects, such as fluid retention. Interestingly, in an animal model it has been shown that the CD36 fatty acid transporter gene is an important determinant of the insulin-sensitizing actions and subsequent metabolic effects of pioglitazone (88). The fatty acid transporter CD36 is one of a number of molecules that mediate the uptake of (free fatty acids) FFA by adipocytes and muscle cells and is a well-known target for PPAR ligands (89,90). Clearly this is an area for future research.

HYPERLIPIDEMIA

Hyperlipidemia, the elevation of lipid concentrations in plasma, is the manifestation of a disorder in the synthesis and degradation of plasma lipoproteins. The major concern in patients with hyperlipidemia is their increased risk of cardiovascular disease. Statins are inhibitors of 3-hydroxy-3-methylglutaryl-coenzyme A (HMG-CoA) reductase, the rate-determining enzyme for cholesterol synthesis. They reduce cholesterol by stimulating an increase in low-density-lipoprotein (LDL) receptors on hepatocyte membranes, thereby increasing the clearance of LDL from the circulation. Their main effect is to reduce LDL-cholesterol (LDL-C), but they may also reduce triglycerides to a modest extent and increase HDL-cholesterol (HDL-C). They are generally considered to be the most effective of all lipid-lowering drugs currently available. Large-scale clinical trials in the primary and secondary prevention of coronary heart disease (CHD) have unequivocally demonstrated the efficacy of statins in reducing the risk of cardiovascular events (91–96).

HMG-CoA reductase inhibitors are a generally well-tolerated class of drug, although in a minority of patients severe adverse effects, such as myopathy or rhabdomyolysis, may occur. The incidence of these potentially life-threatening side effects increases with increasing dose or with the coadminstration of drugs that affect the kinetics or dynamics of statins. The withdrawal of cerivastatin as a result of deaths from rhabdomyolysis illustrates the clinical importance of such interactions. On the other hand, not all patients respond to statin therapy with a reduction in CHD risk. Large clinical trials with statins have demonstrated varying reductions in cardiovascular events associated with similar changes in LDL-C, suggesting that at least some of the benefit of statin therapy may be derived from nonlipid mechanisms of disease attenuation, such as the modification of the inflammatory response, endothelial function, plaque stability, and thrombus formation (97).

Statins Reduce Risk in Specific Populations

Allelic variants in several candidate genes have been identified as markers for CHD, and their relationship with the response to statin therapy (based on metabolic, angiographic, and clinical outcomes) has been evaluated through retrospective analyses in many of the large statin trials. Although treatment with statin therapy results in similar improvements in lipoprotein profiles in all patients (among both carriers and noncarriers of the variant allele), it appears that statins preferentially benefit individuals in terms of the number of cardiovascular events and mortality who carry the high-risk variant genotypes for these risk factors, as compared with the individuals who have the wild-type genotype (98). Several polymorphic candidate genes have been identified as predictors of disease severity; these are summarized in Table 4.

Apolipoprotein E

Apolipoprotein E (ApoE), a constituent of very low-density lipoprotein (VLDL), is derived from the liver and serves in the transport and redistribution of lipids among various tissues throughout the body (99). Carriers of the *ε4* allele have a 40% increased risk of developing CHD when compared with carriers of the *ε2* or *ε3* alleles (100). During the follow-up period of a substudy of the Scandinavian Simvastatin Survival Study (4S), placebo-treated carriers of the *ε4* allele were almost twice as likely to die as noncarriers (15.7% and 9.0%), corresponding to a mortality risk ratio of 1.8 (101). Treatment with simvastatin resulted in a 61% reduction in the number of deaths in carriers of the *ε4* allele (from 15.7% to 6.0%), whereas in non-*ε4* carriers, simvastatin was associated with a 43% decrease in mortality (from 9.0% to 5.1%).

Table 4 Genetic Markers of Statin Response

Marker	Nature	High-risk variant allele	References
Apolipoprotein E (ApoE)	Constituent of liver-derived very low-density lipoprotein Transport and redistribution of lipids	*ε4* (compared with *ε2* and *ε3* alleles)	(100)
ß-Fibrinogen	Deposited in atherosclerotic plaques	*-455G/A* (wild type-*455G/G*)	(105)
Cholesterol ester transfer protein (CETP)	Mediates exchange of lipids between lipoproteins	*Taq1* polymorphism *B1* allele (compared with *B2* allele)	(110)
Hepatic lipase (HL)	Lipolytic enzyme involved in the metabolism of triglycerides, LDL, and HDL	*C* allele (compared with *T* allele)	(114,115)
Lipoprotein lipase (LPL)	Involved in the metabolism of triycerides in lipoproteins	Asp(9)Asn LPL mutation	(116)
Platelet glycoprotein III	Induces neointimal proliferation	PI^{A2} polymorphism	(122)
Stromelysin-1	Associated with connective tissue remodeling in atherogenesis and plaque rupture	*6A* (compared with *5A* allele)	(123)

Abbreviations: VLDL, very low-density lipoproteins; HDL, high-density lipoproteins; LDL, low-density lipoproteins.

ß-Fibrinogen

Polymorphisms in the ß-fibrinogen gene, particularly the *-455G/A* single-nucleotide polymorphism (SNP), have been associated with differences in the plasma levels of fibrinogen and the severity of arterial disease. It has thus been postulated that patients with the *-455A* allele have an increased rate of progression of CHD when compared with the wild type (*-455GG*) because their fibrinogen levels may increase more when the acute-phase response is triggered (102–104). The *-455A* allele was identified in 257 (4% homozygous, 34% heterozygous) out of 697 men enrolled in a study from the Regression Growth Evaluation Statin Study (REGRESS) (105). All patients had similar baseline lipid values and disease history, but the *-455A* homozygotes had significantly higher baseline fibrinogen levels (but less angiographic evidence of CHD) when compared with the other genotypes. However, after a two-year period of follow-up, placebo-treated patients with the *-455AA* genotype experienced a significantly greater progression of CHD as assessed by coronary angiographic parameters when compared with the *-455GA* and *-455GG* genotypes. The authors hypothesize that the *-455A* allele may promote a stronger acute-phase response in fibrinogen and that the resulting higher fibrinogen levels may form the pathogenetic basis for the stronger progression of coronary atherosclerosis. Despite similar reductions in LDL-C in the pravastatin-treated groups, only carriers of the *A* allele demonstrated angiographic regression of the disease. Although carriers of the high-risk allele, particularly the homozygotes, were associated with higher plasma fibrinogen levels and more rapid progression of the atherosclerotic lesions, pravastatin therapy seemed to offset this deleterious effect. The fact that the more rapid progression in the *-455AA* genotype was not apparent in the pravastatin group may be explained by a much larger positive effect of pravastatin treatment than the deleterious influence of the fibrinogen *-455G/A* polymorphism on the development of the disease.

Cholesteryl Ester Transfer Protein

Cholesteryl ester transfer protein (CETP) has a central role in the metabolism of HDL-C, mediating the exchange of lipids between lipoproteins. The CETP-enzyme has a central role in reverse cholesterol transport (RCT), whereby cholesterol from peripheral tissues is transported back to the liver where it is preferentially excreted into bile (106). This results in the net transfer of cholesteryl ester from HDL to other lipoproteins and the subsequent uptake of cholesterol by hepatocytes (107). This is illustrated in Figure 2. The presence of a polymorphism in the CETP gene (which is also called *Taq1B*) is associated with elevated concentrations of CETP, which in turn leads to reduced concentrations of HDL-C, a strong and independent risk factor for the development of CHD (107,109). Individuals with the *Taq1B* polymorphism in the CETP gene may therefore be at higher risk for the development of CHD (110). In the study of 807 men by Kuivenhoven et al. (107), the term *B1* was used to denote the presence of *Taq1*, and *B2* was used to denote absence of *Taq1*. The respective frequencies of the *B1B1*, *B1B2*, and *B2B2* genotypes were 35%, 49%, and 16%, respectively. The *B1* allele was associated with lower HDL-C concentrations and higher CETP concentrations in all patients. Baseline LDL-C concentrations were similar in all genotypes, but on following a 2-year period of follow-up, placebo-treated patients with the *B1B1* genotype showed the most pronounced angiographic progression of atherosclerosis, when compared with the *B1B2* and *B2B2* genotypes. Although patients with each genotype achieved similar reductions in LDL-C from pravastatin therapy, both the *B1* homozygotes and heterozygotes experienced less (angiographically-determined) progression of coronary disease when compared with individuals with the respective genotype who received placebo. Conversely, no significant differences in disease progression were observed between the

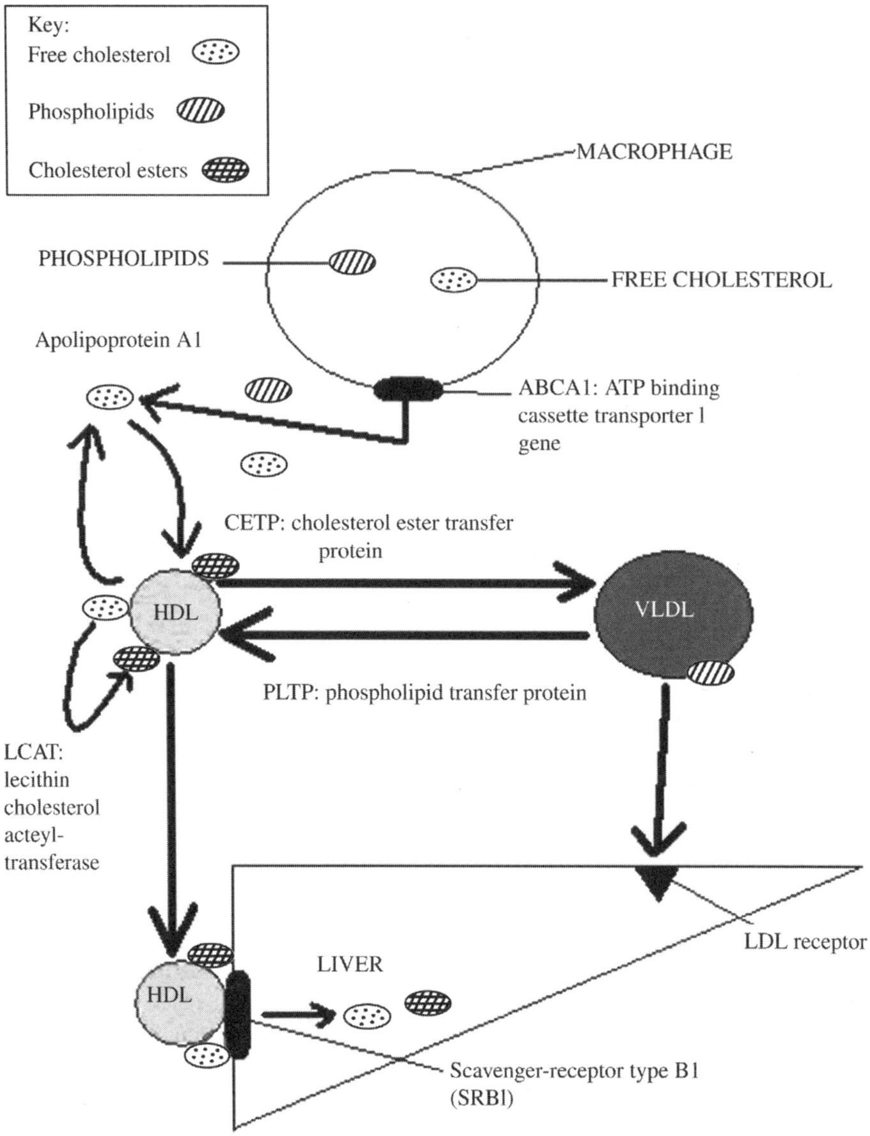

Figure 2 The proteins involved in HDL-mediated reverse cholesterol transport. *Abbreviations*: VLDL, very low-density lipoproteins; HDL, high-density lipoproteins; LDL, low-density lipoproteins; ATP, adenosine triphosphate.

placebo and pravastatin-treated *B2B2* homozygotes. However, there was only a small decrease in plaque regression in the pravastatin-treated group (the decrease in mean luminal diameter was 0.05 ± 0.16 mm for the *B1B1* genotype, 0.07 ± 0.20 mm for the *B1B2* genotype, and 0.09 ± 0.16 mm for the *B2B2* genotype), and whether this leads to a long-lasting clinical benefit is unclear.

Hepatic Lipase

Hepatic lipase (HL) is a plasma lipolytic enzyme that plays an important role in the metabolism of triglycerides, LDL, and HDL. Increased HL activity has been associated with reduced HDL levels and smaller HDL particles, and also an increased number of small, dense LDL particles (111,112). The presence of a C-T substitution at position -514 in the promoter region of the HL gene accounts for approximately one-quarter of the variance in HL activity in men and women (113,114). The presence of the *C* allele has been associated with higher HL activity, more atherogenic LDL particles, and lower levels of anti-atherogenic HDL lipoproteins (115). Results from one study suggest that this promoter region gene polymorphism is responsible for the differential lipoprotein and angiographic response to lipid-lowering therapy (114). In the 49 men included in the analysis, 25 had the *CC* genotype, 20 had the *CT*, and 4 had the *TT* genotype at position -514 of the HL gene promoter. At baseline, men with the *CC* genotype had greater HL activity, lower HDL-C, and lower LDL buoyancy, when compared with those with the TT genotype. Lipid-lowering therapy (lovastatin plus colestipol or niacin plus colestipol) was associated with an 18% decrease in HL activity and a 12% increase in LDL buoyancy in patients with the *CC* genotype, whereas HL activity and LDL buoyancy did not significantly change in patients with the *TT* genotype. Furthermore, lipid-lowering therapy was also associated with a 2.1% reduction in coronary stenosis among men with the *CC* genotype, whereas progression of stenosis was observed in men with the *TT* genotype.

Lipoprotein Lipase

Lipoprotein lipase (LPL) is an enzyme that is involved in the metabolism of triglycerides in lipoproteins, such as chylomicrons and VLDL (111). Common mutations in the LPL gene that lead to deficient LPL activity have been associated with hypertriglyceridemia and low HDL levels, which results in affected individuals being at increased risk for premature CHD (116). In one study, the nature and frequency of the aspartic acid to asparagine substitution at position 9 in exon 2 of the LPL gene (Asp9Asn) has been examined (117). The authors hypothesized that the presence of the Asp9Asn LPL polymorphism in a given patient would increase susceptibility to atherosclerosis and therefore be associated with greater progression of the CHD. Indeed, the Asp9Asn mutation was identified in 4.8% of the population (38 men), and carriers of the polymorphism were more likely to have a positive family history of CHD and a lower HDL-C level at baseline, when compared with patients without the mutation. After a two-year period of follow-up, placebo-treated carriers of the Asp9Asn LPL polymorphism showed greater progression of angiographically significant CHD when compared with the noncarriers. Although the lipid-lowering effect of pravastatin was attenuated in patients carrying the Asp9Asn substitution, the deleterious effects of this polymorphism on the progression of atherosclerosis could apparently be reversed by pravastatin.

Platelet Glycoprotein III

Studies have identified an association between the polymorphism of the gene encoding platelet glycoprotein IIIa (Pl^{A2} polymorphism) and acute coronary syndromes, subacute stent thrombosis, restenosis development following coronary stent implantation, and increased platelet aggregability (118–122). Statin therapy has been shown to reduce the increased rate of restenosis associated with the high risk Pl^{A2} allele and significantly improved clinical outcomes in a consecutive series of patients undergoing coronary stent implantation (122). In a study of 650 patients (78% of whom were homozygous for the Pl^{A1} allele, and 22% of the patients carried the Pl^{A2} allele) by Walter et al. (122), restenosis rates at 6 months were significantly reduced by statin therapy. Although the extent of cholesterol lowering by statin therapy was identical in both carriers of the Pl^{A2} allele and patients homozygous for Pl^{A1} and there were no significant differences in baseline parameters, statin-treated carriers of the Pl^{A2} allele had a 22.3% lower rate of restenosis than PI^{A2} carriers without statin therapy (28.6% vs. 50.9%, respectively; $p = 0.01$). Furthermore, statin-treated patients homozygous for the PI^{A1} allele had a slight reduction in the restenosis rate when compared with the PI^{A1} homozygotes who did not receive statin therapy. In the patients who received placebo, the PI^{A2} allele was associated with an increased rate of restenosis when compared with the PI^{A1} allele (50.9% vs. 34%; $p = 0.01$), although there were no differences in the rate of restenosis observed between statin-treated carriers of either allele. The significantly lower restenosis rate observed in statin-treated carriers of the PI^{A2} allele was associated with a significant improvement in the six-month event-free survival (49.3% in PI^{A2} carriers without statin treatment vs. 28.2% in statin-treated PI^{A2} carriers; $p < 0.01$), whereas statin therapy had a minimal effect on six-month event-free survival among those homozygous for PI^{A1}.

Stromelysin-1

Stromelysin-1, a matrix metalloproteinase, is involved with the connective tissue remodeling processes associated with atherogenesis and atherosclerotic plaque rupture (123). The *6A* allele of the *5A6A* polymorphism in the stromelysin-1 gene promoter region has been linked to a rapidly progressive form of coronary stenosis due to atherosclerosis (124). In a substudy of the REGRESS, de Maat et al. hypothesized that the presence of the stromelysin-1 *6A* allele may be associated with an increased risk of clinical events or requirement for repeat angioplasty due to clinical restenosis (123,125). Greater than 75% of the 494 men evaluated in this analysis carried the variant allele (*6A*) (50% heterozygous and 26% homozygous), and after two years of follow-up, no significant differences in angiographic measures of coronary artery obstruction were found among the three genotypes that were treated with pravastatin or between placebo and pravastatin-treated patients. However, nearly twice as many clinical events [myocardial infarction (MI), CHD death, symptom-driven percutaneous transluminal coronary angioplasty or coronary artery bypass graft surgery, stroke and transient ischemic attack, and death] were observed in the placebo-treated patients with the *5A6A* and *6A6A* genotypes (26% in both groups) when compared with those homozygous for the *5A* allele (12%) ($p < 0.05$). It must be stated, however, that in this study the baseline risk in the *5A5A* group was already lower than for the *5A6A* and *6A6A* groups. Compared with the placebo, treatment with pravastatin was associated with a 48% increase in frequency of clinical events among patients with the *5A5A* genotype, whereas patients with the *5A6A* and *6A6A* genotypes experienced a 71% and a 54% reduction in clinical events, respectively. Pravastatin was also associated with an increase in the frequency of symptom-driven repeat angioplasty among patients with the *5A5A* genotype (from 11% to 28%), whereas patients with the *5A6A* and *6A6A* genotypes experienced reductions in the frequency of repeat angioplasty (from 37.5% to 0%, and 40% to 15%, respectively $p < 0.002$) compared with the placebo.

Thus, it appears that patients with the *5A5A* genotype receive no additional benefit from pravastatin, indicating that the response to pharmacological intervention showed a genotype-specific effect, solely benefiting carriers of the *6A* allele. The results from the Lopid Coronary Angiography Trial (LOCAT), using gemfibrozil, corroborate the findings from REGRESS and suggest that both statins and fibrates offer a protective effect on disease progression solely in carriers of the *6A* allele, whereas the degree of protection in patients with the *5A5A* genotype is marginal (126,127).

Statins and the Genetics of Metabolism and Disposition

Pravastatin is not significantly metabolized by the CYP450 system; the CYP3A family metabolizes lovastatin, simvastatin, atorvastatin, and cerivastatin, whereas CYP2C9 metabolizes fluvastatin (128). Fluvastatin is a synthetic HMG-CoA reductase inhibitor and is a racemic mixture of (−)-3S, 5R-fluvastatin and (+)-3R, 5S-fluvastatin. The latter has a 30-fold higher therapeutic activity (129). Fluvastatin is eliminated from the human body almost entirely by hepatic biotransformation, primarily being metabolized to 5-hydroxy-, 6-hydroxy-, and *N*-deisopropyl-fluvastatin by CYP2C9. In vitro data show that about 50–80% of fluvastatin metabolic clearance is due to CYP2C9 (130). Kirchheiner et al. (130) studied the impact of the two frequent CYP2C9 amino acid polymorphisms on enantio-specific fluvastatin pharmacokinetics and pharmacodynamics in healthy volunteers (130). The pharmacokinetics of both enantiomers of fluvastatin depended on the *CYP2C9* genotype, with a threefold group mean difference in the active enantiomer and even greater differences in the inactive enantiomer. The *CYP2C9*2* variant did not have any significant influence on fluvastatin kinetics. However, differences in plasma concentrations were not reflected in cholesterol-lowering after 14 days of fluvastatin intake in healthy volunteers. The latter result is unsurprising for a number of reasons. First, the baseline cholesterol levels differed between the genotype groups because the study groups were stratified for the *CYP2C9* genotype but not for the baseline cholesterol concentration. Second, fluvastatin steady-state kinetics were not measured after 15 days of treatment, and kinetic differences between genotype groups might have been smaller at steady-state than after a single dose. Third, the sample size of this study was determined for pharmacokinetics analyses, and a larger sample would be necessary to assess the pharmacodynamic impact. As discussed previously, the pharmacodynamic effect of statins is influenced by multiple variables including other pharmacogenomic predictors of HMG-CoA reductase inhibitor efficacy, such as polymorphisms in the LDL receptor, CETP, ApoE, and the β-fibrinogen genes.

Drug transporters are increasingly recognized to be important in drug disposition and response. Polymorphisms in the *MDR1* gene, encoding P-glycoprotein (P-gp), affect the pharmacokinetics of many commonly used drugs, including statins, many of which are substrates for P-gp (131,132). P-gp is a member of the large ATP-binding cassette (*ABCB1*) family of proteins. It is found in the small intestine on the brush border of enterocytes and may thus influence the oral bioavailability of statin therapy (128,133). However, the extent of this has not yet been quantified. It is also evident that many substrates of P-gp are also *CYP3A4* substrates, and this is well demonstrated in the case of statins. The overlap between *CYP3A4* and P-gp substrates may have resulted in part from the coordinated regulation and tissue expression of *CYP3A4* and *MDR1* in organs, such as the liver and intestine. Interestingly, both genes are located on the same chromosome in close proximity, 7q22.1 and 7q21.1 for *CYP3A4* and *MDR1*, respectively (134). Future studies of the relevant statin should therefore take into account both the metabolizing and transport capabilities of individuals, as failure to correct this confounding factor may lead to contradictory data from different studies.

OSTEOPOROSIS

Osteoporosis is a major healthcare problem internationally with significant morbidity and mortality. It is a common problem affecting older women and a large number of older men. The health care costs are estimated at $30 to $50 million per year per million of population across many developed countries (135,136). Furthermore, there is also an increased risk of death in both men and women with all types of osteoporotic fractures (137). The pathophysiology of the disease is complex and involves both endogenous and environmental factors.

Bone mass is influenced by hormonal changes, such as puberty and menopause, and by lifestyle factors, such as smoking and calcium intake. Total bone mass increases approximately threefold over just a few years just before puberty with bone mass remaining stable thereafter until the onset of menopausal and age-related bone loss (138). Age-related bone loss may start in the early forties in both men and women and accelerates with aging (139–141), although androgen deficiency may also result in bone loss in younger men (142–144). There is a considerable amount of variability in the rate of bone loss seen in postmenopausal women. Interestingly, similar variability is also observed with the effects of corticosteroids on bone loss, due to a wide range in sensitivity (145). Such variations in hormonal sensitivity may reflect an interaction between gene(s) and environmental factors.

Osteoporosis and Genes

Family and twin studies have shown that genetic factors play an essential role in bone mass regulation and, apart from rare instances, the heritability of bone mineral density (BMD) and osteoporosis is polygenic. Peak bone mass, as measured by quantitative radiological techniques, also seems to be under genetic control. This has been most clearly shown in studies of MZ and DZ twins (146–148). A positive family history of an osteoporotic fracture has been found to be a risk factor for the development of osteoporotic fracture in numerous epidemiological studies (149–151). Human and animal studies have shown high levels of heritability (45–80% of variance) in the density and structure of bone for any age or group (148–150), and the fact that this heritability is apparent before puberty would suggest that genetic factors are responsible for programming inherent bone structural characteristics.

The twin model has been primarily been used to assess heritability but, twin studies, particularly in MZ twins, can also be used to investigate the impact of the environment and other lifestyle factors (152,153). Environmental factors known to affect bone density, including skeletal loading, calcium intake, smoking, and alcohol use, have been investigated in this manner. Physical loading on the skeleton, ranging from immobilization and microgravity to loading in elite athletic sports, has been shown to affect bone mass (152,154–157). Furthermore, there is considerable debate regarding the most appropriate daily calcium intake. Figures ranging from 800 to more than 1000 mg/day have been recommended (141,158,159). However, in Asian populations where the dairy intake is relatively low, the dietary calcium intake is closer to 400 mg/day, and yet the incidence of osteoporotic fractures is unexpectedly lower than in comparable Caucasian populations (160,161). Although other lifestyle factors may be important, this suggests that ethnic or racial differences in calcium absorption and handling may represent another example of gene–environment interactions.

A Summary of the Management of Osteoporosis

Different approaches to the management of osteoporosis have been advocated, including changes in lifestyle, interventions to reduce falls, the use of drugs to decrease bone resorption, such as calcium, estrogens, calcitonins, and bisphosphonates, and also the administration of drugs to stimulate bone formation, such as sodium fluoride (162–165). Prevention is the most effective method of dealing with osteoporosis because once bone mass has decreased, it is difficult to replace. Optimizing peak bone mass is therefore important. Regular, moderate weight-bearing exercise and adequate dietary calcium during growth have been advocated (138,166). After the third decade of life, interventions should be aimed at reducing the rate of bone loss. In postmenopausal women, hormone replacement therapy (HRT) slows or eliminates postmenopausal bone loss at all skeletal sites. However, the potential value of long-term HRT must be balanced against the potential risks, particularly breast cancer. Alternatives to HRT for the prevention of postmenopausal osteoporosis include the bisphosphonates, alendronate, etidronate, and risedronate. In postmenopausal women, the effects of calcium supplementation (about 1 g of calcium daily by mouth) have been conflicting (167,168).

In postmenopausal women with established osteoporosis, HRT increases bone mass and reduces the incidence of fractures. Alternatively, a bisphosphonate, such as alendronate or etidronate, may be used (169). Improvements in bone mass and fracture rate have also been shown with raloxifene (170). Calcitonins may also have a role. Studies using the vitamin D substance calcitriol for the treatment of osteoporosis have produced conflicting results; although some have reported an increase in spinal bone density and a reduction in the rate of new vertebral fractures, others have found no significant effects (171–173). Vitamin D supplements have beneficial effects in the elderly and may be particularly important in frail or housebound individuals, who are at high risk of vitamin D deficiency and resulting hyperparathyroidism (165,174). The extent of the variability observed, and some of the conflicting findings of studies across this field, may, at least in part, be explained by genetic differences. The influence of drugs on osteoporosis may be another example of the interaction between genes and the environment.

VDR Gene Polymorphism

It has been shown that polymorphisms in the vitamin D receptor (VDR) gene are associated with bone density and that the VDR gene is associated with a particular bone density pattern that varies with chronological age, sex, and anatomical site (175,176). The VDR gene polymorphism is also related to a higher prevalence of vertebral fractures (177,178). Polymorphic alleles of the VDR gene were the first to be associated with bone turnover and bone density in a nonstructural gene (179), though a number of subsequent studies have identified weaker or no effects (180,181). However, two meta-analyses support a role for the VDR gene alleles, though with somewhat less strength than originally reported (182,183). An additional start codon polymorphism of the VDR gene has been associated with differences in bone density in some but not all population groups (181,184). Markers of bone turnover, such as the procollagen type I propeptide, which is cleaved and released when collagen is produced, have also been shown to be genetically linked in some but not all studies (185,186). There may be a relationship between the VDR alleles and the risk of fracture (187), although this has not been found in all studies (188). Several other "candidate" gene loci have been associated with bone density or fractures. These are summarized in Table 5. In each of these cases, the initial positive (association) results have been counterbalanced by some if not several negative (no association) studies. Such contradictory data may be due to several factors, including lack of power, differences in inclusion criteria and clinical phenotyping of patients, and unforeseen population stratification (189). This also makes it difficult to relate any drug effects to genotypes that may be involved in determining the pathogenesis of the disease itself, because the effect of the drug will vary depending on the interaction of the gene with the disease itself.

It is, however, interesting to note that the anti-osteoporotic treatments show significant variability in terms of the gain in BMD. This variability may be a reflection of the

Table 5 Some of the Candidate Gene Loci Associated with Bone Density

Nature	Gene	References
Hormone receptor	Vitamin D receptor	(145)
	Estrogen receptor	(205)
	Calcitonin receptor	(206)
	Parathyroid hormone receptor	(207)
Cytokines	Interleukins-4 and -6	(206,208)
	Interleukin-1 receptor antagonist	(209)
	TGF-1	(210)
	TGF receptor	(211)
	Insulin-like growth factor-I	(212)
Lipoproteins	Apolipoprotein E	(198)

phenomenon of the regression to the mean or the influence of as yet unidentified genetic factors. Dietary calcium intake is an obvious factor that may affect responsiveness of VDR genes. Calcium intake commonly ranges from less than 400 to more than 1000 mg/day in different population groups. In some studies, genotype-related differences in calcium handling have been observed. In one study, homozygous *BB* subjects for the VDR gene did not show an increase in their gut calcium absorption on lower dietary calcium intakes, when compared with the homozygous *bb* subjects, whereas in another study, urinary calcium excretion was higher in the *bb* subjects (190,191). A separate study has also found a 42% difference in gut calcium absorption between alternate homozygotes for the VDR start codon polymorphism (192). Similarly, longitudinal studies have shown differences in the bone density response to calcium intake according to VDR genotype. In one study, VDR gene heterozygotes responded to calcium intake while the alternate homozygotes either gained or lost bone irrespective of calcium intake (193). In contrast, Krall et al. (194) found that the *BB* homozygotes gained some bone when supplemented from a very low basic calcium intake.

Despite apparent differences in gut calcium absorption, this is not reflected in differences in intestinal VDR levels (195). Differences in response of bone density to the vitamin D metabolites and analogs have been reported according to the VDR genotypes, particularly in Japanese studies (196–198). The more common *bb* genotype in Japanese cohorts (about 75% of the subjects) was more responsive, compared with the heterozygotes, who either did not respond or whose bone density actually deteriorated. Given that the heterozygote is the most common genotype in most Caucasian groups, these differences parallel the differences that have been observed in response to the active vitamin D compounds in clinical studies of osteoporosis between Japanese and Caucasian groups. In another study, the response to vitamin D varied according to VDR genotype (199). In the study by Graafman et al. (199), the mean increase in BMD in the vitamin D group—relative to the placebo group, expressed as percentage of baseline BMD—was significantly higher in the *BB* (δBMD: 4.4%) and *Bb* genotype (δBMD: 4.2%), compared with the *bb* genotype (δBMD: -0.3%, $p = 0.61$). The VDR genotype-dependent effect of vitamin D supplementation in the elderly subjects investigated here suggests a functional involvement of the VDR gene variants in determining BMD.

VDR gene polymorphisms have also been shown to modify the BMD response to cyclic etidronate therapy and also HRT (200–202). Palomba et al. (203) demonstrated in postmenopausal women with osteoporosis that the effectiveness of raloxifene on bone metabolism seems to be controlled by different VDR genotypes. Raloxifene is a nonsteroidal drug that inhibits bone resorption and reduces the risk of vertebral fracture in postmenopausal women (170). In this study, the lumbar spine BMD increased significantly more in women homozygous for the *BB* genotype than in those homozygous for the *bb* genotype (203). Serum and urinary levels of bone turnover markers also showed a more significant decrease in women homozygous for *BB* than in those homozygous for *bb*. An intermediate change of lumbar BMD, serum osteocalcin (OC) and urinary deoxypyridinoline (DPD) was observed in heterozygotes, in keeping with a gene dose effect of the *B* allele.

The mechanism by which any changes in the VDR alleles may account for changes in calcium and bone homeostasis is not clear. It is possible that subtle differences may exist in the regulation of the gene or in the stability of the mRNA product. Some initial in vitro studies suggested that change in stability of mRNA product may be responsible (204). However, this finding has not been replicated. Another mechanism may relate to changes in alternative transcripts from the recently reported multiple promoters of the single human VDR gene (204). In any case, the hope is that in the future it may be possible to select the optimal anti-osteoporotic regimen of treatment on the basis of genetic evaluation.

CONCLUSIONS

Metabolic diseases, such as DM, hyperlipidemia, and osteoporosis, are major health problems, responsible for significant morbidity and mortality worldwide. They represent a drain on health care resources internationally, and with the ever-increasing focus on evidence-based medicine, this is only likely to expand, with the requirement to treat a wider, asymptomatic population. DM is a heterogeneous disorder, with a multifactorial etiology. However, the understanding of the pathophysiology and genetic influence of certain specific subtypes of the disease may further our ability to utilize the tools of pharmacogenetics in the wider patient population. In the case of hyperlipidemia, cholesterol-lowering is used as an endpoint, but, more importantly, a reduction in cardiovascular disease progression, morbidity, and mortality is required. There are populations with certain genetic polymorphisms that can be identified to respond well to statin therapy, demonstrating not only a beneficial change in lipid profile but also a reduction in cardiovascular risk. The case of osteoporosis highlights the interaction between genes and environment at all levels, both in terms of physiology and pharmacology. VDR gene polymorphisms result in changes in calcium and bone homeostasis and may modify the response to anti-osteoporotic therapy, but further work is needed in this area not only in relation to the vitamin D receptor gene but also with respect to the many genes that are known to influence bone metabolism and turnover (Table 5).

In the case of metabolic disease, the current understanding of pharmacogenetics extends beyond the knowledge of genetic polymorphism and its role in drug metabolism and disposition. Indeed, these are relatively unimportant in most cases given the relatively wide therapeutic indices and favorable safety profiles of the therapies available and the relative ease of pharmacodynamic monitoring. The challenge for pharmacogenetics in the future is to establish which specific populations are most likely to respond effectively and efficiently to the drugs available. The aim is not to deny treatment to the individual but to ensure that the most appropriate drug is selected for their management—the right drug, at the right dose, and at the right cost.

REFERENCES

1. Zimmet PZ. Kelly West Lecture 1991. Challenges in diabetes epidemiology–from West to the rest. Diabetes Care 1992; 15:232–252.
2. Dinneen S, Gerich J, Rizza R. Carbohydrate metabolism in noninsulin-dependent diabetes mellitus. N Engl J Med 1992; 327:707–713.
3. Firth RG, Bell PM, Marsh HM, Hansen 1, Rizza RA. Postprandial hyperglycemia in patients with noninsulin-dependent diabetes mellitus: role of hepatic and extrahepatic tissues. J Clin Invest 1986; **77**:1525–1532.
4. Butler PC, Rizza RA. Contribution to postprandial hyperglycemia and effect on initial splanchnic glucose clearance of hepatic glucose cycling in glucose-intolerant or NIDDM patients. Diabetes 1991; 40:73–81.
5. Weyer C, Bogardus C, Mott DM, Pratley RE. The natural history of insulin secretory dysfunction and insulin resistance in the pathogenesis of type 2 diabetes mellitus. J Clin Invest 1999; 104:787–794.
6. Kaprio J, Tumiletho J, Koskenvuo M, Romanov K, Renuanen A, Erikson J, Stengaard J, Kesaaniemi YA. Concordance for type 1 (insulin-dependent) and type 2 (non-insulin-dependent) diabetes mellitus in a population-based cohort of twins in Finland. Diabetologia 1992; 35:1060–1067.
7. Kumar D, Gemayel NS, Deapen D, Kapadia D, Yamashita PH, Lee M, Dwyer JH, Roy-Burman P, Bray GA, Mack TM. North-American twins with IDDM: genetic, etiological, and clinical significance of disease concordance according to age, zygosity, and the interval after diagnosis in first twin. Diabetes 1993; 42:1351–1363.
8. Medici F, Hawa M, Ianari A, Pyke DA, Leslie RD. Concordance rate for type II diabetes mellitus in monozygotic twins: actuarial analysis. Diabetologia 1999; 42:146–150.
9. Committee on Diabetic Twins, Japan Diabetes Society. Diabetes mellitus in twins: a cooperative study in Japan. Diabetes Res Clin Pract 1988; **5**:271–280.
10. Radha V, Vimaleswaran KS, Deepa R, Mohan V. The genetics of diabetes mellitus. Indian J Med Res 2003; 117:225–238.
11. Polonsky KS, Sturis J, Bell GI. Seminars in Medicine of the Beth Israel Hospital, Boston. Non-insulin-dependent diabetes mellitus a genetically programmed failure of the beta cell to compensate for insulin resistance. N Engl Med 1996; 334:777–783.
12. Morris RD, Rimm DL, Hartz AJ, Kalkhoff RK, Rimm AA. Obesity and heredity in the etiology of non-insulin-dependent diabetes mellitus in 32,662 adult white women. Am J Epidemiol 1989; 130:112–121.
13. Goldstein JA, de Morais SM. Biochemistry and molecular biology of the human CYP2C subfamily. Pharmacogenetics 1994; 4:285–299.
14. Kirchheiner J, Brockmoller J, Meineke I, Bauer S, Rohde W, Meisel C, et al. Impact of CYP2C9 amino acid polymorphisms on glyburide kinetics and on the insulin and glucose response in healthy volunteers. Clin Pharmacol Ther 2002; 71:286–296.
15. Niemi M, Cascorbi I, Timm R, Kroemer HK, Neuvonen PJ, Kivisto KT. Glyburide and glimepiride pharmacokinetics in subjects with different CYP2C9 genotypes. Clin Pharmacol Ther 2002; 72:326–332.
16. Dunn CJ, Faulds D. Nateglinide. Drugs 2000; 60:607–615.
17. Levien TL, et al. Nateglinide therapy for type 2 diabetes mellitus. Ann Pharmacother 2001; 35:1426–1434.
18. Karara AH, Dunning BE, McLeod JF. The effect of food on the oral bioavailability and the pharmacodynamic actions of the insulinotropic agent A-4166 in healthy subjects. I Clin Pharmacol 1999; 39:172–179.
19. Takesada H, Matsuda K, Ohtake R, et al. Structure determination of metabolites isolated from urine and bile after administration of AY4166, a novel D-phenylalanine-derivative hypoglycemic agent. Bioorg Med Chem 1996; 4:1771–1781.

20. Hanefeld M, Bouter KP, Dickinson S, Guitard C. Rapid and shortacting mealtime insulin secretion with nateglinide controls both prandial and mean glycemia. Diabetes Care 2000; 23:202–207.
21. Horton ES, Clinkingbeard C, Gatlin M, Foley J, Mallows S, Shen S. Nateglinide alone and in combination with metformin improves glycemic control by reducing mealtime glucose levels in type 2 diabetes. Diabetes Care 2000; 23:1660–1665.
22. Schwarz UI. Clinical relevance of genetic polymorphisms in the human CYP2C9 gene. Eur J Clin Invest 2003; 33(suppl 2):23–30.
23. Thomas RC, Ikeda GJ. The metabolic fate of tolbutamide in man and in the rat. J Med Chem 1966; 9:507–510.
24. Nelson E, O'Reilly I. Kinetics of carboxytolbutamide excretion following tolbutamide and carboxytolbutamide administration. J Pharmacol Exp Ther 1961; 132: 103–109.
25. Miners JO, Birkett DJ. Cytochrome P4502C9: an enzyme of major importance in human drug metabolism. Br J Clin Pharmacol 1998; 45:525–538.
26. Lee CR, Pieper JA, Frye RF, Hinderliter AL, Blaisdell JA, Goldstein JA. Tolbutamide, flurbiprofen, and losartan as probes of CYP2C9 activity in humans. J Clin Pharmacol 2003; 43:84–91.
27. Scott J, Poffenbarger PL. Pharmacogenetics of tolbutamide metabolism in humans. Diabetes 1979; 28:41–51.
28. Veronese ME, Miners JO, Rees DLP, Birkett DJ. Tolbutamide hydroxylation in humans: lack of bimodality in 106 healthy subjects. Pharmacogenetics 1993; 3:86–93.
29. Miners JO, Wing LM, Birkett DJ. Normal metabolism of debrisoquine and theophylline in a slow tolbutamide metaboliser. Aust N Z J Medical 1985; 15:348–349.
30. Sullivan-Klose TH, Ghanayem BI, Bell DA, Zhang ZY, Kaminsky LS, Shenfield GM, et al. The role of the CYP2C9-Leu359 allelic variant in the tolbutamide polymorphism. Pharmacogenetics 1996; 6:341–349.
31. Bhasker CR, Miners JO, Coulter S, Birkett DJ. Allelic and functional variability of cytochrome P4502C9. Pharmacogenetics 1997; 7:51–58.
32. Kirchheiner J, Bauer S, Meineke I, Rohde W, Prang V, Meisel C, et al. Impact of CYP2C9 and CYP2C19 polymorphisms on tolbutamide kinetics and the insulin and glucose response in healthy volunteers. Pharmacogenetics 2002; 12:101–109.
33. Shon JH, Yoon YR, Kim KA, Lim YC, Lee KJ, Park JY, et al. Effects of CYP2C19 and CYP2C9 genetic polymorphisms on the disposition of and blood glucose lowering response to tolbutamide in humans. Pharmacogenetics 2002; 12:111–119.
34. Lee CR, Pieper JA, Hinderliter AL, Blaisdell JA, Goldstein JA. Evaluation of cytochrome P4502C9 metabolic activity with tolbutamide in CYP2C9*1 heterozygotes. Clin Pharmacol Ther 2002; 72:562–571.
35. Miners J. CYP2C9 polymorphism. Impact on tolbutamide pharmacokinetics and response. Pharmacogenetics 2002; 12:91–92.
36. Niemi M, Leathart JB, Neuvonen M, Backman JT, Daly AK, Neuvonen PJ. Polymorphism in CYP2C8 is associated with reduced plasma concentrations of repaglinide. Clin Pharmacol Ther 2003; 74:380–387.
37. Leslie RDG, Pyke DA. Chlorpropamide-alcohol flushing: a dominantly inherited trait associated with diabetes. BMJ 1978; 2:1519–1521.
38. Pyke DA, Leslie RDG. Chlorpropamide-alcohol flushing: a definition of its relation to non-insulin-dependent diabetes. BMJ 1978; 2:1521–1522.
39. Jerntorp P, Almer LO. Chlorpropamide-alcohol flushing in relation to macroangiopathy and peripheral neuropathy in non-insulin dependent diabetes. Acta Med Scand Suppl 1981; 656:33–36.
40. Ohlin H, Jerntorp P, Bergstrom B, Almer LO. Ohlin H, Jerntorp P, Bergstrom B, Almer LO. Chlorpropamide-alcohol flushing, aldehyde dehydrogenase activity, and diabetic complications. Br Med J 1982; 285:838–840.

41. Bonisolli L, Pontiroli AE, De Pasqua A, Calderara A, Maffi P, Gallus G, Radaelli G, Pozza G. Association between chlorpropamide-alcohol flushing and fast acetylator phenotype in type I and type II diabetes. Acta Diabetol Lat 1985; 22:305–315.
42. de Silva NE, et al. Low incidence of chlorpropamide-alcohol flushing in diet-treated, non-insulin-dependent diabetes. Lancet 1981; i:128–131.
43. Fui SNT, Keen H, Jarrett RJ, Strakosch C, Murrells T, Marsden P, Stott R. Epidemiological study of prevalence of chlorpropamide alcohol flushing in insulin dependent diabetes, non-insulin dependent diabetics, and non-diabetics. BMJ 1983; 287:1509–1512.
44. Fui SNT, et al. Test for chlorpropamide-alcohol flush becomes positive after prolonged chlorpropamide treatment in insulin-dependent and non-insulin-dependent diabetics. N Engl J Med 1983; 309:93–96.
45. Lao B, Czyzyk A, Szutowski M, Szczepanik Z. Alcohol tolerance in patients with non-insulin-dependent (type 2) diabetes treated with sulphonylurea derivatives. Arzneimittelforschung 1994; 44:727–734.
46. Tattersall RB. Mild familial diabetes with dominant inheritance. QJM 1974; 43:339–357.
47. Ehtisham S, Barrett TG. The emergence of type 2 diabetes in childhood. Ann Clin Biochem 2004; 41:10–16.
48. Frayling TM, Lindgren CM, Chevre JC, Menzel S, Wishart M, Benmezroua Y, Brown A, Evans JC, Rao PS, Dina C, et al. A genome-wide scan in families with maturity-onset diabetes of the young: evidence for further genetic heterogeneity. Diabetes. 2003; 52(3):872–881.
49. Owen K, Hattersley AT. Maturity-onset diabetes of the young: From clinical description to molecular genetic characterization. Bailliere's Best Practice and Research in Clinical Endocrinology and Metabolism 2001; 15/3:309–323.
50. Pearson ER, Velho G, Clark P, Stride A, Shepherd M, Frayling TM, Bulman MP, Ellard S, Froguel P, Hattersley AT. Beta-cell genes and diabetes: quantitative and qualitative differences in the pathophysiology of hepatic nuclear factor-1alpha and glucokinase mutations. Diabetes 2001; 50:S101-S107.
51. Lambert AP, Ellard S, Allen LI, Gallen IW, Gillespie KM, Bingley PJ, Hattersley AT. Identifying hepatic nuclear factor 1alpha mutations in children and young adults with a clinical diagnosis of type 1 diabetes. Diabetes Care 2003; 26:333–337.
52. Owen KR, Stride A, Ellard S, Hattersley AT. Etiological investigation of diabetes in young adults presenting with apparent type 2 diabetes. Diabetes Care 2003; 26:2088–2093.
53. Richter S, Shih DQ, Pearson ER, Wolfrum C, Fajans SS, Hattersley AT, Stoffel M. Regulation of apolipoprotein M gene expression by MODY3 gene hepatocyte nuclear factor-1alpha: haploinsufficiency is associated with reduced serum apolipoprotein M levels. Diabetes 2003; 52:2989–2995.
54. Yamagata K, Oda N, Kaisaki PJ, Menzel S, Furuta H, Vaxillaire M, Southam L, Cox RD, Lathrop GM, Boriraj VV, et al. Mutations in the hepatocyte nuclear factor-1alpha gene in maturity-onset diabetes of the young (MODY3). Nature 1996; 384:455–458.
55. Hattersley AT, Turner RC, Permutt MA, Patel P, Tanizawa Y, Chiu KC, O'Rahilly S, Watkins PJ, Wainscoat JS. Linkage of type 2 diabetes to the glucokinase gene. Lancet 1992; 339:1307–1310.
56. Vaxillaire M, Boccio V, Philippi A, Vigouroux C, Terwilliger J, Passa P, Beckmann JS, Velho G, Lathrop GM, Froguel P. A gene for maturity onset diabetes of the young (MODY) maps to chromosome 12q. Nat Genet 1995; 9(4):418–423.
57. Frayling TM, Evans JC, Bulman MP, Pearson E, Allen L, Owen K, Bingham C, Hannemann M, Shepherd M, Ellard S, Hattersley AT. Beta-cell genes and diabetes: molecular and clinical characterization of mutations in transcription factors. Diabetes 2001; 50:S94-S100.
58. Heiervang E, Folling I, Sovik O, et al. Maturity-onset diabetes of the young: studies in a Norwegian family. Acta Paediatr Scand 1989; 78:74–80.
59. Sovik O, Njolstad P, Folling I, Sagen J, Cockburn BN, Bell GI. Hyperexcitability to sulphonylurea in MODY3. Diabetologica 1998; 41:607–608.
60. Hathout EH, Cockburn BN, Mace JW, Sharkey J, Chen-Daniel J, Bell GI. A case of hepatocyte nuclear factor-1 alpha diabetes/MODY3 masquerading as type 1 diabetes in a

Mexican-American adolescent and responsive to a low dose of sulphonylurea. Diabetes Care 1999; 22:867–868.
61. Pearson ER, Liddell WG, Shepherd M, Corrall RJ, Hattersley AT. Sensitivity to sulphonylureas in patients with hepatocyte nuclear factor-1alpha gene mutations: evidence for pharmacogenetics in diabetes. Diabetic medicine {Diabet-Med} 2000; 17(7):543–545.
62. Hansen T, Eiberg H, Rouard M, et al. Novel MODY3 mutations in the hepatic nuclear factor-1α gene: evidence for a hyperexcitability of pancreatic ß-cells to intravenous secretagogues in a glucose-tolerant carrier of a P447L mutation. Diabetes 1997; 46:726–730.
63. Pearson ER, Starkey BJ, Powell RJ, Gribble FM, Clark PM, Hattersley AT. Genetic cause of hyperglycaemia and response to treatment in diabetes. Lancet. 2003; 362:1275–1281.
64. Ashcroft FM, Gribble FM. Tissue-specific effects of sulphonylureas: lessons from studies of cloned K (ATP) channels. J Diabetes Complications 2000; 14:192–196.
65. Pontoglio M, Barra J, Hadchouel M, Doyen A, Kress C, Bach JP, Babinet C, Yaniv M. Hepatocyte nuclear factor 1 inactivation results in hepatic dysfunction, phenylketonuria, and renal Fanconi syndrome. Cell 1996; 84:575–585.
66. Lee YH, Sauer B, Gonzalez FJ. Laron dwarfism and non-insulin dependent diabetes mellitus in the HNF-1alpha knockout mouse. Mol Cell Biol 1998; 18:3059–3068.
67. Boileau P, Wolfrum C, Shih DQ, Yang TA, Wolkoff AW, Stoffell M. Decreased glibenclamide uptake in hepatocytes of hepatocyte nuclear factor-1(alpha)-deficient mice: A mechanism for hypersensitivity to sulfonylurea therapy in patients with maturity-onset diabetes of the young, type 3 (MODY3). Diabetes 2002; 51(3):S343-S348.
68. Wang H, Antinozzi PA, Hagenfeldt KA, Maechler P, Wollheim CB. Molecular targets of a human HNF-1apha mutation responsible for pancreatic beta-cell dysfunction. Embo J 2000; 19:4257–4264.
69. Shih DQ, Screenan S, Munoz KN, Philipson L, Pontoglio M, Yaniv M, Polonsky KS, Stoffel M. Loss of HNF-1alpha function in mice leads to abnormal expression of genes involved in pancreatic islet development and metabolism. Diabetes 2001; 50:2472–2480.
70. Willson TM, Brown PJ, Sternbach DD, Henke BR. The PPARs: from orphan receptors to drug discovery. J Med Chem 2000; 43:527–550.
71. Marx N, Sukhova G, Murphy C, Libby P, Plutzky J. Macrophages in human atheroma contain PPAR[gamma]: differentiation-dependent peroxisomal proliferator-activated receptor gamma (PPAR[gamma]) expression and reduction of MMP-activity through PPAR[gamma] activation in mononuclear phagocytes in vitro. Am J Pathol 1998; 153:17–23.
72. Watanabe-I, Tomita-A, Shimizu-M, Sugawara-M, Yasumo-H, Koishi-R, Takahashi-T, Miyoshi-K, Nakamura-K, Izumi-T, Matsushita-Y, Furukawa-H, Haruyama-H, Koga-T. A study to survey susceptible genetic factors responsible for troglitazone-associated hepatotoxicity in Japanese patients with type 2 diabetes mellitus. Clinical Pharmacology and Therapeutics 2003; 73:435–455.
73. Inzucchi SE, Maggs DG, Spollett GR, Page SL, Rife FS, Walton V, Shulman GI. Efficacy and metabolic effects of metformin and troglitazone in type II diabetes mellitus. N Engl J Med 1998; 338:867–887.
74. Schwartz S, Raskin P, Fonseca V, Graveline JF. Effect of troglitazone in insulin-treated patients with type II diabetes mellitus: Troglitazone and Exogenous Insulin Study Group. N Engl J Med 1998; 338:861–866.
75. Kumar S, Boulton AJ, Beck-Nielsen H, Berthezene F, Muggeo M, Persson B, Spinas GA, Donoghue S, Lettis S, Stewart-Long P. Troglitazone, an insulin action enhancer, improves metabolic control in NIDDM patients: Troglitazone Study Group. Diabetologia 1996; 39:701–709.
76. Antonucci T, Whitcomb R, McLain R, Lockwood D, Norris RM. Impaired glucose tolerance is normalized by treatment with the thiazolidinedione troglitazone. Diabetes Care 1997; 20:188–193.
77. Masugi J, Tamori Y, Kasuga M. Inhibition of adipogenesis by a COOH-terminally truncated mutant of PPARγ2 in 3T3–L1 cells. Biochem Biophys Res Commun 1999; 264:93–99.

78. Yen CJ, Beamer BA, Negri C, Silver K, Brown KA, Yarnall DP, Burns DK, Roth J, Shuldiner AR. Molecular scanning of the human peroxisome proliferator-activated receptor γ (PPAR-) gene in diabetic Caucasians: identification of a Pro12Ala PPAR2 missense mutation. Biochem Biophys Res Commun 1997; 240:270–276.
79. Deeb SS, Fajas L, Nemoto M, Pihlajamaki J, Mykkanen C, Kuusisto J, Laakso M, Fujimoto W, Auwerx J. Pro12Ala substitution in PPARγ2 associated with decreased receptor activity, lower body mass index and improved insulin sensitivity. Nat Genet 1998; 20:284–287.
80. Hamann A, Münzberg H, Buttron P, Busing P, Hinney A, Mayer H, Siegfried W, Hebebrand J, Greten H. Missense variants in the human peroxisome proliferator-activated receptor-γ2 gene in lean and obese subjects. Eur J Endocrinol 1999; 141:90–92.
81. Beamer BA, Yen CJ, Andersen RE, Muller D, Elahi D, Cheskin LJ, Andres R, Roth J, Shuldiner AR. Association of the Pro12Ala variant in the peroxisome proliferator-activated receptor-γ2 gene with obesity in two Caucasian populations. Diabetes 1998; 47:1806–1808.
82. Ek J, Urhammer SA, Sorensen TIA, Andersen T, Auwerx J, Pedersen O. Homozygosity of the Pro12Ala variant of the peroxisome proliferator-activated receptor-γ2 (PPARγ-2): divergent modulating effects on body mass index in obese and lean Caucasian men. Diabetologia 1999; 42:892–895.
83. Koch M, Rett K, Maerker E, Volk A, Haist K, Deninger M, Renn W, Haring HU. The PPAR-γ2 amino acid polymorphism Pro12Ala is prevalent in offspring of type II diabetic patients and is associated to increased insulin sensitivity in a subgroup of obese subjects. Diabetologia 1999; 42:758–762.
84. Ristow M, Müller-Wieland D, Pfeiffer A, Krone W, Kahn CR. Human obesity associated with a mutation in PPARγ2, a regulator of adipocyte differentiation. N Engl J Med 1998; 339:953–959.
85. Barroso I, Gurnell M, Crowley VE, Agostini M, Schwabe JW, Soos MA, Soos MA, Maslen GL, Williams TD, Lewis H, Schafer AJ, Chatterjee VK, O'Rahilly S. Dominant negative mutations in human PPAR associated with severe insulin resistance, diabetes mellitus and hypertension. Nature 1999; 402:880–883.
86. Shuldiner AR, Nguyen W, Kao WH, Beamer BA, Andersen RE, Pratley R, Brancati FL. Pro115Gln peroxisome proliferator-activated receptor-γ and obesity. Diabetes Care 2000; 23:126–127.
87. Blüher M, Lübben G, Paschke R. Analysis of the relationship between the Pro12Ala variant in the PPAR-γ2 gene and the response rate to therapy with pioglitazone in patients with type 2 diabetes. Diabetes Care 2003; 26: 825–831.
88. Qi N, Kazdova L, Zidek V, Landa V, Kren V, Pershadsingh HA, Lezin ES, Abumrad NA, Pravenec M, Kurtz TW. Pharmacogenetic evidence that cd36 is a key determinant of the metabolic effects of pioglitazone. J Biol Chem 2002; 277:48501–48507.
89. Tontonoz P, Nagy L, Alvarez JG, Thomazy VA, Evans RM. PPARgamma promotes monocyte/macrophage differentiation and uptake of oxidized LDL. Cell 1998; 93:241–252.
90. Abumrad NA, el-Maghrabi MR, Amri EZ, Lopez E, Grimaldi PA. Cloning of a rat adipocyte membrane protein implicated in binding or transport of long-chain fatty acids that is induced during preadipocyte differentiation. Homology with human CD36. J Biol Chem 1993; 268:17665–17668.
91. Downs JR, Clearfield M, Weis S, et al. Primary prevention of acute coronary events with lovastatin in men and women with average cholesterol levels. JAMA 1998; 279:1615–1622.
92. Shepherd J, Olsson AG, Sacks FM, Black DM, Orloff DG, Bilheimer DW. Should separate endpoint trials be required for all lipid-lowering drugs acting by the same mechanism? Am J Cardiol 1998; 81:88F-94F.
93. Shepherd J, Cobbe SM, Ford I, et al. Prevention of coronary heart disease with pravastatin in men with hypercholesterolemia. New Eng J Med 1995; 333:1301–1307.
94. Scandinavian Simvastatin Survival Study Group. Randomised trial of cholesterol lowering in 4444 patients with coronary heart disease: The Scandinavian Simvastatin Survival Study (4S). Lancet 1994; 344:1383–1389.

95. Sacks FM, Pfeffer MA, Moye LA, et al. The effect of pravastatin on coronary events after myocardial infarction in patients with average cholesterol levels. New Eng J Med 1996; 335:1001–1009.
96. The Long-Term Intervention with Pravastatin in Ischaemic Disease (LIPID) Study Group. Prevention of cardiovascular events and death with pravastatin in patients with coronary heart disease and a broad range of initial cholesterol levels. New Eng J Med 1998; 339:1349–1357.
97. Rosenson RS, Tangney CC. Antiatherothrombotic properties of statins. JAMA 1998; 279:1643–1650.
98. Dornbrook-Lavender KA, Pieper JA. Genetic polymorphisms in emerging cardiovascular risk factors and response to statin therapy. Cardiovasc Drugs Ther 2003; 17:75–82.
99. Mahley RW. Apolipoprotein E: cholesterol transport protein wit expanding role in cell biology. Science 1988; 240:622–640.
100. Wilson PWF, Schaefer EJ, Larson MG, et al. Apolipoprotein E alleles and risk of coronary disease: a meta-analysis. Arterioscler Thromb Vasc Biol 1996; 16:1250–1255.
101. Gerdes LU, Gerdes C, Kervinen K, et al. The apolipoprotein €4 allele determines prognosis and the effect on prognosis of simvastatin in survivors of myocardial infarction – A Substudy of the Scandinavian Simvastatin Survival Study. Circulation 2000; 101:1366–1371.
102. Green F, Hamsten A, Blomback M, et al. The role of ß-fibrinogen genotype in determining plasma fibrinogen levels in young survivors of myocardial infarction and healthy controls from Sweden. Thrombosis and Hemostasis 1993; 70:915–920.
103. Humphries SE, Cook M, Dubowitz M, et al. Role of genetic variation at the fibrinogen locus in determination of plasma fibrinogen concentrations. Lancet 1987; 1:1452–1455.
104. Behague I, Poirier O, Nicaud V, et al. ß-fibrinogen gene polymorphisms are associated with plasma fibrinogen and coronary artery disease in patients with myocardial infarction - The ECTIM Study. Circulation 1996; 93:440–449.
105. de Maat, Kastelein JPJ, Jukema JW, et al. -455G/A polymorphism of the ß-fibrinogen gene is associated with the progression of coronary atherosclerosis in symptomatic men - proposed role for an acute-phase reaction pattern of fibrinogen. Arterioscler Thromb Vasc Biol 1998; 18:265–271.
106. Tall AR, Wang N. Tangier disease as a test of the reverse cholesterol transport hypothesis. J Clin Invest 2000; 106:1205–1207.
107. Kuivenhoven JA, Jukema JW, Zwinderman AH, et al. The role of a common variant of the cholesteryl ester transfer protein gene in the progression of coronary atherosclerosis. N Engl J Med 1998; 338:86–93.
108. Maitland-van der Zee AH, Klungel OH, Stricker BH, Monique Verschuren WM, Kastelein JJ, Leufkens HG, et al. Genetic polymorphisms: importance for response to HMG-CoA reductase inhibitors. Atherosclerosis 2002; 163:213–222.
109. Gordon DJ, Rifkind BM. High-density lipoprotein - The clinical implications of recent studies. N Engl J Med 1989; 321:1311–1316.
110. Hannuksela ML, Liinamaa MJ, Kesaniemi YA, et al. Relation of polymorphisms in the cholesteryl ester transfer protein gene to transfer protein activity and plasma lipoprotein levels in alcohol drinkers. Atherosclerosis 1994;110:35–44.
111. Jin W, Marchandier D, Rader DJ. Lipases and HDL metabolism. Trends in Endocrinology and Metabolism 2002; 13:174–178.
112. Zambon A, Austin MA, Brown BG, et al. Effect of hepatic lipase on LDL in normal men and those with coronary artery disease. Arterioscler Thromb 1993; 13:147–153.
113. Austin MA, Breslow JL, Hennekens CH, et al. Low-density lipoprotein subclass patterns and risk of myocardial infarction. JAMA 1988; 260:1917–1921.
114. Zambon A, Deeb SS, Brown BG, et al. Common hepatic lipase gene promoter variant determines clinical response to intensive lipid-lowering treatment. Circulation 2001; 103:792–798.
115. Zambon A, Deeb SS, Hokanson JE, et al. Common variants in the promoter of the hepatic lipase gene are associated with lower levels of hepatic lipase activity, buoyant LDL, and higher HDL cholesterol. Arterioscler Thromb Vasc Biol 1998; 18:1723–1729.

116. Gehrisch S. Common mutations of the lipoprotein lipase gene and their clinical significance. Curr Atheroscler Rep 1999; 1:70–78.
117. Jukema JW, van Boven AJ, Groenmeijer B, et al. The Asp(9)Asn mutation in the lipoprotein lipase gene is associated with increased progression of coronary atherosclerosis. Circulation 1996; 94:1913–1918.
118. Weiss EJ, Bray PF, Tayback M, et al. A polymorphism of a platelet glycoprotein receptor as an inherited risk factor for coronary thrombosis. N Eng J Med 1996; 334:1090–1094.
119. Walter DH, Schachinger V, Elsner M, et al. Platelet glycoprotein IIIa polymorphisms and risk of coronary stent thrombosis. Lancet 1997; 350:1217–1219.
120. Kastrati A, Schomig A, Seyfarth M, et al. PIA polymorphism of platelet glycoprotein IIIa and risk of restenosis after coronary stent placement. Circulation 1999; 99:1005–1010.
121. Feng D, Lindpainter K, Larson MG, et al. The Framingham offspring study. Increased platelet aggregability associated with platelet GPIIIa PIA2 polymorphism. Arterioscler Thromb Vasc Biol 1999; 19:1142–1147.
122. Walter DH, Schachinger V, Elsner M, et al. Statin therapy is associated with reduced restenosis rates after coronary stent implantation in carriers of the PIA2 allele of the platelet glycoprotein IIIa gene. Eur Heart J 2001; 22:587–595.
123. de Maat MPM, Jukema JW, Ye S, et al. Effect of the stromelysin-1 promoter on efficacy of pravastatin in coronary atherosclerosis and restenosis. Am J Cardiol 1999; 83:852–856.
124. Ye S, Watts GF, Mandalia S, et al. Preliminary report: genetic variation in the human stromelysin promoter is associated with progression of coronary atherosclerosis. Br Heart J 1995; 73:209–215.
125. Jukema JW, Bruschke AVG, van Boven AJ, et al. Effects of lipid lowering by pravastatin on disease progression and regression of coronary artery disease in symptomatic men with normal to moderately elevated serum cholesterol levels-The Regression Growth Evaluation Statin Study (REGRESS). Circulation 1995; 91:2528–2540.
126. Humphries SE, Luong L, Talmud PJ, et al. The 5A/6A polymorphism in the promoter of the stromelysin-1 (MMP-3) gene predicts progression of angiographically determined coronary artery disease in men in the LOCAT gemfibrozil study. Atherosclerosis 1998; 139:49–56.
127. Syvanne M, Taskinen MR, Nieminen MS, et al. A study to determine the response of coronary atherosclerosis to raising low high-density lipoprotein cholesterol with a fibric-acid derivative in men after coronary bypass surgery. The rationale, design, and baseline characteristics of the LOCAT study. Control Clin Trials 1997; 18:93.
128. Williams D, Feely J. Pharmacokinetic-pharmacodynamic drug interactions with HMG-CoA reductase inhibitors. Clin Pharmacokinet 2002; 41:343–370.
129. Kathawala FG. HMG-CoA reductase inhibitors: an exciting development in the treatment of hyperlipoproteinemia. Med Res Rev 1991; 11:121–146.
130. Kirchheiner J, Kudlicz D, Meisel C, Bauer S, Meineke I, Roots I, Brockmoller J. Influence of CYP2C9 polymorphisms on the pharmacokinetics and cholesterol-lowering activity of (-)-3S,5R-fluvastatin and (+)-3R,5S-fluvastatin in healthy volunteers. Clin Pharmacol Ther 2003; 74:186–194.
131. Ambudkar SV, Kimchi-Sarfaty C, Sauna ZE, Gottesman MM. P-glycoprotein: from genomics to mechanism. Oncogene 2003; 22:7468–7485.
132. Marzolini C, Paus E, Buclin T, Kim RB. Polymorphisms in human MDR1 (P-glycoprotein): recent advances and clinical relevance. Clin Pharmacol Ther 2004; 75:13–33.
133. Thiebaut F, Tsuruo T, Hamada H, Gottesman MM, Pastan I, Willingham MC. Cellular localization of the multidrug-resistance gene product P-glycoprotein in normal human tissues. Proc Natl Acad Sci USA 1987; 84:7735–7738.
134. Kim R, Wilkinson G. Pharmacogenetics of drug transporters. In: Kalow W, Meyer UA, Tyndale RF, eds. Pharmacogenomics. New York: Marcel Dekker, 2001:81–108.
135. Randell A, Sambrook PN, Nguyen TV, Lapsley H, Jones G, Kelly PJ, Eisman JA. Direct clinical and welfare costs of osteoporotic fractures in elderly men and women. Osteoporos Int 1995; 5:427–432.

136. Ray NF, Chan JK, Thamer M, Melton LJR. Medical expenditures for the treatment of osteoporotic fractures in the United States in 1995: Report from the National Osteoporosis Foundation. J Bone Miner Res 1997; 12:24–35.
137. Cooper C, Atkinson EJ, Jacobsen SJ, O'Fallon WM, Melton LJD. Population-based study of survival after osteoporotic fractures. Am J Epidemiol 1993; 137:1001–1005.
138. Johnston CJ, Miller JZ, Slemenda CW, Reister TK, Hui S, Christian JC, Peacock M. Calcium supplementation and increases in bone mineral density in children. N Engl J Med 1992; 327:82–87.
139. Hui SL, Slemenda CW, Johnston CC Jr. The contribution of bone loss to postmenopausal osteoporosis. Osteoporos Int 1990; 1:30–34.
140. Johnston CC Jr, Slemenda CW. Changes in skeletal tissue during the aging process. Nutr Rev 1992; 50:385–387.
141. Tuppurainen M, Honkanen R, Kroger H, Saarikoski S, Alhava E. Osteoporosis risk factors, gynaecological history and fractures in perimenopausal women: the results of the baseline postal enquiry of the Kuopio Osteoporosis Risk Factor and Prevention Study. Maturitas 1993; 17:89–100.
142. Seeman E. The dilemma of osteoporosis in men. Am J Med 1995; 98:76S-88S.
143. Soule SG, Conway G, Prelevic GM, Prentice M, Ginsburg J, Jacobs HS. Osteopenia as a feature of the androgen insensitivity syndrome. Clin Endocrinol 1995; 43:671–675.
144. Slemenda CW, Longcope C, Zhou L, Hui SL, Peacock M, Johnston CC. Sex steroids and bone mass in older men. Positive associations with serum estrogens and negative associations with androgens. J Clin Invest 1997; 100:1755–1759.
145. Eisman JA. Pharmacogenetics of the vitamin D receptor and osteoporosis. Drug Metab Dispos 2001; 29:505–512.
146. Slemenda CW, Christian JC, Williams CJ, Norton JA, Johnston CC Jr. Genetic determinants of bone mass in adult women: a re-evaluation of the twin model and the potential importance of gene interaction on heritability estimates. J Bone Miner Res 1991; 6:561–567.
147. Kelly PJ, Nguyen T, Hopper J, Pocock N, Sambrook P, Eisman J. Changes in axial bone density with age: A twin study. J Bone Miner Res 1993; 8:11–17
148. Nguyen TV, Howard GM, Kelly PJ, Eisman J. Bone mass, lean mass, and fat mass: Same genes or same environments? Am J Epidemiol 1998; 147:3–16.
149. Sowers MR, Boehnke M, Jannausch ML, Crutchfield M, Corton G, Burns TL. Familiality and partitioning the variability of femoral bone mineral density in women of child-bearing age. Calcif Tissue Int 1992; 50:110–114.
150. Diaz MN, O'Neill TW, Silman AJ. The influence of family history of hip fracture on the risk of vertebral deformity in men and women: The European Vertebral Osteoporosis Study. Bone 1997; 20:145–149.
151. Evans RA, Marel GM, Lancaster EK, Kos S, Evans M, Wong SY. Bone mass is low in relatives of osteoporotic patients. Ann Intern Med 1998; 109:870–873.
152. Pocock N, Eisman J, Gwinn T, Sambrook P, Kelly P, Freund J, Yeates M. Muscle strength, physical fitness, and weight but not age predict femoral neck bone mass. J Bone Miner Res 1989; 4:441–448.
153. Young D, Hooper JL, Nowson CA, Green RM, Sherwin AJ, Kaymakci B, Smid M, Guest CS, Larkins RG, Wark JD. Determinants of bone mass in 10- to 26-year-old females: a twin study. J Bone Miner Res 1995; 10:558–567.
154. Sessions ND, Halloran BP, Bikle DD, Wronski TJ, Cone CM, Morey-Holton E. Bone response to normal weight bearing after a period of skeletal unloading. Am J Physiol 1989; 257:E606-E610.
155. Kroger H, Tuppurainen M, Honkanen R, Alhava E, Saarikoski S. Bone mineral density and risk factors for osteoporosis: a population-based study of 1600 perimenopausal women. Calcif Tissue Int 1994; 55:1–7.
156. Lonzer MD, Imrie R, Rogers D, Worley D, Licata A, Secic M. Effects of heredity, age, weight, puberty, activity, and calcium intake on bone mineral density in children. Clin Pediatr (Phila) 1996; 35:185–189.

157. Ulrich CM, Georgiou CC, Snow-Harter CM, Gillis DE. Bone mineral density in mother-daughter pairs: Relations to lifetime exercise, lifetime milk consumption and calcium supplements. Am J Clin Nutr 1996; 63:72–79.
158. Kelly PJ, Pocock NA, Sambrook PN, Eisman JA. Dietary calcium, sex hormones, and bone mineral density in men. Br Med J 1990; 300:1361–1364.
159. Jackman LA, Millane SS, Martin BR, Wood OB, McCabe GP, Peacock M, Weaver CM. Calcium retention in relation to calcium intake and postmenarcheal age in adolescent females. Am J Clin Nutr 1997; 66:327–333.
160. Nakamura T, Turner CH, Yoshikawa T, Slemenda CW, Peacock M, Burr DB, Mizuno Y, Orimo H, Ouchi Y, Johnston CJ. Do variations in hip geometry explain differences in hip fracture risk between Japanese and white Americans? J Bone Miner Res 1994; 9: 1071–1076.
161. Xu L, Lu A, Zhao X, Chen X, Cummings SR. Very low rates of hip fracture in Beijing, People's Republic of China the Beijing Osteoporosis Project. Am J Epidemiol 1996; 144:901–907.
162. Peel N, Eastell R. Osteoporosis. BMJ 1995; 310:989–992.
163. Kanis JA, et al. Guidelines for diagnosis and management of osteoporosis. Osteoporosis Int 1997; 7:390–406.
164. Riggs BL, Melton LJ. The prevention and treatment of osteoporosis. N Engl J Med 1992; 327:620–627.
165. Gibaldi M. Prevention and treatment of osteoporosis: does the future belong to hormone replacement therapy? J Clin Pharmacol 1997; 37:1087–1099.
166. Lloyd T, et al. Calcium supplementation and bone mineral density in adolescent girls. JAMA 1993; 270:841–844.
167. Reid IR, et al. Effect of calcium supplementation on bone loss in postmenopausal women. N Engl J Med 1993; 328:460–464.
168. Riis B, et al. Does calcium supplementation prevents postmenopausal bone loss? N Engl J Med 1987; 316:173–177.
169. Altkorn D, Vokes T. Treatment of postmenopausal osteoporosis. JAMA 2001; 285:1415–1418.
170. Clemett D, Spencer CM. Raloxifene: a review of its use in post-menopausal osteoporosis. Drugs 2000; 60:379–411.
171. Gallagher JC, Goldgar D. Treatment of postmenopausal osteoporosis with high doses of synthetic calcitriol: a randomized controlled study. Ann Intern Med 1990; 113:649–655.
172. Tilyard MW, et al. Treatment of postmenopausal osteoporosis with calcitriol or calcium. N Engl J Med 1992; 326:357–362.
173. Ott SM, Chesnut CH. Calcitriol treatment is not effective in postmenopausal osteoporosis. Ann Intern Med 1989; 110:267–274.
174. Compston JE. Osteoporosis: management of established disease. Prescribers' J 1997; 37:119–124.
175. Morrison NA, Qi JC, Tokita A, Kelly PJ, Crofts L, Nguyen TV, Sambrook PN, Eisman JA. Prediction of bone density from vitamin D receptor alleles. Nature 1994; 367:284–287.
176. Gong G, Stern HS, Cheng SC, Fong N, Mordeson J, Deng HW, Recker RR. The association of bone mineral density with vitamin D receptor gene polymorphisms. Osteoporosis Int 1999; 9:55–64.
177. Gomez C, Naves ML, Barrios Y, Diaz JB, Fernandez JL, Salido E, Torres A, Cannata JB. Vitamin D receptor gene polymorphisms, bone mass, bone loss and prevalence of vertebral fracture: differences in postmenopausal women and men. Osteoporosis Int 1999; 10:175–182.
178. Uitterlinden AG, Weel AE, Burger H, Fang Y, van Duijn CM, Hofman A, van Leeuwen JP, Pols HA. Interaction between the vitamin D receptor gene and collagen type I alpha1 gene in susceptibility for fracture. J Bone Miner Res 2001; 16:379–385.
179. Eisman J. Genetics of osteoporosis, in Osteoporosis 996. In: Papapoulos SEA, ed., New York: Elsevier Science Publishing Co., Inc., pp 131–135.

180. Hauache OM, Lazaretti-Castro M, Andreoni S, Gimeno SG, Brandao C, Ramalho AC, Kasamatsu TS, Kunii I, Hayashi LF, Dib SA, Vieira JG.Vitamin D receptor gene polymorphism: Correlation with bone mineral density in a Brazilian population with insulin-dependent diabetes mellitus. Osteoporos Int 1998; 8:204–210.
181. Eccleshall TR, Garnero P, Gross C, Delmas PD, Feldman D. Lack of correlation between start codon polymorphism of the vitamin D receptor gene and bone mineral density in premenopausal French women: The OFELY study. J Bone Miner Res 1998; 13:31–35.
182. Cooper GS, Umbach DM. Are vitamin D receptor polymorphisms associated with bone mineral density? A meta-analysis [see comments]. J Bone Miner Res 1996; 11:1841–1849.
183. Gong G, Stern H, Cheng S, Fong N, Mordeson J, Deng H, Recker R. The association of bone mineral density with vitamin D receptor gene polymorphisms. Osteoporos Int 1999; 9:55–64.
184. Sainz J, Van Tornout JM, Loro ML, Sayre J, Roe TF, Gilsanz V. Vitamin D-receptor gene polymorphisms and bone density in prepubertal American girls of Mexican descent. N Engl J Med 1997; 337:77–82.
185. Tokita A, Matsumoto H, Morrison NA, Tawa T, Miura Y, Fukamauchi K, Mitsuhashi N, Irimoto M, Yamamori S, Miura M, et al. Vitamin D receptor alleles, bone mineral density and turnover in premenopausal Japanese women [see comments]. J Bone Miner Res 1996; 11:1003–1009.
186. Hustmyer FG, Peacock M, Hui S, Johnston CC, Christian J. Bone mineral density in relation to polymorphism at the vitamin D receptor gene locus. J Clin Invest 1994; 94:2130–2134.
187. Feskanich D, Hunter DJ, Willett WC, Hankinson SE, Hollis BW, Hough HL, Kelsey KT, Colditz GA.Vitamin D receptor genotype and the risk of bone fractures in women. Epidemiol 1998; 9:535–539.
188. Ensrud K, Stone K, Cauley J, White C, Zmuda J, Nguyen T, Eisman J, Cummings S. Vitamin D receptor gene polymorphisms and the risk of fractures in older women. J Bone Miner Res 1999; 14:1637–1645.
189. Nguyen TV, Morrison NA, Sambrook PN, Kelly PJ, Eisman JA. Vitamin D receptor gene and osteoporosis. J Clin Endocrinol Metab 1996; 81:1674–1675.
190. Dawson-Hughes B, Harris SS, Finneran S. Calcium absorption on high and low calcium intakes in relation to vitamin D receptor genotype. J Clin Endocrinol Metab 1995; 80:3657–3661.
191. Ongphiphadhanakul B, Rajatanavin R, Chanprasertyothin S, Chailurkit L, Piaseu N, Teerarungsikul K, Sirisriro R, Komindr S, Puavilai G. Vitamin D receptor gene polymorphism is associated with urinary calcium excretion but not with bone mineral density in postmenopausal women. J Endocrinol Invest 1997; 20:592–596.
192. Ames S, Ellis K, Gunn S, Copeland K, Abrams S. Vitamin D receptor gene Fok1 polymorphism predicts calcium absorption and bone mineral density in children. J Bone Miner Res 1999; 14:740–746.
193. Ferrari S, Rizzoli R, Chevalley T, Slosman D, Eisman JA, Bonjour JP. Vitamin-D-receptor-gene polymorphisms and change in lumbar-spine bone mineral density. Lancet 1995; 345:423–424.
194. Krall EA, Dawson-Hughes B. Soft tissue body composition: Familial resemblance and independent influences on bone mineral density. J Bone Miner Res 1995; 10:1944–1950.
195. Barger-Lux MJ, Heaney RP, Hayes J, DeLuca HF, Johnson ML, Gong G. Vitamin D receptor gene polymorphism, bone mass, body size and vitamin D receptor density. Calcif Tissue Int 1995; 57:161–162.
196. Tokita A, Kelly PJ, Nguyen TV, Qi JC, Morrison NA, Risteli L, Risteli J, Sambrook PN, Eisman JA. Genetic influences on type I collagen synthesis and degradation: Further evidence for genetic regulation of bone turnover. J Clin Endocrinol Metab 1994; 78:1461–1466.
197. Yamagata Z, Miyamura T, Iijima S, Asaka A, Sasaki M, Kato J, Koizumi K. Vitamin D receptor gene polymorphism and bone mineral density in healthy Japanese women. Lancet 1994; 344:1027.
198. Shiraki M, Shiraki Y, Aoki C, Hosoi T, Inoue S, Kaneki M, Ouchi Y. Association of bone mineral density with apolipoprotein E phenotype. J Bone Miner Res 1990; 12:1438–1445.

199. Graafmans WC, Lips P, Ooms ME, van Leeuwen JP, Pols HA, Uitterlinden AG. The effect of vitamin D supplementation on the bone mineral density of the femoral neck is associated with vitamin D receptor genotype. J Bone Miner Res 1997; 12:1241–1245.
200. Marc J, Prezelj J, Komel R, Kocijancic A. VDR genotype and response to etidronate therapy in late postmenopausal women. Osteoporos Int 1999; 10:303–306.
201. Deng HW, Li J, Li JL, Johnson M, Gong G, Davis KM, Recker RR. Change of bone mass in postmenopausal Caucasian women with and without hormone replacement therapy is associated with vitamin D receptor and estrogen receptor genotypes. Hum Genet 1998; 103:576–585.
202. Kurabayashi T, Tomita M, Matsushita H, Yahata T, Honda A, Takakuwa K, Tanaka K. Association of vitamin D and estrogen receptor gene polymorphism with the effect of hormone replacement therapy on bone mineral density in Japanese women. Am J Obstet Gynecol 1999; 180:1115–1120.
203. Palomba S, Numis FG, Mossetti G, Rendina D, Vuotto P, Russo T, Zullo F, Nappi C, Nunziata V. Raloxifene administration in post-menopausal women with osteoporosis: effect of different BsmI vitamin D receptor genotypes. Hum Reprod 2003; 18:192–198.
204. Arai H, Miyamoto K, Taketani Y, Yamamoto H, Iemori Y, Morita K, Tonai T, Nishisho T, Mori S, Takeda E. A vitamin D receptor gene polymorphism in the translation initiation codon: Effect on protein activity and relation to bone mineral density in Japanese women. J Bone Miner Res 1997; 12:915–921.
205. Gennari L, Becherini L, Masi L, Mansani R, Gonnelli S, Cepollaro C, Martini S, Montagnani A, Lentini G, Becorpi AM, Brandi ML. Vitamin D and estrogen receptor allelic variants in Italian postmenopausal women: Evidence of multiple gene contribution to bone mineral density. J Clin Endocrinol Metab 1998; 83:939–944.
206. Duncan EL, Brown MA, Sinsheimer JS, Carr JA, Wordsworth BP, Wass JAH. Candidate gene linkage screen in osteoporosis. Bone 1998; 23:S160.
207. Masi L, Becherini L, Colli E, Gennari L, Mansani R, Falchetti A, Becorpi AM, Cepollaro C, Gonnelli S, Tanini A, Brandi ML. Polymorphisms of the calcitonin receptor gene are associated with bone mineral density in postmenopausal Italian women. Biochem Biophys Res Commun 1998; 248:190–195.
208. Tsukamoto K, Yoshida H, Watanabe S, Suzuki T, Miyao M, Hosoi T, Orimo H, Emi M. Association of radial bone mineral density with CA repeat polymorphism at the interleukin 6 locus in postmenopausal Japanese women. J Hum Genet 1999; 44:148–151.
209. Keen RW, Woodford-Richens KL, Lanchbury JS, Spector TD. Allelic variation at the interleukin-1 receptor antagonist gene is associated with early postmenopausal bone loss at the spine. Bone 1998; 23:367–371.
210. Keen RW, Snieder H, Daniels J, Davies H, Chiano M, MacGregor AJ, Gewert D, Spector TD. A novel TGF-1 gene polymorphism is linked and associated with hip BMD in female twins. Bone 1998; 23:S161.
211. Langdahl BL, Knudsen JY, Jensen HK, Gregersen N, Eriksen EF. A sequence variation: 713–8delC in the transforming growth factor-beta 1 gene has higher prevalence in osteoporotic women than in normal women and is associated with very low bone mass in osteoporotic women and increased bone turnover in both osteoporotic and normal women. Bone 1997; 20:289–294.
212. Rosen CJ, Donahue LR. Insulin-like growth factors and bone: The osteoporosis connection revisited. Proc Soc Exp Biol Med 1998; 219:1–7.

13
Pharmacogenetics in Gastroenterology

Guruprasad Padur Aithal
Queen's Medical Centre University Hospital, Nottingham, U.K.

INTRODUCTION

A subgroup of patients receiving a drug may fail to respond to the medication or develop adverse reactions. Such interindividual variability in drug response has a major impact in both clinical practice and drug development. Several host factors, including the patient's age, gender, smoking habit, alcohol consumption, renal and liver function, and disease factors are likely to influence drug response. In addition to this, genetic factors may also be important (1–4). This chapter reviews the evolving concepts and potential applications of such genetic factors, a field of study termed pharmacogenetics, and more recently pharmacogenomics (5), in gastrointestinal and liver diseases. Much of the focus of pharmacogenetics is on single-nucleotide polymorphisms (SNPs) which are the most common source of variation in the human genome, occurring at approximately 1 in 1000 base pairs (6).

APPLICATION OF PHARMACOGENETICS IN CLINICAL GASTROENTEROLOGY AND HEPATOLOGY

The liver has a complex detoxification system in which several enzymes participate in the metabolism of a large number of xenobiotics. Essentially, all of the major human drug metabolizing enzymes (DMEs) responsible for phase I (modification of functional groups of the xenobiotics) or phase II reactions (conjugation with endogenous substrates) exhibit common polymorphisms at the genomic level (1). The clinical relevance of these polymorphisms depends on how they affect individual susceptibility to disease or response to therapy (efficacy and toxicity). The potential applications of pharmacogenetics in various aspects of clinical gastroenterology and hepatology are summarized in Table 1.

Association of Polymorphisms in DME and Drug Transporters with Disease Susceptibility and Progression

The association of DME polymorphisms with disease susceptibility has mainly been explored in models of environmental carcinogenesis (7). In theory, genetic polymorphisms could

Table 1 Application of Pharmacogenetics in Clinical Gastroenterology and Hepatology

Disease susceptibility and phenotype
DME polymorphism in alcoholic liver disease
mEH polymorphism in HCV-related liver disease
mEH and *GSTM1 polymorphism* in hepatocellular carcinoma
MDR1 gene polymorphism in inflammatory bowel disease
Efficacy of therapy
Drug metabolism and disposal
TPMT genotype in treatment of IBD with azathioprine
CYP2C19 genotype and efficacy of proton pump inhibitors
Drug targets
SERT polymorphism and treatment of IBS with alosetron
Mutations in the ISDR and treatment of HCV-1B infection
Adverse drug reaction
Adverse gastrointestinal reactions
Irinotecan toxicity
Adverse hepatic reactions
Gilbert's syndrome and Indinavir-induced hyperbilirubinemia
NAT2 polymorphism and isoniazid-induced hepatotoxicity
HLA association of co-amoxiclav-induced jaundice

Abbreviations: DME, drug-metabolizing enzymes; HCV, hepatitis C virus; TPMT, thiopurine methyl transferase; HLA, human leukocyte antigen; IBD, inflammatory bowel disease; IBS, irritable bowel syndrome; SERT, serotonin transporter gene; ISDR, interferon sensitivity-determining region.

account for heterogeneity in disease progression and also in the predisposition to complications. They may therefore assist in identifying phenotypic subgroups of common diseases.

Alcoholic Liver Disease

Deaths from chronic liver disease have increased threefold in the United Kingdom during the last three decades (8). The mortality can largely be attributed to alcoholic liver disease and viral hepatitis. Two-thirds of deaths from liver cirrhosis occur in patients under the age of 65 years (8). Alcohol is a major contributor to death, injuries, and illness, accounting for 10.3% of disability adjusted life years among established market economies, compared with 11.7% for tobacco and 2.3% for illicit drugs. The U.S. Veterans Administration Twin Panel Study showed a higher concordance for cirrhosis in monozygotic twins (17%) compared with dizygotic twins (5%), indicating that genetic factors contribute to susceptibility although most of the liability for cirrhosis occurs due to the shared risk for alcoholism (9,10). The strongest genetic association with alcoholism has been shown to be with genes encoding alcohol-metabolizing enzymes.

Ethanol is rapidly absorbed from the gastrointestinal tract with most being metabolized in the liver. Hepatic oxidation of ethanol to acetaldehyde is carried out by the alcohol dehydrogenase (ADH) in the cytosol, with variable contribution by cytochrome P450 2E1 (CYP2E1) in microsomes and catalase in peroxisomes (Fig. 1). Aldehyde dehydrogenases (ALDH), especially the mitochondrial form ALDH2, convert acetaldehyde to acetate. The resultant production of acetaldehyde and reactive oxygen species may lead to liver injury either by inducing lipid peroxidation or by formation of protein adducts, which in turn leads to liver injury through an immune-mediated mechanism (11). Polymorphisms in the alcohol and aldehyde dehydrogenase genes result in considerable interindividual variation in the rate at which both ethanol and acetaldehyde are metabolized.

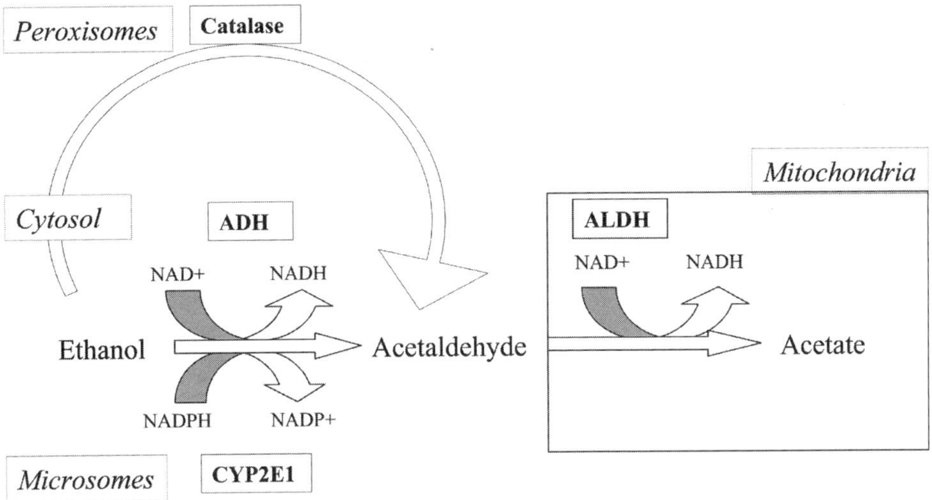

Figure 1 Pathways of alcohol metabolism. *Abbreviations*: ADH, alcohol dehydrogenase; NAD, nicotinamide-adenine dinucleotide; NADH, nicotinamide-adenine dinucleotide, reduced; NADPH, nicotinamide-adenine dinucleotide phosphate, reduced; NADP, nicotinamide-adenine dinucleotide phosphate; ALDH, aldehyde dehydrogenase.

Humans have two polymorphic ADH gene loci, *ADH2* and *ADH3* (12). Alleles with high enzyme activity (*ADH2*2* and *ADH3*1*) appear to be less frequent in alcohol-dependent subjects as these are associated with a high acetaldehyde concentration, which has an aversive effect. Possession of the *ADH2*2* allele has been associated with increased susceptibility to alcoholic liver disease in the Japanese (13). However, the evidence for such an association in Caucasians has been inconsistent, with two small studies suggesting an association of *ADH3*1* with advanced liver disease (14,15), whereas three other studies found no difference in ADH genotype frequencies between cases and controls (16–18). A polymorphism in *ALDH2* is common in Asians, and individuals homozygous for the variant allele (*ALDH2*2*) lack mitochondrial ALDH2 enzyme activity. Accumulation of acetaldehyde in these subjects leads to facial flushing, tachycardia, nausea, and vomiting even with moderate alcohol consumption. As the point mutation acts as a dominant negative, those heterozygous for the variant *ALDH2* allele have a marked reduction in the activity of ALDH2. Asians with the *ALDH2*2* allele have an increased susceptibility to advanced liver disease, presumably through the accumulation of acetaldehyde (19). There is currently no evidence for the existence of similar polymorphisms in the *ALDH2* gene in Caucasians.

CYP2E1 is associated with NADPH-CYP450 reductase in the microsomal membrane and oxidizes ethanol to acetaldehyde (20). CYP2E1 has a high K_m for ethanol but is inducible by chronic drinking. Metabolism of ethanol by CYP2E1 generates reactive oxygen species including the hydroxyl radical (OH^-), superoxide anion (O_2^-), and hydrogen peroxide (H_2O_2), and hence could induce lipid peroxidation. Several restriction fragment length polymorphisms (RFLPs) in the upstream and noncoding regions of CYP2E1 have been identified. Although individual studies have found an association of the variant *CYP2E1*5* allele with advanced liver disease among Caucasians (17,21), a meta-analysis of published studies did not confirm the association with alcoholic liver disease (22).

Viral Hepatitis

An estimated 0.5% to 1% of the U.K. population and 170 million people worldwide are infected with the hepatitis C virus (HCV). Chronic hepatitis related to HCV is the most common cause of cirrhosis and hepatocellular carcinoma in Europe and the United States. Overall, about 20% of the infected individuals develop cirrhosis or hepatocellular carcinoma over a 20- to 30-year period (23). Several environmental, host, and viral factors are likely to interact in determining individual susceptibility to progressive disease. Risk factors, such as male gender, age at infection, mode of transmission, alcohol consumption, and hepatitis B virus coinfection, are associated with more rapid disease progression, although these account for only a small part of the variability in the disease.

Epoxide hydrolase catalyzes the irreversible hydration of highly reactive alkene epoxides and arene oxides generated by CYP450-dependent oxidation to yield metabolites that can be readily conjugated and excreted (24). In the liver, the distribution of epoxide hydrolase parallels that of CYP450 being located in the centrilobular region (zone 3). The enzyme plays an important role in detoxifying electrophilic epoxides that might otherwise bind to proteins and nucleic acids and cause cellular toxicity and genetic mutation. Microsomal epoxide hydroxylase (mEH) is involved in the metabolism of a wide variety of xenobiotics and has been found in virtually all tissues, including liver, kidney, lung, and testis (25). Two point mutations in exons 3 and 4 lead to the amino acid changes, Tyr113His and His139Arg, respectively, which affect mEH activity by influencing protein stability (26,27). In a study involving 394 patients at different stages of HCV-related liver disease, patients homozygous for the exon 3 variant allele (113 His/His) were overrepresented in advanced stages of the disease (28), being associated with a threefold increased risk of cirrhosis and a fivefold increased risk of hepatocellular carcinoma. The association was stronger in men. When the exon 3 and exon 4 genotypes were combined to express the metabolic phenotype, very slow metabolizers were highly prevalent among patients with cirrhosis and hepatocellular carcinoma (28). The independent role of mEH polymorphisms in cancer risk suggests that the reduced disposal of specific classes of compounds, such as aflatoxin B1, may be important in the pathogenesis.

Aflatoxin B1 is considered to be a hepatocarcinogen in humans. It has been postulated that aflatoxin B1 induces carcinogenesis by causing a mutation in the tumor suppressor gene p53 at codon 249 (29,30). An individual's capacity to detoxify the mutagenic metabolite aflatoxin 8,9-epoxide by mEH and glutathione-*S*-transferase (GST) M1 could determine the amount of epoxide available to bind to DNA. In two populations in Ghana and China, a significant association was found between the mEH exon 3 variant allele and presence of the aflatoxin B1-albumin adduct (indicative of exposure to aflatoxin B1) and hepatocellular carcinoma (31). In addition, a synergistic relationship between the mEH variant allele and hepatitis B surface antigen was demonstrated. Thus, individuals with only the mEH variant allele had a threefold increased risk, those with hepatitis B infection had a 15-fold increased risk, whereas subjects with both the hepatitis B surface antigen and the mEH variant allele had a 77-fold risk of hepatocellular carcinoma, whereas compared with individuals without either of the risk factor. The frequency of the *GSTM1* null genotype, which abolishes GSTM1 enzyme activity (32), was also greater in patients with hepatocellular carcinoma, although the association was not as strong. The p53 codon 249 mutation was observed only among hepatocellular carcinoma patients with one or more of the high-risk genotype for either mEH or GSTM1 (31).

Inflammatory Bowel Disease

Crohn's disease and ulcerative colitis are common causes of gastrointestinal morbidity in Western countries, with a combined prevalence of 100 to 200 cases per 100,000 population (33).

Microbial, immunologic, and genetic factors are thought to be involved in the pathogenesis of inflammatory bowel disease. An experimental model of UC in mice deficient for the multidrug resistant 1 (*mdr 1a*) gene product P-glycoprotein (Pgp) showed that adenosine triphosphate (ATP)-binding cassette transporters probably have an important barrier function in protecting against xenobiotics, bacteria, and their toxins (34,35). In humans, Pgp (ABCB1) is localized to the apical membrane of epithelial cells in both the small and large intestines (36). The exon 26 C3435T polymorphism in the *MDR1* gene affects Pgp expression in the intestine, with individuals homozygous for the *T* allele having the lowest expression (37). Presumably, impairment of barrier function in these subjects makes them more susceptible to the development of ulcerative colitis (38). In contrast, high Pgp expression may be associated with poor response to medical therapy in patients with inflammatory bowel disease (39). In addition, the *MDR1* C3435T polymorphism may also play an important role in determining the disease phenotype. In a case-control study, subjects with the CC genotype had a higher prevalence of penetrating or stricturing Crohn's disease (38). The 3435CC genotype was also found to have a higher prevalence in patients with Crohn's disease requiring azathioprine or 6-mercaptopurine (38).

Association of Genetic Polymorphisms with Drug Efficacy

A patient's response to a drug depends on many factors, including absorption and distribution of the drug, drug metabolism and elimination, concentration of the drug at the target site, and the number and function of the target receptors. It is possible to identify genetic polymorphisms in all of these processes, which could theoretically influence the drug response phenotype in individual patients, and allow identification of those patients with a greater chance of responding to the particular medication.

Genetic Polymorphisms in Drug Metabolism and Disposal

Studies investigating associations between specific drug metabolizing enzyme genotypes with drug response have sometimes reached different and, at times, apparently conflicting conclusions. There may be many reasons for this, including differences in ethnic populations studied, heterogeneous disease phenotypes, differences in the endpoints used to define response, and the polygenic nature of many drug effects.

Azathioprine in Inflammatory Bowel Disease. Immunomodulatory therapy with azathioprine and 6-mercaptopurine has been shown to be effective in both steroid-dependent and resistant cases of inflammatory bowel disease, achieving and maintaining remission in 70% of the patients (40). However, a delay of 7 to 14 weeks before the onset of therapeutic benefit and concern regarding toxicity have limited their use in inflammatory bowel disease. Azathioprine is a prodrug, which is converted to 6-mercaptopurine by non-enzymatic cleavage (Fig. 2) (41). 6-mercaptopurine is rapidly taken up by erythrocytes and other tissues. Intracellular biotransformation of 6-mercaptopurine occurs via two competing routes. The drug is catabolized into the inactive 6-methylmercaptopurine by thiopurine methyl transferase (TPMT) or anabolized to the active thioguanine nucleotides by hypoxanthine phosphoribosyltransferase. Incorporation of 6-thioguanine nucleotides into lymphocyte DNA induces cytotoxicity and immunosuppression.

Interindividual and interethnic variability in TPMT activity is caused by polymorphisms in the gene (42). Measurement of TPMT activity in erythrocytes has shown that about 1 in 300 of various European populations have undetectable activity (homozygous for variant alleles $TPMT^{L}$), 11% inherit intermediate levels (heterozygous $TPMT^{H}/TPMT^{L}$), whereas 89% have high enzyme activity (homozygous for wild-type $TPMT^{L}$) (43). The molecular basis of the variation in enzyme activity has been studied. Although a number of variant TPMT alleles have been described, the most common polymorphisms

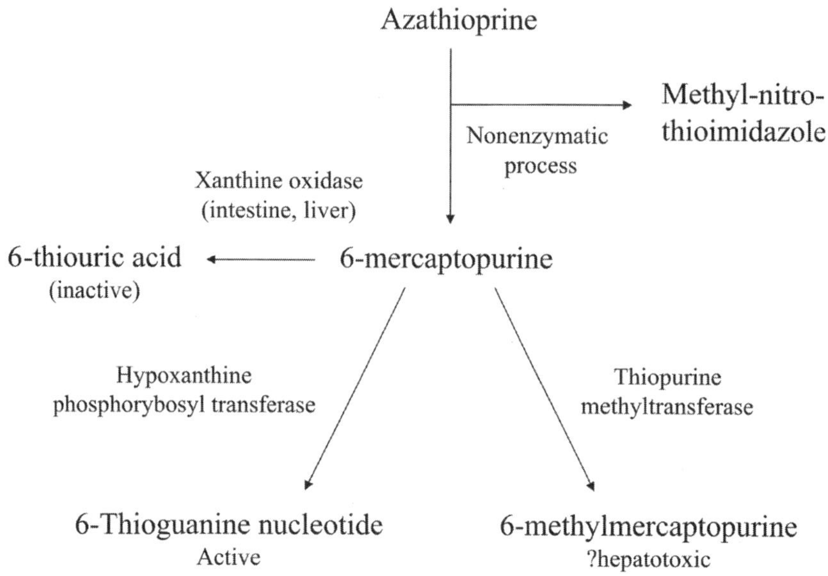

Figure 2 Metabolism of azathioprine and 6-mercaptopurine.

result from two substitutions at position 460 (G460A, Ala-to-Thr) and at position 719 (A719G, Tyr-to-Cys), resulting in the *TPMT*3A* (both G460A and A719G) and *TPMT*3B* (only G460A) genotypes (44–46). These genotypes account for 75% of the variant alleles associated with absence of catalytic activity.

Both measurement of erythrocyte TPMT activity and genotyping have been used in optimizing azathioprine or 6-mercaptopurine therapy in patients with inflammatory bowel disease. Dubinsky et al. (47) in a study of 92 pediatric IBD (inflammatory bowel disease) patients (79 with Crohn's disease) reported higher 6-thioguanine levels in patients heterozygous for TPMT ($TPMT^H/TPMT^L$), all of whom responded to therapy. A prospective study thereafter demonstrated that measurement of 6-thioguanine levels could be used to achieve remission in patients with Crohn's disease who had initially failed to respond to conventional dosing with azathioprine (48). However, a large study of 170 patients (130 with Crohn's disease) found no correlation between 6-thioguanine nucleotide levels and disease activity, as measured by an inflammatory bowel disease questionnaire. However, the study design led to the inclusion of only those who had responded to and tolerated the treatment and hence would not have allowed evaluation of the role of measuring 6-thioguanine levels in the management of inflammatory bowel disease (49). Overall, the strength of the observed correlation between 6-thioguanine nucleotide levels and therapeutic efficacy suggests that monitoring metabolites may identify those patients not responding to azathioprine or 6-mercaptopurine because of either inadequate dosing or noncompliance (41).

Metabolic variability also appears to influence the prevalence of adverse reactions. Reduced TPMT activity and high 6-thioguanine levels have been associated with azathioprine-induced leukopoenia (47,50). Variant TPMT allele can be found in up to 27% of the patients with Crohn's disease who develop myelosuppression, and the toxicity appears early in the course of treatment (within six weeks) in subjects homozygous for the variant allele (51). In a subgroup of patients with inflammatory bowel disease who fail to respond to azathioprine/6-mercaptopurine therapy, dose escalation does not result in optimal 6-thioguanine nucleotide production but rather results in the preferential production of 6-methyl mercaptopurine ribonucleotide, which has been associated with hepatotoxicity (47,52).

CYP2C19 Polymorphism and Efficacy of Proton Pump Inhibitors. Proton pump inhibitors, such as omeprazole and lansoprazole, are mainly metabolized by CYP2C19 in the liver. Rabeprazole is nonenzymatically converted largely to thioether-rabeprazole and partially metabolized to demethyl rabeprazole by CYP2C19. The variant alleles *CYP2C19m1* (G to A substitution in exon 5 at position 681, which produces a cryptic splice site resulting in a truncated nonfunctional protein) and *CYP2C19m2* (G to A substitution in exon 4 at position 636, which creates a premature stop codon) are responsible for the CYP2C19 poor metabolizer phenotype (53,54). *CYP2C19m1* is found in both Asians and Caucasians, but *CYP2C19m2* is not found in Caucasians. The effects of lansoprozole, omeprazole, and rabeprazole on intragastric pH have been shown to dependent on the CYP2C19 genotype (55,56). Studies in small groups of patients have shown that *Helicobacter pylori* eradication rate on dual therapy (combination of proton pump inhibitor and amoxicillin) was significantly higher in those homozygous for the poor metabolizer genotypes (57,58). However, the CYP2C19 genotype did not significantly affect cure rates for *H. pylori* infection by triple therapy (combination of proton pump inhibitor, amoxicillin, and clarithromycin) (59). CYP2C19 genotype also seems to partly determine the efficacy of lansoprazole in gastroesophageal reflux disease: patients homozygous for the extensive metabolizer genotype had the lowest plasma lansoprazole levels and the lowest cure rate (60). Overall, however, the influence of the CYP2C19 genotype on efficacy of proton pump inhibitor therapy is likely to be greatest in Asians, where the frequency of the poor metabolizer phenotype is five times greater compared with the Caucasians.

Genetic Polymorphisms in Drug Targets

Drugs usually exert their effects via an interaction with membrane receptors (about 50% of drugs), enzymes (about 30%), or ion channels (about 5%) (61). Many of the genes encoding these drug targets exhibit genetic polymorphisms, which alter their sensitivity to the medication and thereby response to therapy. Mutations in transporters involved in the reuptake of neurotransmitters may alter neurotransmitter levels within the synaptic cleft and thereby lead to an altered response to both agonists and antagonists.

Serotonin-Transporter Polymorphism and Response to Alosetron. Irritable bowel syndrome affects about 15% of the adults (62). Diarrhea-predominant irritable bowel syndrome is associated with an accelerated transit and rectal hypersensitivity. Serotonin (5-HT) modulates the sensorimotor function in the digestive tract with the 5-HT type 3 receptors, in particular, mediating the postprandial colonic motor response (63), which is often associated with cramping, urgency, and diarrhea in patients with the syndrome. Alosetron, a 5-HT3 receptor antagonist, results in the relief of pain and normalization of bowel function in women with diarrhea-predominant irritable bowel syndrome (64,65).

5-HT undergoes reuptake by a transporter protein (SERT), which controls its activity locally. A 44-base pair insertion/deletion polymorphism, approximately 1-kb upstream of the serotonin transporter gene SERT, has been identified (66). Homozygosity for the short variant results in less transcript, less protein expression, and hence less reuptake of serotonin (66,67). In a study involving 30 patients, the SERT polymorphism was associated with the colonic transit response to alosetron (68) with the long homozygous patients showing greater response (slowing of colonic transit) to alosetron, compared with the heterozygous patients.

Polymorphisms in HCV and Response to Interferon. The efficacy of interferon therapy in HCV infection varies depending on viral genotype; infection with genotype 1b is associated with a sustained virologic response in 10% to 25% of the patients (69). The efficacy of interferon therapy in HCV1b infection can be predicted based on the HCV RNA levels and the number of amino acid mutations in the interferon sensitivity-determining region (ISDR in the 2209 to 2248 region of NS5A gene) (70–72). A recent study using a decision analysis model showed that interferon therapy was not useful in patients aged 50 to 60 years with HCV-1b infection without mutations in the interferon sensitivity-determining region and HCV RNA levels exceeding 1.0 mEq/mL (73).

Genetic Susceptibility to Adverse Drug Reactions

An adverse drug reaction (ADR) is defined as any response to a drug that is noxious, unintended, and occurs at doses normally used in humans for the prophylaxis, diagnosis, or therapy of disease (74). ADRs result in significant morbidity, mortality, and excess medical care costs. In the United States, more than two million hospitalized patients suffer serious ADRs annually (75). There are many different types of ADRs (chap. 5). "Idiosyncratic," or type B, ADRs are not predictable from a knowledge of the pharmacology of the drug, and mechanisms are not clearly understood. A postulated mechanism involves covalent binding of reactive metabolites to proteins, which then either directly interferes with cellular function resulting in cytotoxicity or induces an immune response (76,77). Susceptibility to ADRs could therefore theoretically depend on genetic factors that determine the metabolism and also on the biochemical and immunological responses to the metabolites. It is therefore likely that drug therapy based on an individual's genetic make-up may result in a clinically important reduction in ADRs (4).

Gastrointestinal Adverse Drug Reactions

Of the many different types of adverse reactions that can be induced by drugs, gastrointestinal ADRs are the commonest cause of hospital admission (78), accounting for about 18% of cases (79,80). Although gastrointestinal bleeding, nausea, vomiting, and antibiotic-induced diarrhea account for the majority of the events, a wide variety of other drug-induced gastrointestinal adverse effects have also been reported.

Irinotecan Toxicity. Irinotecan (7-ethyl-10-[4-(1-piperidino)-1-piperidino] carbonyloxy camptothecin or CPT-11) is an anticancer agent that inhibits topoisomerase I activity (81). Clinical trials have established the role of irinotecan (in combination with 5-fluorouracil/leucovorin) in the treatment of metastatic colorectal cancer (82,83). The most common adverse effects of irinotecan are bone marrow toxicity and ileocolitis leading to diarrhea (84). These adverse effects may lead to the discontinuation of an otherwise effective anticancer treatment.

Irinotecan is a prodrug—metabolism by tissue and serum carboxylesterases generates the more active metabolite 7-ethyl-10-hydroxycamptothecin (SN-38) (85). Metabolism of SN-38 by glucuronidation and subsequent elimination through biliary excretion is the primary route of detoxification (Fig. 3) (86). Diarrhea due to irinotecan therapy is due to the toxic actions of unconjugated SN-38 on the intestinal mucosa. SN-38 can be absorbed into epithelial cells from both the basolateral (blood) and apical (luminal side) surfaces, targeted for glucuronidation, and effluxed back into the lumen (87). There is an inverse relationship between SN-38 glucuronidation rates and severity of diarrhea in patients treated with irinotecan (88,89). Two major hepatic

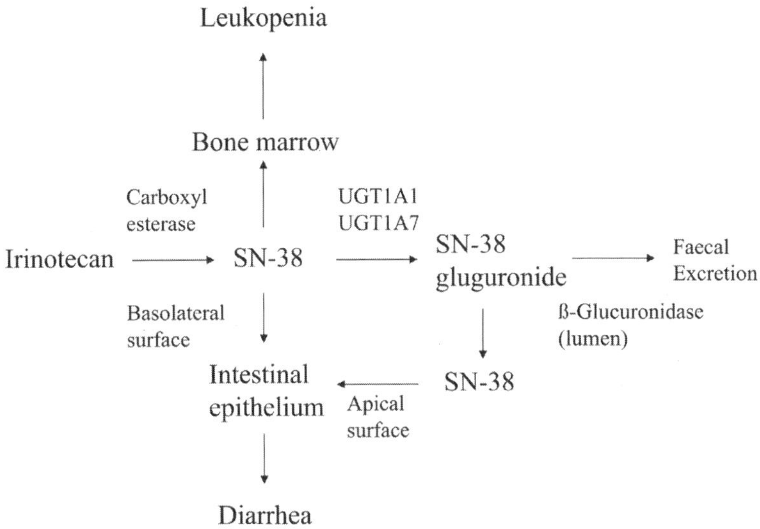

Figure 3 Biotransformation of irinotecan.

UDP-glucuronosyltransferases (UGT), UGT1A1 and UGT1A9, and the extrahepatic UGT1A7, are involved in SN-38 glucuronidation (90).

More than 50 variants have been reported in *UGT1A1*; many of these are found in patients with Gilbert's syndrome, an inherited condition of impaired bilirubin conjugation, occurring in 5% to 10% of the general population (91). One of the most common genotypes leading to Gilbert's syndrome is *UGT1A1*28*, wherein the promoter contains a sequence of [A(TA)$_7$TAA] compared with the wild-type *UGT1A1* with a sequence of [A(TA)$_6$ TAA]. The *UGT1A1*28* polymorphism is present in about 40% of the Caucasians of whom 8% have Gilbert's syndrome (92). *UGT1A1*28* is associated with a 70% reduction in transcriptional activity compared with the wild-type *UGT1A1*. In a case-control study, 46% (12/26) of the patients with severe toxicity due to irinotecan (leukocyte count $\leq 0.9 \times 10/l$ or diarrhea >5 days/bloody diarrhea/diarrhea with dehydration) were carrying the *UGT1A1*28* allele (either heterozygous or homozygous), compared with 14% (13/92) of the controls (93). Multivariate analysis suggested that subjects carrying *UGT1A1*28* were seven times more likely to get irinotecan toxicity. All three patients heterozygous for *UGT1A1*27* also suffered adverse effects, whereas there was no association with *UGT1A1*6*. None of the subjects in the study had *UGT1A1*7* or *UGT1A1*29* alleles, and hence their role could not be evaluated (93).

UGT1A7 is the most efficient of the UGTs in metabolizing SN-38 (90). The influence of the UGT1A7 genotype in predisposing to irinotecan toxicity may be different to that due to Gilbert's syndrome (87). UGT1A7 is not expressed in the small or large intestine, unlike UGT1A1 (94). Thus, the majority of the SN-38 in the intestine results from cleavage of SN-38 glucuronide by bacterial β-glucuronidase allowing reabsorption of SN-38 (86). Therefore, extensive metabolizers with a *UGT1A7*1* or *UGT1A7*2* genotype may have reduced plasma SN-38 levels but may still be at increased risk of gastrointestinal toxicity because of increased fecal SN-38 after deconjugation of SN-glucuronide (87). Common variants of *UGT1A7, UGT1A7*3* ($N^{129}K;R^{131}K;W^{208}R$), and *UGT1A7*4* ($W^{208}R$) could be at risk of bone marrow suppression as they are associated with reduced SN-38 glucuronidation. However, a recent case-control study has not shown any association between the *UGT1A7* genotype and irinotecan-induced adverse reactions (95).

Adverse Reactions Involving the Liver

Because the liver is central to the biotransformation of virtually all drugs and foreign substances, drug-induced liver injury is a potential complication of nearly every medication that is prescribed. The liver is the most common target organ for toxicity encountered during the course of drug development (96). Despite considerable progress in toxicological studies, the correlation between liver toxicity in animals and man remains poor (97). As the "high-risk" agents have been replaced, relatively rare reactions to commonly prescribed "low-risk" agents have contributed to the total burden of the drug-induced liver disease (98). The incidence of symptomatic hepatic ADRs is estimated to be 14 per 100,000 population, 16 times greater than the number noted by spontaneous reporting to the regulatory authorities (99). Adverse hepatic drug reactions have been the leading cause of postmarketing withdrawals in the last four decades (98,100).

The basic mechanism underlying drug-induced hepatotoxicity is considered to be metabolic or immunologic idiosyncrasy. Metabolic idiosyncrasy implies that the patient developing the adverse reaction metabolizes the drug in a different way than most individuals or lacks adequate protective mechanisms to neutralize any reactive metabolites that are formed. Immunologic idiosyncrasy implies that the susceptible individual has an immune system that would more readily recognize any formed neoantigens. Genetic factors influencing the development of drug-hepatotoxicity can be grouped into factors affecting the amount of reactive metabolite formed and therefore the levels of the protein adduct, and factors affecting the immune response to the adducts.

Metabolic Idiosyncrasy. Initial studies investigating the role of DME polymorphisms in drug-induced liver disease used phenotyping experiments in small groups of patients. Polymorphism in debrisoquine oxidation (CYP 2D6) has been shown to result in accumulation of perhexiline, leading to liver injury in poor metabolizers (101), and to increase the formation of reactive metabolites, leading to chlorpromazine hepatotoxicity in extensive metabolizers (102). Defective hepatic sulfoxidation has also been shown to contribute to chlorpromazine jaundice (102). Polymorphism in mephenytoin hydroxylation (CYP 2C19) has been associated with Atrium (phenobarbital, febarbamate, and difebarbamate)-induced hepatotoxicity, with poor metabolizers being at increased risk (103). More recently, genotyping for drug metabolizing enzyme gene polymorphisms has been used to study genetic susceptibility to drug-induced liver disease.

Isoniazid hepatotoxicity. The growing prevalence of drug-resistant *Mycobacterium tuberculosis* strains and the increasing number of patients with acquired immunodeficiency syndrome (AIDS) has lead to the worldwide resurgence of tuberculosis. Regimens containing isoniazid, rifampicin, ethambutol, and pyrazinamide are used as first-line therapy for tuberculosis. The incidence of antituberculosis drug-induced hepatotoxicity varies from 13% to 36% in different populations (104–107), with a 1% to 10% case-fatality rate. Isoniazid is the major drug incriminated, and liver injury secondary to this drug continues to be reported worldwide (108–111).

The enzyme *N*-acetyltransferase (NAT) is responsible for the metabolism of isoniazid to acetylisoniazid, which in turn is hydrolyzed to acetyl hydrazine (Fig. 4) (112). The latter could be oxidized by CYP2E1 to form *N*-hydroxy-acetylhydrazine, which further dehydrates to yield acetyldiazene. Acetyldiazene may itself be the toxic metabolite or may break down to the reactive acetylonium ion, acetyl radical, and ketene, which could bind covalently to hepatic macromolecules resulting in liver injury (112–114). NAT is also responsible for further acetylation of acetylhydrazine to the nontoxic diacetylhydrazine. Therefore, slow acetylation results not only in accumulation of the parent compound but also of monoacetylhydrazine. Acetylation of acetylhydrazine is further suppressed by isoniazid itself. In addition, direct hydrolysis of isoniazid without acetylation

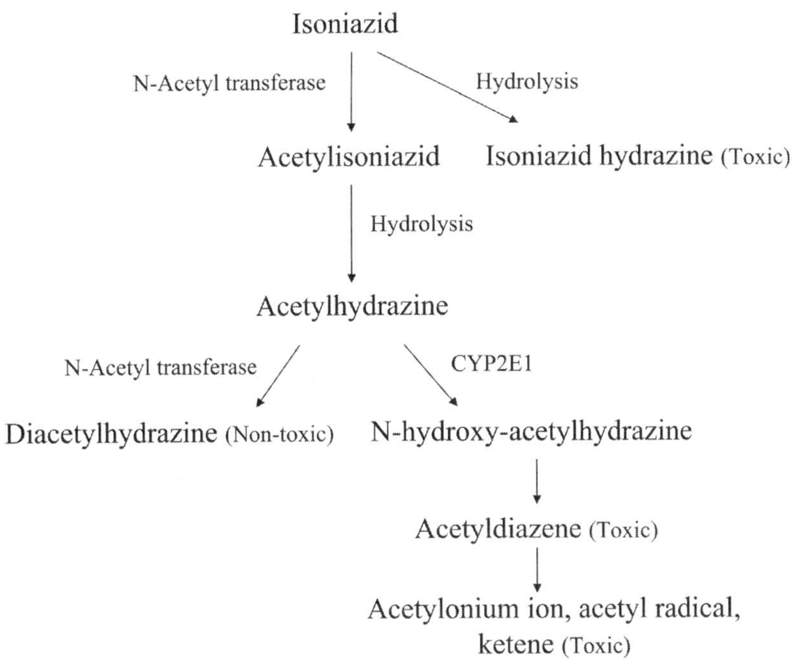

Figure 4 Metabolism of isoniazid.

produces hydrazine that could cause liver injury (115). Metabolism of isoniazid through this minor pathway is increased 10-fold in slow acetylators, especially when given with rifampicin (116).

Two human NAT functional genes (*NAT1* and *NAT2*) and one pseudogene (*NATP*) have been cloned (117). *NAT2* is polymorphic in humans and has a 10-times lower K_m for aromatic amines than that of *NAT1*. The presence of any two of the several variant alleles of the *NAT2* gene leads to the slow acetylator phenotype, whereas fast acetylators have one or more wild-type *NAT2*4* alleles (117). Acetylation activity in vitro is progressively reduced in association with the *NAT2*4* > *NAT2*7* > *NAT2*6* > *NAT2*5* alleles (118). In a recent study involving 224 patients who received antituberculosis therapy, patients possessing the *NAT2* genotypes associated with slow acetylation were four times more likely to develop isoniazid-induced hepatotoxicity (105). In addition, the hepatic injury in slow acetylators was more severe than that seen in rapid acetylators. Patients with the *NAT2*6/6* and *NAT2*6/7* genotypes had a significantly higher risk than those with other genotypes.

Indinavir-induced hyperbilirubinemia. Indinavir is a viral protease inhibitor used in the treatment of HIV infection. Indinavir therapy is associated with unconjugated hyperbilirubinemia in 6% to 25% of the subjects (119,120). This could lead to unnecessary investigations and inappropriate withdrawal of the medication. Although indinavir is predominantly metabolized by the CYP450 enzyme system, the drug is also a substrate for UGT (121). Indinavir competitively inhibits conjugation of bilirubin by UGT1A1 in rat hepatoma cell culture (122). In experiments with Gunn rats, a strain deficient in hepatic bilirubin-conjugating activity caused by a mutation in the *UGT1A1* gene, administration of indinavir results in a greater elevation of serum bilirubin in heterozygous ($j/+$) animals than in wild-type controls ($+/+$) (122). Consistent with this, an increase in serum bilirubin following indinavir therapy has been found to be more pronounced in patients with one or more variant *UGT1A1* alleles (122). Therefore, hyperbilirubinemia secondary indinavir is likely to be most pronounced in individuals with reduced hepatic UGT activity, such as those with Gilbert's syndrome.

Immunologic Idiosyncrasy. The second group of genetic factors influencing susceptibility to immune-mediated hepatic drug reactions are those involved in immune regulation. Genetic polymorphisms in the major histocompatibility complex (MHC) are the most obvious example. The presence or absence of a given human leukocyte antigen (HLA) molecule may determine the efficient presentation of an alkylated immunogenic peptide. Associations have been reported between HLA A11 and hepatotoxicity due to halothane, tricyclic antidepressants and diclofenac; HLA DR6 and liver injury secondary to chlorpromazine and nitrofurantoin, and HLA B8; and clometacine-induced hepatitis (123). However, patients with liver injury due to a heterogeneous group of drugs were included in this study, and, hence, the association of the genotype with the liver injury should be considered to be preliminary and requires replication.

Co-amoxiclav-induced jaundice. Co-amoxiclav is a commonly used antibiotic, that causes cholestatic jaundice. The frequency of this ADR is about one case per 5000–80,000 prescriptions, and the risk increases with advancing age (124–126). Clavulanic acid rather than amoxicillin has been considered to be responsible for immunoallergic hepatitis. Two case-control studies involving Caucasians have demonstrated that co-amoxiclav-induced jaundice is strongly associated with the HLA *DRB1*1501-DRB5*0101-DQB1*0602* haplotype (126,127). Subjects carrying the extended haplotype had a ninefold higher risk of cholestasis (126). These findings suggest that HLA class II molecules are important in presenting the drug-metabolite to the T-cell receptor of CD4+ helper T-cells with the subsequent stimulation of B-cells and cytotoxic T-cells and development of the immune reaction.

CANDIDATE GENE CASE–CONTROL ASSOCIATION STUDIES

Until recently, genetic polymorphisms in drug metabolism were typically described on the basis of phenotypic differences among individuals in a population. With recent advances in molecular sequencing technology, SNPs, especially in the regulatory or coding regions, are being discovered and are followed by biochemical studies assessing the phenotypic effects. Ultimately, clinical studies may allow the elucidation of polymorphisms in DME genes that have important consequences in patients. Such a framework may permit the elucidation of polymorphisms in DME that have more subtle, yet clinically important consequences for interindividual variability in drug response.

Population-based case-control studies with appropriately matched cases and controls are a widely used method for detecting genetic associations. The first step in designing a case-control study is to decide on the candidate gene or genes to be studied. The relevance of the candidate gene in the pathogenesis of the particular disease or ADR, and the functional effects of a particular polymorphism may indicate the importance of the association that is detected (128,129). With the availability of data from the human genome project, many studies now attempt to relate the phenotype to polymorphisms in multiple genes. The study of the genetic susceptibility to diclofenac-induced hepatotoxicity is an example where "both metabolic" and "immune" factors potentially involved in the development of liver injury have been investigated.

Diclofenac is a widely used nonsteroidal anti-inflammatory drug that can rarely cause potentially serious hepatotoxicity. Severe liver injury occurs in 3.6 per 100,000 users, and 8% of those who are jaundiced die of hepatic failure (130). Because of its common use, diclofenac hepatotoxicity has been one of the common causes of hepatic ADRs with 180 confirmed cases reported to Food and Drug Administration during the first three years of marketing in the United States (131). The major pathway of metabolism of diclofenac is through 4′-hydroxylation by CYP2C9 (Fig. 5) (132,133). Minor pathways include the formation of 5-hydroxydiclofenac catalyzed by a number of P450s, including CYP3A4, CYP2C8, CYP2C18, and CYP2C19 (134–136), and 3′-hydroxydiclofenac catalyzed by CYP2C9 (134). Both diclofenac and its metabolites undergo glucuronidation and sulfate conjugation, with acylglucuronide appearing to be the most common glucuronic acid conjugate. Conversion of diclofenac to diclofenac acylglucuronide is mediated by UGT2B7 (137). Diclofenac acylglucuronide can form adducts with hepatocellular proteins (138–140), resulting in immune-mediated destruction of hepatocytes (141). There is some in vitro evidence to suggest that 5-hydroxydiclofenac can also bind covalently, leading to the formation of protein adducts (135).

It has been hypothesized that susceptibility to diclofenac-induced hepatotoxicity may be genetically determined by factors affecting the amount of the reactive metabolite and, therefore, protein adduct formed and factors affecting the immune response to those adducts (142). Impaired 4′-hydroxylation or increased metabolism via the minor pathways of metabolism could lead to increased formation of the diclofenac reactive metabolites and hence, adduct formation. Polymorphisms in the *CYP2C9* gene, which is responsible for the 4′-hydroxylation of diclofenac, have not been found to be a risk factor for the development of hepatic injury (143). A recent study has found an association between an upstream (C-161T) UGT2B7 polymorphism and diclofenac-induced liver injury (144). Preliminary results indicate that individuals carrying at least one variant *-161T* allele, which is associated with increased glucuronidation, are at ninefold increased risk of developing an adverse hepatic reaction to diclofenac (144). Therefore, formation of high levels of

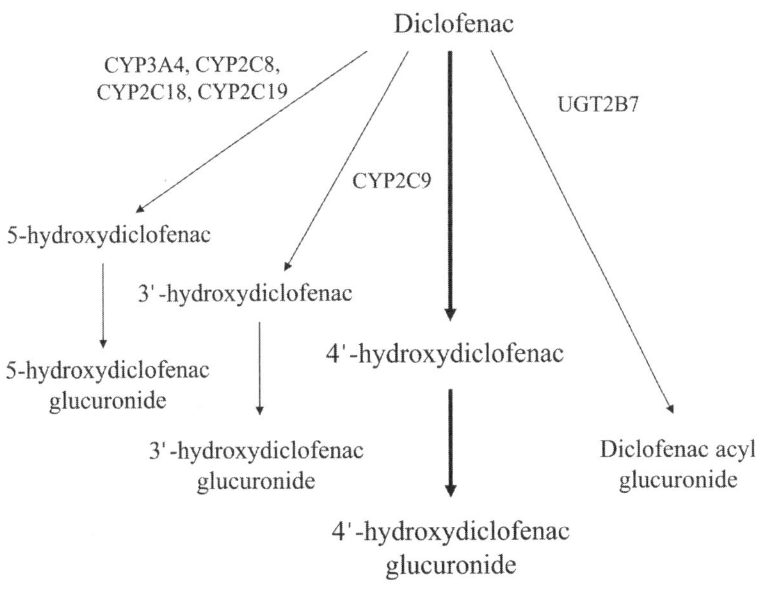

Figure 5 Metabolism of diclofenac in humans.

diclofenac acylglucuronide in hepatocytes may be an important step in the production of antigenic covalent drug-protein adducts.

The pattern and magnitude of the immune response to drug-protein adducts is likely to vary between individuals, potentially explaining differences in susceptibility to hepatotoxicity. A major determinant of interindividual variation in immune reactions is likely to be interindividual variation in the production of immunoregulatory cytokines, such as interleukin-10 (IL-10) and -4 (IL-4), both of which are encoded by polymorphic genes. A small case-control study has shown an association between diclofenac-hepatotoxicity and the *-627*A* allele in the IL-10 gene (which reduces transcription) and *-590T* allele in the IL-4 gene, which increases transcription (145). Low IL-10 and high IL-4 levels would favor a Th-2-mediated antibody response to neoantigenic stimulation and hence could be associated with disease susceptibility. The risk of hepatotoxicity was increased by fivefold in subjects carrying variant alleles for both the IL-10 and IL-4 genes (145).

FUTURE DEVELOPMENTS

Cross-sectional association studies are a crude method to assess the role of low-penetration genetic traits in polygenic disorders (146), because they are biased by the lack of controls for disease duration, disease expression, and timing of diagnosis. In addition, the overall effect of xenobiotics is determined by the interplay of several genes encoding proteins involved in the multiple pathways of drug metabolism, disposition, and effects. The high degree of complexity and redundancy in the metabolic pathways, combined with the limitations of hypothesis-driven research, may delay the discovery of novel pathways (147). Therefore, more comprehensive pharmacogenomic studies are required to define traits that are determined by multiple polymorphic genes. The Human Genome Project, coupled with DNA array technology, high-throughput screening systems, and advanced bioinformatics may allow rapid elucidation of the complex genetic components of human disease and drug response (1). In contrast to the candidate gene approach, a new pharmacogenomic paradigm is emerging in which the entire human genome is screened for SNPs that may be associated with drug response (148). SNP maps could be used to correlate genetic information with the response to a drug. It would thus not be necessary to identify actual genes involved in determining the response to a drug, but the pattern of SNP markers would suffice (149). The hypothesis-free approach to pharmacogenomics may also allow the identification of new drug targets for further exploration.

REFERENCES

1. Evans WE, Relling MV. Pharmacogenomics: translating functional genomics into rational therapeutics. Science 1999; 286:487–491.
2. Roses AD. Pharmacogenetics and the practice of medicine. Nature 2000; 405:857–865.
3. Meyer UA. Pharmacogenetics and adverse drug reactions. Lancet 2000; 356:1667–1671.
4. Phillips KA, Veenstra DL, Oren E, Lee JK, Sadee W. Potential role of pharmacogenomics in reducing adverse drug reactions. A systematic review. J Am Med Assoc 2001; 286:2270–2279.
5. Kalow W. Pharmacogenetics, pharmacogenomics, and pharmacobiology. Clin Pharmacol Ther 2001; 70:1–4.
6. Brookes AJ. The essence of SNPs. Gene 1999; 234:177–186.
7. Vineis P, Malats N, Lang M, d'Errico A, Caporaso N, Cuzick J, Boffetta P. Metabolic polymorphisms and susceptibility to cancer. IARC Sci Publ (148). Lyon: IARC, 1999.

8. Donaldson M. Annual Report of the Chief Medical Officer. London: Department of Health, 2001.
9. Hrubec Z, Omenn GS. Evidence of genetic predisposition to alcoholic cirrhosis and psychosis—twin concordances for alcoholism and its biological end-points by zygosity among male veterans. Alcohol Clin Exp Res 1981; 5:207–215.
10. Crabb DW. Alcoholic liver disease: new concepts in pathogenesis. In: Suchy FJ, Fitz JG, Maher JJ, eds. Mechanisms of Acute & Chronic Liver Diseases: Implications for Diagnosis, Pathogenesis & Treatment. Boston: American Association for the Study of Liver Diseases, 2002:104–112.
11. Morimoto M, Hagbjork AL, Wan YJY, Fu PC, Clot P, Albano E, Ingelman-Sundberg M, French SW. Modulation of experimental alcohol-induced liver-disease by cytochrome-P450 2E1 inhibitors. Hepatology 1995; 21:1610–1617.
12. Bosron WF, Li T-K. Genetic polymorphism of human liver alcohol and aldehyde dehydrogenases, and their relationship to alcohol metabolism and alcoholism. Hepatology 1986; 6:502–510.
13. Tanaka F, Shiratori Y, Yokosuka O, Imazeki F, Tsukada Y, Omata M. Polymorphism of alcohol-metabolizing genes affects drinking behavior and alcoholic liver disease in Japanese men. Alcohol Clin Exp Res 1997; 21:596–601.
14. Day CP, Bashir R, James OFW, Bassendine MF, Crabb DW, Thomasson HR, Li TK, Edenberg HJ. Investigation of the role of polymorphisms at the alcohol and aldehyde dehydrogenase loci in genetic predisposition to alcohol-related end-organ damage. Hepatology 1991; 14:798–801.
15. Poupon RE, Nalpas B, Outelle C, Leury B, Ouzigou P, Higueret D. Polymorphism of alcohol-dehydrogenase, alcohol and aldehyde dehydrogenase-activities—implication in alcoholic cirrhosis in white patients. Hepatology 1992; 15:1017–1022.
16. Couzigou P, Fleury B, Roppi A, Assaigne A, Egueret J, Ron A. Genotyping study of alcohol-dehydrogenase class-I polymorphism in French patients with alcoholic cirrhosis. Alcohol Alcohol 1990; 25:623–626.
17. Grove J, Brown ASM, Daly AK, Bassendine MF, James OFW, Day CP. The RsaI polymorphism of CYP2E1 and susceptibility to alcoholic liver disease in Caucasians: effect on age of presentation and dependence on alcohol dehydrogenase genotype. Pharmacogenetics 1998; 8:335–342.
18. Borras E, Coutelle C, Rosell A, Fernandez-Muixi F, Broch M, Crosas B, Hjelmqvist L, Lorenzo A, Gutierrez C, Santos M, Szczepanek M, Heilig M, Quttrocchi P, Farres J, Vidal F, Richart C, Mach T, Bogdal J, Jornvall H, Seitz H, Couzigou P, Pares X. Genetic polymorphism of alcohol dehydrogenase in Europeans: the ADH2*2 allele decreases the risk for alcoholism and is associated with ADH3*1. Hepatology 2000; 31:984–989.
19. Enomoto N, Takase S, Takada N, Takada A. Alcoholic liver-disease in heterozygotes of mutant and normal aldehyde dehydrogenase-2 genes. Hepatology 1991; 13:1071–1075.
20. Lieber CS. Microsomal ethanol-oxidizing system (MEOS): the first 30 years (1968–1998)—a review. Alcohol Clin Exp Res 2002; 23:991–1007.
21. Pirmohamed M, Kitteringham NR, Quest LJ, Allott RL, Green VJ, Gilmore IT, Park BK. Genetic polymorphism of cytochrome P4502E1 and risk of alcoholic liver disease in Caucasians. Pharmacogenetics 1995; 5:351–357.
22. Wong N, Rae F, Simpson KJ, Murray GD, Harrison DJ. Genetic polymorphisms of cytochrome P4502E1 and susceptibility to alcoholic liver disease and hepatocellular carcinoma in a white population: a study and literature review, including meta-analysis. Mol Pathol 2000; 53:88–93.
23. Kiyosawa K, Sodeyama T, Tanaka E, Gibo Y, Yoshizawa K, Nakano Y, Furuta S, Akahane Y, Nishioka K, Purcell RH. Interrelationship of blood transfusion, non-A, non-B hepatitis and hepatocellular carcinoma: analysis by detection of antibody to hepatitis C virus. Hepatology 1990; 12:671–675.
24. Parkinson A. Biotransformation of xenobiotics. In: Klaassen CD, ed. Casarett & Doull's Toxicology: The Basic Science of Poisons. Kansas: McGraw-Hill, Inc., 1996:113–186.

25. Guengerich FP. Epoxide hydrolase: properties and metabolic roles. Rev Biochem Toxicol 1982; 4:5–30.
26. Hassett C, Aicher L, Sidhu JS, Omiecinski CJ. Human microsomal epoxide hydrolase genetic polymorphism and functional expression in vitro of amino acid variants. Hum Mol Genet 1994; 3:421–428.
27. Omiecinski CJ, Hassett C, Hosagrahara V. Epoxide hydrolase-polymorphism and role in toxicology. Toxicol Lett 2000; 112–113:365–370.
28. Sonzogni L, Silvestri L, De Silvestri A, Gritti C, Foti L, Zavaglia C, Bottelli R, Mondelli MU, Civardi E, Silini EM. Polymorphisms of microsomal epoxide hydrolase gene and severity of HCV-related liver disease. Hepatology 2002; 36:195–201.
29. Hsu IC, Metcalf RA, Sun T, Wesh JA, Wang NJ, Harris CC. Mutational hotspot in the p53 gene in human hepatocellular carcinoma. Nature 1991; 350:427–428.
30. Bressac B, Kew M, Wands J, Ozturk M. Selective G to T mutations of p53 gene in hepatocellular carcinoma from southern Africa. Nature 1991; 350:429–431.
31. McGlynn KA, Rosvold EA, Lustbader ED, Hu Y, Clapper ML, Zhou T, Wild CP, Xia X-L, Baffoe-Bonnie A, Ofori-Adjei D, Chen G-C, London WT, Shen F-M, Buetow KH. Susceptibility to hepatocellular carcinoma is associated with genetic variation in the enzymatic detoxification of aflatoxin B_1. Proc Natl Acad Sci USA 1995; 92:2384–2387.
32. Brockmoller J, Kerb R, Drakoulis N, Nitz M, Roots I. Genotype and phenotype of glutathione S-transferase class mu isoenzymes mu and psi in lung cancer patients and controls. Cancer Res 1993; 53:1004–1011.
33. Farrokyar F, Swarbrick ET, Irvine EJ. A critical review of epidemiological studies in inflammatory bowel disease. Scand J Gastroenterol 2001; 36:2–15.
34. Panwala CM, Jones JC, Viney JL. A novel model of inflammatory bowel disease: mice deficient for the multiple drug resistance gene, mdr1a, spontaneously develop colitis. J Immunol 1998; 161:5733–5744.
35. Maggio-Price L, Shows D, Waggie K, Burich A, Zeng W, Escobar S, Morrissey P, Viney JL. Helicobacter bilis infection accelerates and H. hepaticus infection delays the development of colitis in multiple drug resistance-deficient (mdr1a-/-) mice. Am J Pathol 2002; 160:739–751.
36. Thiebaut F, Tsuruo T, Hamada H, Gottesman MM, Pastan I, Willingham MC. Cellular localization of the multidrug-resistance gene product P-glycoprotein in normal human tissues. Proc Natl Acad Sci USA 1987; 84:7735–7738.
37. Hoffmeyer S, Burk O, von Richter O, Arnold HP, Brockmoller J, Johne A, Cascorbi I, Gerloff T, Roots I, Eichelbaum M, Brinkmann U. Functional polymorphisms of the human multidrug-resistance gene: multiple sequence variations and correlation of one allele with P-glycoprotein expression and activity in vivo. Proc Natl Acad Sci USA 2000; 97:3473–3478.
38. Schwab M, Schaeffeler E, MarX C, Fromm MF, Kaskas B, Metzler J, Stange E, Herfarth H, Schoelmerich J, Gregor M, Walker S, Cascorbi I, Roots I, Brinkmann U, Zanger UM, Eichelbaum M. Association between the C3435T MDR1 gene polymorphism and susceptibility for ulcerative colitis. Gastroenterology 2003; 124:26–33.
39. Farrell JR, Murphy A, Long A, Donnelly S, Cherikuri A, O'Toole D, Mahmud N, Keeling PWN, Weir DG, Kelleher D. High multidrug resistance (P-glycoprotein 170) expression in inflammatory bowel disease patients who fail medical therapy. Gastroenterology 2000; 118:279–288.
40. Pearson DC, May GR, Fick GH, Sutherland LR. Azathioprine and 6-mercaptopurine in Crohn's disease. A meta-analysis. Ann Intern Med 1995; 123:132–142.
41. Aithal GP, Hoffman BJ. Steering azathioprine safely: lessons from pharmacogenetics. Am J Gastroenterol 2001; 96:3002–3003.
42. Weinshilboum R. Thiopurine pharmacogenetics: clinical and molecular studies of thiopurine methyl transferase. Drug Metab Dispos 2001; 29:601–605.
43. Weinshilboum R, Sladck SL. Mercaptopurine pharmacogenetics: monogenic inheritance of erythrocyte thiopurine methyltransferase activity. Am J Hum Genet 1980; 32:651–662.

44. Krynetski EY, Schuetz JD, Galpin AJ, Pui C-H, Relling MV, Evans WE. A single point mutation leading to loss of catalytic activity in human thiopurine S-methyltransferase. Proc Nat Acad Sci USA 1995; 92:949–953.
45. Szumlanski C, Otterness D, Her C, Lee D, Brandriff B, Kelsell D, Spurr N, Lennaed L, Wieben E, Weinshilboum R. Thiopurine methyltransferase pharmacogenetics: human gene cloning and characterization of common polymorphism. DNA Cell Biol 1996; 15:17–30.
46. Tai -L, Krynetski EY, Yates CR, Loennechen T, Fessing MY, Krynetskala NF, Evans WE. Thiopurine S-methyltransferase deficiency. Two nucleotide transitions define the most prevalent mutant allele associated with loss of catalytic activity in Caucasians. Am J Hum Genet 1996; 58:694–702.
47. Dubinsky MC, Lamothe S, Yang HY, Targan SR, Sinnett D, Theoret Y, Seidman EG. Pharmacogenomics and metabolite measurement for 6-mercaptopurine therapy in inflammatory bowel disease. Gastroenterology 2000; 118:705–713.
48. Cuffari C, Hunt S, Bayless T. Utilisation of erythrocyte 6-thioguanine metabolite levels to optimise azathioprine therapy in patients with inflammatory bowel disease. Gut 2001; 48:642–646.
49. Lowry PW, Franklin CL, Weaver AL, Gennett Pike M, Mays DC, Tremaine WJ, Lipsky JJ, Sandborn WJ. Measurement of thiopurine methyltransferase activity and azathioprine metabolites in patients with inflammatory bowel disease. Gut 2001; 49:665–670.
50. Campbell S, Kingstone K, Ghosh S. Relevance of thiopurine methyltransferase activity in inflammatory bowel disease patients maintained on low-dose azathioprine. Aliment Pharmacol Ther 2002; 16:389–398.
51. Colombel J-F, Ferrari N, Debuyscre H, Marteau P, Gendre J-P, Bonaz B, Soule J-C, Modigliani R, Groupe d'Etudes Therapeutique des Affections Inflammataires Digestives (GETAID), Touze Y, Catala P, Libersa C, Broly F. Genotyping analysis of thiopurine S-methyltransferase in patients with Crohn's disease and severe myelosuppression during azathioprine therapy. Gastroenterology 2000; 119:1025–1030.
52. Dubinsky MC, Yang H, Hassard PV, Seidman EG, Kam LY, Abreu MT, Targan SR, Vasiliauskas EA. 6-MP metabolite profiles provide a biochemical explanation for 6-MP resistance in patients with inflammatory bowel disease. Gastroenterology 2002; 122: 904–915.
53. de Morais SMF, Wilkinson GR, Blaisdell J, Nakamura K, Meyer UA, Goldstein JA. The major genetic defect responsible for the polymorphism of S-mephenytoin metabolism in humans. J Biol Chem 1994; 269:15419–15422.
54. de Morais SMF, Wilkinson GR, Blaisdell J, Meyer UA, Nakamura K, Goldstein JA. Identification of a new genetic defect responsible for the polymorphism of (S)-mephenytoin metabolism in Japanese. Mol Pharmacol 1994; 46:594–598.
55. Furuta T, Shirai N, Xiao F, Ohashi K, Ishizaki T. Effect of high-dose lansoprozole on intragastric pH in subjects who are homozygous extensive metabolizers of cytochrome P4502C19. Clin Pharmacol Ther 2001; 70:484–492.
56. Shirai N, Furuta T, Moriyama Y, Okochi H, Kobayashi K, Takashina M, Xino F, Kosuge K, Nakagawa K, Hanai H, Chiba K, Ohashi K, Ishizaki T. Effects of CYP2C19 genotypic differences in the metabolism of omeprazole and rabeprazole on intragastric pH. Aliment Pharmacol Ther 2001; 15:1929–1937.
57. Aoyama N, Tanigawara Y, Kita T, Sakai T, Shirakawa K, Shirasaka D, Kodama F, Okumura K, Kasuga M. Sufficient effect of 1-week omeprazole and amoxacillin dual treatment for Helicobacter pylori eradication in cytochrome P450 2C19 poor metabolizers. J Gastroenterol 1999; 34:80–83.
58. Furuta T, Shirai N, Takashima M, Xiao F, Hanai H, Nakagawa K, Sugimura H, Ohashi K, Ishizaki T. Effects of genotypic differences in CYP2C19 status on cure rates for Helicobacter pylori by dual therapy with rabeprazole plus amoxicillin. Pharmacogenetics 2001; 11:341–348.
59. Furuta T, Shirai N, Takashima M, Xiao F, Hanai H, Sugimura H, Ohashi K, Ishizaki T, Kaneko E. Effect of genotypic differences in CYP1C19 on cure rates for Helicobacter

pylori infection by triple therapy with a proton pump inhibitor, amoxicillin, and clarithromycin. Clin Pharmacol Ther 2001; 69:158–168.

60. Furuta T, Shirai N, Watanabe F, Honda S, Takeuchi K, Lida T, Sato Y, Kajimura M, Futami H, Takayanagi S, Yamada M, Ohashi K, Ishizaki T, Hanai H. Effect of cytochrome P4502C19 genotypic differences on cure rates for gastroesophageal reflux disease by lansoprozole. Clin Pharmacol Ther 2002; 72:453–460.
61. Drews J, Ryser S. The role of innovation in drug development. Nat Biotech 1997; 15:1318–1319.
62. Everhart JE, Renault PF. Irritable bowel syndrome in office-based practice in the United States. Gastroenterology 2002; 123:425–432.
63. von der Ohe MR, Harison RB, Camilleri M. Serotoninergic mediation of postprandial colonic tonic and phasic response in humans. Gut 1994; 35:536–541.
64. Camilleri M, Northcutt AR, Kong S, Dukes GE, McSorley D, Mangel AW. Efficacy and safety of alosetron in women with irritable bowel syndrome: a randomised, placebo-controlled trial. Lancet 2000; 355:1035–1040.
65. Camilleri M, Chey WY, Mayer EA, Northcutt AR, Heath A, Dukes GE, McSorley D, Mangel AW. A randomized controlled clinical trial of serotonin type 3 receptor antagonist aloserton in women with diarrhea predominant irritable bowel syndrome. Arch Intern Med 2001; 161:1733–1740.
66. Heils A, Teufel A, Petri S, Stober G, Riederer P, Bengel D, Lesch KP. Allelic variation of human serotonin transporter gene expression. J Neurochem 1996; 66:2621–2624.
67. Lesch KP, Bengel D, Heils A, Sabol SZ, Greenberg BD, Petri S, Benjamin J, Muller CR, Hamer DH, Murphy DL. Association of anxiety-related traits with a polymorphism in the serotonin transporter gene regulatory region. Science 1996; 274:1527–1531.
68. Camilleri M, Atanasova E, Carlson PJ, Ahmad U, Kim HJ, Viramontes BE, McKinzie S, Urrutia R. Serotonin-transporter polymorphism pharmacogenetics in diarrhoea-predominant irritable bowel syndrome. Gastroenterology 2002; 123:425–432.
69. Herion D, Hoofnagle JH. The interferon sensitivity determining region: all hepatitis C virus isolates are not the same. Hepatology 1997; 25:769–771.
70. Enomoto N, Sakuma I, Asahina Y, Kurosaki M, Murakami T, Yamamoto C, Ogura Y, Izumi N, Marumo F, Sato C. Mutations in the nonstructural protein 5A gene and response to interferon in patients with chronic hepatitis C virus 1b infection. New Engl J Med 1996; 334:77–81.
71. Chayama K, Tsubota A, Kobayashi M, Okamoto K, Hashimoto M, Miyano Y, Koike H, Kobayashi M, Koida I, Arase Y, Saitoh S, Suzuki Y, Murashima M, Ikeda K, Kumada H. Pretreatment virus load and multiple amino acid substitution in the interferon sensitivity-determining region predict the outcome of interferon treatment in patients with chronic genotype 1b hepatitis C virus infection. Hepatology 1997; 25:745–749.
72. Kurosaki M, Enomoto N, Murakami T, Sakuma I, Asahina Y, Yamamoto C, Ikeda T, Tozuka S, Izumi N, Marumo F, Sato C. Analysis of genotypes and aminoacid residues 2209 to 2248 of the NS5A region of hepatitis C virus in relation to the response to interferon-beta therapy. Hepatology 1997; 25:750–753.
73. Moriguchi H, Uemura T, Kobayashi M, Chung RT, Sato C. Management strategies using pharmacogenomics in patients with severe HCV-1b infection: a decision analysis. Hepatology 2002; 36:177–185.
74. Zatonski WA, Lowenfels AB, Boyle P, Maisonneuve P, Bueno, de Mesquita HB, Ghadirian P, Jain M, Przewozniak K, Baghurst P, Moerman, CJ, Simard A, Howe GR, McMichael AJ, Hsieh CC, Walker AM. Epidemiologic aspects of gallbladder cancer: a case-control study of the SEARCH Program of the International Agency for Research on Cancer. J Natl Cancer Inst 1997; 89:1132–1138.
75. Lazarou J, Pomeranz B, Corey P. Incidence of adverse drug reactions in hospitalized patients: a meta-analysis of prospective studies. J Am Med Assoc 1998; 279:1200–1205.
76. Knowles SR, Uetrecht J, Shear NH. Idiosyncratic drug reactions: the reactive metabolite syndrome. Lancet 2000; 356:1587–1591.

77. Park B, Pirmohamed M, Kitteringham N. Role of drug disposition in drug hypersensitivity: a chemical, molecular, and clinical perspective. Chem Res Toxicol 1998; 11:969–988.
78. Pouyanne P, Haramburu F, Imbs JL, Begaud B. Admissions to hospital caused by adverse drug reactions: cross sectional incidence study. French Pharmacovigilance Centres. Br Med J 2000; 320:1036.
79. Bowman L, Carlstedt BC, Black CD. Incidence of adverse drug reactions in adult medical inpatients. Can J Hosp Pharm 1994; 47:209–216.
80. Bates DW, Spell N, Cullen DJ, Burdick E, Laird N, Petersen LA, Small SD, Sweitzer BJ, Leape LL. The costs of adverse drug events in hospitalized patients. Adverse Drug Events Prevention Group. J Am Med Assoc 1997; 277:307–311.
81. Creemers GJ, Lund B, Verweij J. Tropoisomerase I inhibitors topotecan and irenotecan. Cancer Treat Rev 1994; 20:73–96.
82. Saltz LB, Cox JV, Blanke C, Rosen LS, Fehrenbacher L, Moore MJ, Maroun JA, Ackland SP, Locker PK, Pirotta N, Elfring GL, Miller LL. Irinotecan plus fluorouracil and leucovorin for metastatic colorectal cancer. Irinotecan Study Group. New Engl J Med 2000; 343: 905–914.
83. Rothenberg ML. Irinotecan (CPT-11): recent developments and future directions-colorectal cancer and beyond. Oncologist 2001; 6:66–80.
84. Sasaki Y, Hakusui H, Mizuno S, Morita M, Miya T, Eguchi K, Shinkai T, Tamura T, Ohe Y, Saijo N. A pharmacokinetic and pharmacodynamic analysis of CPT-11 and its active metabolite SN-38. Jpn J Cancer Res 1995; 86:101–110.
85. Kawato Y, Aonuma M, Hirota Y, Kuga H, Sato K. Intracellular roles of SN-38, a metabolite of the camptothecin derivative CPT-11, in the antitumor effect of CPT-11. Cancer Res 1991; 51:4187–4191.
86. Atsumi R, Suzuki W, Hakusui H. Identification of the metabolites of irinotecan, a new derivative of camptothecin, in rat bile and its biliary excretion. Xenobiotica 1991; 21:1159–1169.
87. Tukey RH, Strassburg CP, Mackenzie PI. Pharmacogenomics of human UDP-glucuronosyltransferases and irinotecan toxicity. Mol Pharmacol 2002; 62:446–450.
88. Gupta E, Lestingi TM, Mick R, Ramirez J, Vokes EE, Ratain MJ. Metabolic rate of irinotecan in humans: correlation of glucuronidation with diarrhea. Cancer Res 1994; 54:3723–3725.
89. Iyer L, Hall D, Das S, Mortell MA, Radmirez J, Kim S, Di Rienzo, Ratain MJ. Phenotype-genotype correlation of in vitro SN-38 (active metabolite of irinotecan) and bilirubin glucuronidation in human liver tissue with UGT1A1 promoter polymorphism. Clin Pharmacol Ther 1999; 65:576–582.
90. Gagne J-F, Montminy V, Belanger P, Journault K, Gaucher G, Guillemette C. Common human UGT1A polymorphisms and altered metabolism of irinotecan active metabolite 7-ethyl-10-hydroxycamptothecin (SN-38). Mol Pharmacol 2002; 62:608–617.
91. Strassburg CP, Manns MP. Jaundice, genes and promoters. J Hepatol 2000; 33:476–479.
92. Lampe JW, Bigler J, Horner NK, Potter JD. UDP-Glucuronosyltransferase (UGT1A1*28 and UGT1A6*2) polymorphisms in Caucasians and Asians: relationships in serum bilirubin concentrations. Pharmacogenetics 1999; 9:341–349.
93. Ando Y, Saka H, Ando M, Sawa T, Muro K, Ueoka H, Yokoyama A, Saitoh S, Shimokata K, Hasegawa Y. Polymorphisms of UDP-glucuronosyltransferase gene and irinotecan toxicity: a pharmacogenetic analysis. Cancer Res 2000; 60:6921–6926.
94. Strassburg CP, Nguyen N, Manns MP, Tukey RH. UDP-glucuronosyl-transferase activity in human liver and colon. Gastroenterology 1999; 116:149–160.
95. Ando M, Ando Y, Sekido Y, Ando M, Shimokata K, Hasegawa Y. Genetic polymorphisms of the UDP-glucuronosyltransferase 1A7 gene and irinotecan toxicity in Japanese cancer patients. Jpn J Cancer Res 2002; 93:591–597.
96. de Groen PC, Gores GJ, LaRusso NF, Gunderson LL, Nagorney DM. Biliary tract cancers. New Engl J Med 1999; 341:1368–1378.
97. Lumley C. Clinical toxicity: could it have been predicted? Pre-marketing experience. In: Lumley CE, Walker SR, eds. Animal Toxicity Studies. Their Relevance to Man. Lancaster: Quay Publishing, 1990:49–57.

98. Aithal GP, Day CP. Hepatic adverse drug reactions. In: Andrews EB, Mann RD, eds. Pharmacovigilance. 1st ed. Chichester: John Wiley & Sons Ltd, 2002:459–474.
99. Sgro C, Clinard F, Ouazir K, Chanay H, Allard C, Guilleminet C, Lenoir C, Lemoine A, Hillon P. Incidence of drug-induced hepatic injuries: a French population-based study. Hepatology 2002; 36:451–455.
100. Spriet-Pourra C, Auriche M. Drug withdrawal from sales. 2nd ed. Richmond: PJB Publications Ltd, 1994.
101. Morgan MY, Reshef R, Shah RR, Oates NS, Smith RL, Sherlock S. Impaired oxidation of debrisoquine in patients with perhexiline liver injury. Gut 1984; 25:1057–1064.
102. Watson RG, Olomu A, Clements D, Waring RH, Mitchell S, Elias E. A proposed mechanism for chlorpromazine jaundice-defective hepatic sulphoxidation combined with rapid hydroxylation. J Hepatol 1988; 7:72–78.
103. Horsmans Y, Lannes D, Pessayre D, Larrey D. Possible association between poor metabolism of mephenytoin and hepatotoxicity caused by Atrium, a fixed combination preparation containing phenobarbital, febarbamate and difebarbamate. J Hepatol 1994; 21:1075–1079.
104. Wong WM, Wu PC, Yuen MF, Cheng CC, Yew WW, Wong PC, Tam CM, Leung CC, Lai CL. Antituberculosis drug-related liver dysfunction in chronic hepatitis B infection. Hepatology 2000; 31:201–206.
105. Huang Y-S, Chern H-D, Su W-J, Wu J-C, Lai S-L, Yang S-Y, Chang F-Y, Lee S-D. Polymorphism of the N-acetyltransferase 2 gene as a susceptibility risk factor for antituberculosis drug-induced hepatitis. Hepatology 2002; 35:883–889.
106. Hwang SJ, Wu Jc, Lee CN, Yen FS, Lu CJ, Lin TP, Lee SD. A prospective clinical study of isoniazid-rifampicin-pyrazinamide-induced liver injury in an area endemic for hepatitis B. J Gastroenterol Hepatol 1997; 12:87–91.
107. Yamamoto T, Suou T, Hirayama C. Elevated serum aminotransferase induced by isoniazid in relation to isoniazid acetylator phenotype. Hepatology 1986; 6:295–298.
108. Acharya SK, Dasarathy S, Kumer TL, Shuma S, Prasanna KS, Tandon A, Sreenivas V, Nijhawan S, Panda SK, Nanda SK, Irshad M, Joshi YK, Duttagupta S, Tandon RK, Tandon BN. Fulminant hepatitis in a tropical population: clinical course, cause, and early predictors of outcome. Hepatology 1996; 23:1448–1455.
109. Lucena MI, Camargo R, Andrade RJ, Perez-Sanchez CJ, Cuesta FSDL. Comparison of two clinical scales for causality assessment in hepatotoxicity. Hepatology 2001; 33:123–130.
110. Spahr L, Villeneuve J-P, Dufresne M-P, Tasse D, Bui B, Willems B, Fenyves D, Pomier-Layrargues G. Gastric antral vascular ectasia in cirrhotic patients: absence of relation with portal hypertension. Gut 1999; 44:739–742.
111. Littlewood ER, Barrison IG, Murray-Lyon IM, Paradinas FJ. Cholangiocarcinoma and oral contraceptives. Lancet 1980; 1:310–311.
112. Mitchell JR, Zimmerman HJ, Ishak KG, Thorgeirsson UP, Timbrell JA, Snodgrass WR, Nelson SD. Isoniazid liver injury: clinical spectrum, pathology and probable pathogenesis. Ann Intern Med 1976; 84:181–192.
113. Ellard GA, Gammon PT. Pharmacokinetics of isoniazid in humans. J Pharmacokinet Biopharm 1976; 4:83–113.
114. Lauterburg BH, Smith CV, Todd EL, Mitchell JR. Pharmacokinetics of the toxic hydrazine metabolites formed from isoniazid in humans. J Pharmacol Exp Ther 1985; 235: 566–570.
115. Scales MD, Timbrell JA. Studies on hydrazine hepatotoxicity. 1. Pathological findings. J Toxicol Environ Health 1982; 10:941–953.
116. Sarma GR, Immanuel C, Kailasam S, Narayana AS, Venkatesan P. Rifampin-induced release of hydrazine from isoniazid. A possible cause of hepatitis during treatment of tuberculosis with regimens containing isoniazid and rifampicin. Am Rev Resp Dis 1986; 133:1072–1075.
117. Blum M, Grant DM, McBride W, Heim H, Meyer UA. Human arylamine *N*-acetyltransferase genes: isolation, chromosomal localization and functional expression. DNA Cell Biol 1990; 9:193–203.

118. Hein DW, Doll MA, Rustan TD, Ferguson RJ. Metabolic activation of N-hydroxyarylamines and N-hydroxyarylamides by 16 recombinant human NAT2 allozymes: effects of 7 specific NAT2 nucleic acid substitutions. Cancer Res 1995; 55:3531–3536.
119. Hammer SM, Squires KE, Hughes MD, Grimes JM, Demeter LM, Currier JS, Eron JJ Jr, Feinberg JE, Balfour HH Jr, Deyton LR, Chodakewitz JA, Fischl MA. A controlled trial of two nucleoside analogues plus indinavir in persons with human immunodeficiency virus infection and CD4 cell counts of 200 per cubic millimeter or less. AIDS Clinical Trials Group 320 Study Team. New Engl J Med 1997; 337:725–733.
120. Kaul DR, Cinti SK, Carver PL, Kazanjian PH. HIV protease inhibitors: advances in therapy and adverse reactions, including metabolic complications. Pharmacotherapy 1999; 19:281–298.
121. Balani SK, Woolf EJ, Hoagland VL, Sturgill MG, Deutsch PJ, Yeh KC, Lin JH. Disposition of indinavir, a potent HIV-1 protease inhibitor, after an oral dose in humans. Drug Metab Dispos 1996; 24:1389–1394.
122. Zucker SD, Qin X, Rouster SD, Yu F, Green RM, Keshavan P, Feinberg J, Sherman KE. Mechanism of indinavir-induced hyperbilirubinemia. Proc Natl Acad Sci USA 2001; 98:12671–12676.
123. Berson A, Freneaux E, Larrey D, Lepage V, Douay C, Mallet C, Fromenty, Benhamou JP, Pessayre D. Possible role of HLA in hepatotoxicity. an exploratory study in 71 patients with drug-induced idiosyncratic hepatitis. J Hepatol 1994; 20:336–342.
124. Larrey D, Vial T, Micaleff A, Babany G, Morichau-Beauchant M, Michel H, Benhamou JP. Hepatitis associated with amoxicillin-clavulanic acid combination: report of 15 cases. Gut 1992; 33:368–371.
125. Garcia Rodriguez LA, Stricker BH, Zimmerman HJ. Risk of acute liver injury associated with the combination of amoxycillin and clavulanic acid. Arch Intern Med 1996; 156:1327–1332.
126. O'Donohue J, Oien KA, Donaldson P, Underhill J, Clare M, MacSween RN, Mills PR. Co-amoxiclav jaundice: clinical and histological features and HLA class II association. Gut 2000; 47:717–720.
127. Hautekeete ML, Horsmans Y, Waeyenberge CV, Demanet C, Henrion J, Verbist L, Brenard R, Sempoux C, Michielsen PP, Yap PSH, Rahier J, Geubel AP. HLA association of amoxicillin-clavulanate-induced hepatitis. Gastroenterology 1999; 117:1181–1186.
128. Daly AK, Day CP. Candidate gene case-control association studies: advantages and potential pitfalls. Br J Clin Pharmacol 2001; 52:489–499.
129. Risch NJ. Searching for genetic determinants in the new millenium. Nature 2000; 405: 847–856.
130. Rodriguez LAG, Williams R, Derby LE, Dean AD, Jick H. Acute liver injury associated with non-steroidal anti-inflammatory drugs and the role of risk factors. Arch Intern Med 1994; 154:311–316.
131. Banks AT, Zimmerman HJ, Ishak KG, Harter JG. Diclofenac-associated hepatotoxicity. Analysis of 180 cases reported to the Food and Drug Administration as adverse reactions. Hepatology 1995; 22:820–827.
132. Leemann T, Transon C, Dayer P. Cytochrome P450TB (CYP2C): a major monooxygenase catalyzing diclofenac 4′-hydroxylation in human liver. Life Sci 1993; 52:29–34.
133. Transon C, Lecoeur S, Leemann T, Beaune P, Dayer P. Interindividual variability in catalytic activity and immunoreactivity of three major human liver cytochrome P450 isozymes. Eur J Clin Pharmacol 1996; 51:79–85.
134. Bort R, Mace K, Boobis A, Gomez-Lechon M-J, Pfeifer A, Castell J. Hepatic metabolism of diclofenac: role of human CYP in the minor oxidative pathways. Biochem Pharmacol 1999; 58:787–796.
135. Shen S, Marchick MR, Davis MR, Doss GA, Pohl LR. Metabolic activation of diclofenac by human cytochrome P450 3A4: role of 5-hydroxydiclofenac. Chem Res Toxicol 1999; 12:214–222.
136. Tang W, Stearns RA, Wang RW, Chiu S-HL, Baillie TA. Roles of human hepatic cytochrome P450s 2C9 and 3A4 in the metabolic activation of diclofenac. Chem Res Toxicol 1999; 12:192–199.

137. King C, Tang W, Ngui J, Tephly T, Braun M. Characterization of rat and human UDP-glucuronosyltransferases responsible for the in vitro glucuronidation of diclofenac. Toxicol Sci 2001; 61:49–53.
138. Kretz-Rommel A, Boelsterli UA. Diclofenac covalent protein binding is dependent on acyl glucuronide formation and is inversely related to P450-mediated acute cell injury in cultured rat hepatocytes. Toxicol Appl Pharmacol 1993; 120:155–161.
139. Kretz-Rommel A, Boelsterli UA. Selective protein adducts to membrane proteins in cultured rat hepatocytes exposed to diclofenac: radiochemical and immunochemical analysis. Mol Pharmacol 1994; 45:237–244.
140. Hargus SJ, Amouzedeh HR, Pumford NR, Myers TG, McCoy SC, Pohl LR. Metabolic activation and immunochemical localization of liver protein adducts of the nonsteroidal anti-inflammatory drug diclofenac. Chem Res Toxicol 1994; 7:575–582.
141. Kretz-Rommel A, Boelsterli UA. Cytotoxic activity of T cells and non-T cells from diclofenac-immunised mice against cultured syngenic hepatocytes exposed to diclofenac. Hepatology 1995; 22:213–222.
142. Aithal GP. Hepatotoxicity: accuracy of diagnosis, long term outcome and the role of genetic polymorphism in drug metabolism and adverse drug reactions. PhD dissertation, University of Newcastle, Newcastle upon Tyne 2000.
143. Aithal GP, Day CP, Leathart JB, Daly AK. Relationship of polymorphism in CYP2C9 to genetic susceptibility to diclofenac-induced hepatitis. Pharmacogenetics 2000; 10:511–518.
144. Aithal GP, Leathart JB, Dang TS, Day CP, Daly AK. Association of UDP-glucuronyltransferase (UGT) 2B7 genotype with diclofenac-induced hepatotoxicity (abstr). Hepatology 2002; 36(4):333A.
145. Aithal GP, Ramsay L, Daly AK, Sonchit N, Leathart JBS, Alexander G, Kenna JG, Coldwell J, Day CP. Hepatic adults, circulating antibodies and cytokine polymorphisms in patients with diclofenac hepatotoxicity. Hepatology 2004; 39:1430–1440.
146. Lander ES, Schork NJ. Genetic dissection of complex traits. New Engl J Med 2002; 265:2037–2048.
147. Schreiber S, Hampe J, Eickhoff H, Lehrach H. Functional genomics in gastroenterology. Gut 2000; 47:601–607.
148. Lander ES. Array of hope. Nat Genet 1999; 21:3–4.
149. Roses AD. Pharmacogenetics and future drug development and delivery. Lancet 2000; 355:1358–1361.

14

The Genetics of Antipsychotic Response: Pharmacogenetic and Pharmacogenomic Investigations and Clinical Applications

Maria J. Arranz, Dalu Mancama, and Robert W. Kerwin
Section of Clinical Neuropharmacology, Institute of Psychiatry—King's College, London, U.K.

INTRODUCTION

Antipsychotic drugs constitute the mainstay of treatment for schizophrenia; they are used to treat acute psychotic episodes and reduce risk of relapse (1). However, a significant proportion of treated patients (25–50%) fail to show satisfactory recovery, and 80% will have a relapse within five years (2,3). In addition, between 50% and 70% of the patients develop severe and lasting side effects as a result of long-term antipsychotic treatment (4). Failure to find an appropriate treatment is associated with poor prognosis and may reduce chances of recovery. Early and effective treatment is therefore important. There are two major classes of antipsychotics, classical and atypical drugs, with different pharmacological profiles and varied success in the treatment of the disease. However, at present it is not possible to determine, other than by a trial of treatment, which individuals will respond to which drugs. Pharmacogenetic and pharmacogenomic research approaches aim to identify genetic factors that influence response variability and to use that information for treatment prediction and selection. Pharmacogenetic research has produced in recent years interesting results that have been translated into useful clinical applications (i.e., determination of metabolic status). Pharmacogenomic research is producing a wealth of information on response-related factors, although the clinical utility of this approach will only become apparent over the next decade.

PHARMACOGENETIC AND PHARMACOGENOMIC RESEARCH

Treatment variability in response to antipsychotic treatment has been hypothesized to be a result of genetic and environmental factors. Nongenetic observations, such as demographic or clinical measurements, have been investigated as indicators of therapeutic outcome. Female gender and early onset have been associated with unsatisfactory response to treatment with the antipsychotic clozapine, whereas the history of drug-induced side effects and paranoid symptoms predict good response (5). Weight gain during clozapine and olanzapine treatment predicts satisfactory improvement (6,7). Duration of episodes and severity of illness can predict neuroleptic response (8), and a combination of clinical measurements was reported to predict clinical response with more than 90% success using a mathematical model (9). These findings illustrate the contribution of nongenetic and environmental factors to treatment variability. However, their predictive capability is of limited value, and most observations are obtained during drug treatment.

Genetic research provides a different approach towards the prediction of treatment response. The main aim of pharmacogenetics and pharmacogenomics is to provide response predictors at early stages of the illness, before chemical intervention is started. Initially, research focused on a selected number of genes and their influence on treatment response (pharmacogenetics). However, the development of high-throughput techniques for the rapid examination of gene sequence and expression facilitates the simultaneous study of differences in a large number of genes and individuals (pharmacogenomics). Pharmacogenetic research has produced important information on factors determining treatment response, which has already translated into clinically applicable tests (i.e., detection of metabolic polymorphisms), and research on prediction tests for a number of antipsychotic drugs is underway. Pharmacogenomic research is producing a wealth of information on sequence and expression differences between individuals that will accelerate the identification of genetic influence on treatment variability. These genetic strategies have succeeded in the identification of response-related factors in metabolic pathways and neurotransmitter systems. The following sections summarize the findings in metabolic enzymes, in neurotransmitter receptors and transporters, and in signal transduction genes.

Metabolic Enzymes

The absorption, distribution, and elimination of antipsychotic drugs require a series of metabolic processes that take place mostly in the liver. Phase I (oxidation and hydrolysis) and Phase II (conjugation with glucuronic acid, glycine, glutathione or with acetate, sulfate, and methyl groups) reactions are the main mechanisms whereby antipsychotic drugs are metabolized. Most antipsychotics are converted to hydrophilic compounds [mainly by cytochrome P450 (CYP) enzymes] and are then conjugated [mainly by *N*-acetyltransferases, UDP-glucuronosyltransferases (UGT), and thiopurine methyltransferases (TPMT)] to facilitate renal excretion. Alterations of these processes may influence the serum and tissue concentrations of antipsychotics and their metabolites and modify their therapeutic effect. Functional mutations have been described that render metabolic enzymes inactive or ultra-active, resulting in accumulation or rapid elimination of the drug and metabolites. Subjects presenting slow (poor metabolizers, PM) or fast (ultrarapid metabolizers, UM) metabolizing phenotypes will not be responsive to therapeutic doses or will present toxic reactions due to accumulated drug metabolites. The frequency of metabolic alterations varies considerably among populations, a fact that is considered to contribute to response variability. Pretreatment genotyping of metabolic variants can help to identify patients who will not respond to average therapeutic doses of antipsychotics and who may, as a result of poor metabolism, develop adverse reactions. Genetic identification of individuals with altered metabolic enzymes constitutes one of the first and most important clinical applications of pharmacogenetics in psychiatry and will be discussed later in the chapter. In this section we are going to review polymorphisms described in cytochrome P450 (CYP) and *N*-acetyltransferase (NAT) genes, as these enzymes are involved in the metabolism of the vast majority of commonly used antipsychotics.

CYP Enzymes

The metabolism of most antipsychotics is initiated by CYP enzymes. Four families of CYP enzymes (CYP1–CYP4) are directly involved in drug metabolism, each divided into subfamilies and subtypes (10). In particular, the CYP1A2, CYP2D6, and CYP3A4 subtypes are the most important for the metabolism of psychotropic drugs (Table 1), and several functional polymorphisms have been described in their genes that determine blood drug concentrations.

CYP1A2. The CYP1A2 subfamily accounts for nearly 15% of the liver cytochromes and is one of the major metabolic pathways of the antipsychotics clozapine, olanzapine, and haloperidol (Table 1) (11,12). CYP1A2 PM are relatively frequent in the population (5–10%), although significant ethnic variations are known (13). Several variants with a functional effect on metabolic rate have been described in the promoter region of the *CYP1A2* gene (**1C*, **1F*) (14,15). The *CYP1A2 *F* variant has been associated with drug-induced tardive dyskinesia (16). Although this finding is yet to be confirmed, it illustrates the clinical effect of alterations in metabolic rates.

CYP2D6. Genetically determined metabolic alterations were first discovered in the 1970s when several individuals treated with debrisoquine, a substrate for CYP2D6, and presenting with adverse reactions were found to possess a mutation in the gene that rendered the enzyme inactive (17). Since then, several genetically determined forms of the enzyme have been described with different levels of activity, including poor, intermediate, extensive, and UM (18). The frequency of these phenotypes varies greatly among populations: PMs constitute 5% to 10% of Caucasian populations and 1% to 2% of Asian populations (18,19). However, the greatest variation is observed among African populations, ranging from 0% to 19% of the PMs (20). The antipsychotics olanzapine, risperidone, chlorpromazine, and haloperidol are metabolized, at least partially, by this enzyme (18,19). However, although several reports have associated *CYP2D6* genetic mutations with drug blood levels and drug-induced side effects (21–23), no clear relation with general therapeutic response has been reported (24,25).

Table 1 List of Metabolic Polymorphisms in CYP Enzymes and Their Associations with Antipsychotic Response Traits

Enzyme	Substrate(s)	Functional polymorphism	Reported association
CYP1A2	Clozapine, olanzapine, haloperidol	**1F*	Tardive dyskinesia (16)
CYP2D6	Olanzapine, risperidone, chlorpromazine, haloperidol	**3, *4, *5, *10*	Susceptibility to tardive dyskinesia (21–23)
CYP3A4	Chlorpromazine, clozapine, haloperidol, risperidone, sertindole, ziprasidone	**4, *5, *6, *17, *18*	No reported association

Abbreviation: CYP, cytochrome P450.

CYP3A4. This subtype is one of the most abundant forms of CYP in the human liver (26) and participates in the metabolism of the antipsychotics chlorpromazine, clozapine, haloperidol, risperidone, sertindonle, and ziprasidone, among others (Table 1). Numerous mutations have been described in the *CYP3A4* gene, and several have been reported to cause functional alterations of the enzyme activity (27,28). However, few studies have investigated the potential implications of these polymorphisms on treatment variability and their influence on clinical response remains to be elucidated.

Phase II Enzymes

Conjugation reactions with an exogenous substance or group to facilitate renal excretion are catabolised by phase II enzymes, such as NAT, TPMT, and UGT. These enzymes are known to exist in different forms with variable levels of activity.

NAT enzymes catalyze the acetylation of drugs and their metabolites. Two NAT subtypes, NAT1 and NAT2, have been described, of which several forms with variable activity levels are known (29,30). As is the case with other metabolic polymorphisms, the frequency distribution of these variants is subject to geographical differences. In particular, NAT2 slow acetylators constitute 40% of the Caucasians but less than 10% of the Japanese and 30% of other Asian populations.

Several polymorphisms (**2*, **3A*, **3C*) have been described in individuals with slow TPMT metabolism, which present ethnic variations (31,32). Similarly, several naturally occurring mutations in the UGT gene have been described that may alter enzyme activity (33,34). As in the case of NAT polymorphisms, their influence on antipsychotic response is yet to be investigated.

Clinical Relevance of Metabolic Polymorphisms

Given the high frequency in the population and the detrimental effects of metabolic polymorphisms, their importance in the success of antipsychotic treatment cannot be underestimated. As many as 70% of the successfully treated patients develop side effects that may be partially caused by metabolic polymorphisms (4). In addition, normal metabolizing individuals may still experience toxic reactions due to simultaneous treatment with drug acting as substrates for the same metabolic enzyme. Pretreatment genotyping of CYP polymorphisms could be helpful to avoid extra-pyramidal side effects caused by toxic accumulation of drug metabolites and also provide information on the appropriate therapeutic doses for each individual according to their metabolic rate.

Neurotransmitter Systems

Aside from the pharmacokinetic influence of metabolic polymorphisms, therapeutic efficacy of antipsychotic drugs is determined by their interaction with neurotransmitter systems. Dopaminergic, serotonergic, histaminergic, muscarinic, glutamergic, and adrenergic receptors are targeted to a variable extent by antipsychotic compounds. The two major classes of antipsychotic drugs, conventional and atypical antipsychotics, have a marked difference in their sites of action. Classical conventional antipsychotics, such as chlorpromazine and haloperidol, have dopaminergic receptors as their main targets, whereas atypical antipsychotics have a wider range of receptor targets (35). Clozapine, the archetypal atypical antipsychotic, displays high affinities for histamine, serotonin, dopamine (D), muscarinic, and adrenergic receptors (35,36). Different pharmacological properties may translate into different therapeutic characteristics: classical antipsychotics are reported to improve positive psychotic symptoms (e.g., hallucinations, delusions) and induce severe extra-pyramidal side effects (EPS), whereas atypical antipsychotics are reported to improve positive and negative (loss of energy and motivation) symptoms with low induction of EPS. Drug–receptor interactions may be altered by mutations in receptor genes, a fact that can be reflected in the clinical outcome. This hypothesis has been extensively tested during the last decade. Drug-targeted receptor genes have been systematically screened for naturally occurring mutations. Reported mutations were investigated in groups of treated patients differing in their response traits (e.g., general response, presence of side effects) in the search of response-related variants. Difference in the frequency representation of a mutation between groups would indicate a direct or indirect relation with response variability. This strategy has proven the therapeutic value of D and serotonin receptor targeting and has identified variants in neurotransmitter transporters that contribute to individual variability. Further investigations in other neurotransmitter systems and in signal transduction genes are likely to produce information on additional contributing factors. The following sections summarize the most relevant findings in the area.

Dopaminergic Receptors

The D hypothesis of schizophrenia suggests that enhanced dopaminergic activity is partly responsible for the etiology of the disease (37,38). This hypothesis is supported by studies suggesting that blockade of D receptors relieves psychotic symptoms (36,39). Most conventional antipsychotics display high affinities for D receptors, particularly the type 2 (D2) receptors (40). However, antagonism of D2 receptors is also associated with severe and long-lasting EPSs (4,40). Type 3 (D3) and type 4 (D4) receptors are also targeted by conventional and atypical antipsychotics, although their exact contribution to antipsychotic activity is still being debated (41–43).

Genetic variation has been suggested to influence the clinical efficacy and side effects associated with D antagonism. This hypothesis is supported by reports of association between D2 receptor variants and early response to treatment with the antipsychotic haloperidol (Table 2) (44). Response to the atypical antipsychotic clozapine is allegedly influenced by D2 and D3 receptor variants (45,46).

Investigation of more specific traits, such as symptom variability or side-effect induction, may facilitate the finding of related factors. According to a recent study, D3 polymorphisms are associated with improvement in positive symptoms after treatment with the atypical antipsychotic clozapine (47), a fact that supports the mediation of the dopaminergic system in schizophrenia symptomatology. As interesting as the prediction of response is the forecast of adverse reactions: several studies have reported association between a D3 polymorphic variant, Ser9Gly, and tardive dyskinesia (48–50). Although several studies fail to repeat this finding, a recent meta-analysis confirmed the validity of the association (51). Studies on Japanese schizophrenia patients have shown that D2 mutations may be related to neuroleptic malignant syndrome (NMS) (52), although this finding was not repeated in an independent study (53) and needs further investigation. In general, therefore, it seems that an increased frequency of D2 and D3 mutations is observed in patients presenting tardive dyskinesia (54,55).

It is important to mention that inconsistent findings such as those summarized here have been reported in many other disease areas (56). Genetic association studies are prone to produce false-positive or false-negative results, and reports with seemingly opposite findings are frequently found in pharmacogenetic research. Contradictory reports may be the result of experimental error, small study size, or a reflection of differences in clinical

Table 2 List of Polymorphisms in Dopamine Receptor Genes and Their Association with Antipsychotic Response Traits

Receptor	Targeted by	Polymorphism	Reported association
D2	Haloperidol, chlorpromazine, risperidone, ziprasidone, amisulpride	−141-C *Ins/Del*	Early response to clozapine (45)
		Taq I	Early response to haloperidol (44)
			Related to neuroleptic malignant syndrome (52)
D3	Haloperidol, chlorpromazine, risperidone, olanzapine, ziprasidone, amisulpride	Ser9Gly	Tardive dyskinesia (48–51)
			Improvement in positive symptoms after olanzapine treatment (47)
		−205-G/A	Improvement in positive symptoms after olanzapine treatment (47)

Abbreviations: D2, dopamine type 2 receptor; D3, dopamine type 3 receptor.

or demographical characteristics of the patients investigated (57). Nevertheless, repeated association reports should be considered as reliable evidence. Therefore, dopaminergic mediation of antipsychotic activity is supported by pharmacogenetic results and suggests that genotyping of D variants may help to predict treatment outcome and adverse responses.

Serotonergic Receptors

Dysfunction of the serotonergic system has been implicated in the etiology of mood disorders and in schizophrenia symptomatology (58–60). Because of this involvement, serotonin (5-HT) receptors are candidate targets for antipsychotic activity. In particular, atypical antipsychotics strongly target serotonin type 2 (5-HT2) receptors, a characteristic that has been suggested to mediate their success in the treatment of negative symptoms of schizophrenia (36,60,61).

As in the case of the D research, studies investigating 5-HT polymorphisms and therapeutic response have produced inconsistent results. A number of reports suggesting association between 5-HT2A variants and response to a variety of antipsychotics, clozapine, and risperidone have been published (61–66), and also studies with contradicting findings (Table 3) (67–69). 5-HT2A mediation of therapeutic activity seems to be proved by a meta-analysis of association studies indicating a strong relation between the presence of genetic variants in the receptor gene and variability in response to the antipsychotic clozapine (70). Other 5-HT receptors have been less studied, although associations between 5-HT2C polymorphisms and clozapine response (71) and tardive dyskinesia (72), and 5-HT6 variants and clozapine response (73) have been suggested. 5-HT2C variants have also been related to weight-gain, a drug-induced side effect of particular relevance following treatment with the atypical antipsychotics clozapine and olanzapine (74,75).

Taken together, these studies strengthen the hypothesis of serotonin involvement in the mechanisms of antipsychotic action. As it will be discussed later, genotyping of serotonin polymorphisms greatly contribute to the pretreatment prediction of antipsychotic response.

Table 3 List of Polymorphisms in Serotonergic Receptors and Their Associations with Antipsychotic Response Traits

Receptor	Targeted by	Polymorphism	Reported association
5-HT2A	Chlorpromazine, clozapine, risperidone, olanzapine, ziprasidone	102-T/C & −1438-G/A	Response to clozapine (61,63,65) Response to risperidone (66)
		His452Tyr	Response to clozapine (62,64)
5-HT2C	Clozapine, risperidone, olanzapine, ziprasidone	Cys23Ser	Response to clozapine (71) Related to tardive dyskinesia (72)
		−759-C/T	Associated to clozapine-induced weight gain (74)
5-HT6	Clozapine, olanzapine, ziprasidone	267-C/T	Response to clozapine (73)

Abbreviations: 5-HT2, serotonin type 2; 5-HT6, serotonin type 6.

Adrenergic Receptors

Adrenergic transmission is implicated in cognitive and emotional behavior. Dysfunction of this system is observed in patients suffering mood disorders, depression, or schizophrenia. Therefore, targeting of adrenergic receptors is thought to have therapeutic properties. However, pharmacogenetic studies have only produced a scarce number of reports showing no association between adrenergic polymorphisms and treatment response (76,77), although adrenergic variants may be involved in drug-induced weight gain (75). Given the involvement of the adrenergic system in the symptomatology of mental disorders, analyses of the influence of adrenergic mutations on defined traits, such as depression and negative symptoms, will likely produce more definite results.

Other Neurotransmitter Receptors

Histaminergic, muscarinic, and glutamate receptors are drug-targeted for their involvement in the etiology of mental disorders. Dysfunction of these systems has been strongly related with the etiology of schizophrenia, although investigations of the genetic contribution of alterations in these genes towards the development of mental disorders are still underway. Systematic screening for the genes coding for histamine receptors (H1, H2, H3), muscarinic receptors (M1, M2, M3, M4, M5), and several genes of the glutamate system has revealed the presence of numerous mutations, but their full contribution to clinical outcome is yet to be investigated (78,79). Nevertheless, several reports have suggested that mutations in histamine receptors contribute to determine clozapine response (80,81).

Neurotransmitter Transporters

Transporter proteins regulate the availability of neurotransmitter for brain transmission. Therefore, they exert an important role in the control and regulation of neurotransmitter systems. In particular, D and serotonin transporter genes have been investigated, and a series of interesting associations have been reported. D transporter type 1 (*DAT1*) allelic variants have been associated with poor response to methylphenidate, a drug used for the treatment of children with attention-deficit and hyperactivity disorders

(ADHD) (82,83). Functional and nonfunctional polymorphisms of the serotonin transporter (*5-HTT*) gene have been associated with clozapine response (84), a result not found in a later study on a variety of antipsychotics (85). However, the strong associations detected between *5-HTT* polymorphisms and response to antidepressants (86,87) support the mediating role of this transporter protein in the mechanism of action of psychotropic drugs.

Signal Transduction

The efficacy of antipsychotic drugs is mediated by neurotransmitter receptor targets linked to downstream cellular responses through an intricate network of signaling pathways. Receptor-linked heterotrimeric G-proteins play a particularly important role in this process, by stimulating effector molecules that activate or inhibit second messenger molecules. These responses in turn regulate key biological functions, including gene transcription, cell proliferation, differentiation, and development. G-proteins consist of three subunits (α, β, and γ), for which there are known to be $16G\alpha$, $5G\beta$, and $12G\gamma$ human genes. Functionally important genetic variants have been identified throughout these genes, and growing evidence implicates their involvement in the etiology of depression and its treatment (88,89). However, the extent to which these mutations contribute to the treatment of psychiatric disorders remains to be fully determined.

CLINICAL APPLICATIONS OF PHARMACOGENETICS AND PHARMACOGENOMICS

The previous sections described a number of genetic factors influencing treatment response identified through genetic association studies. However, these individual findings have had no immediate application in clinical practice, because they do not provide a sufficiently high degree of prediction as they account for a relatively small fraction of response variability. This fact may be a reflection of the multitarget profile of most drugs. Antipsychotics interact with several neurotransmitter systems to a different extent, and alterations in all/most of the genes controlling drug–target interactions may contribute to response variability. Pharmacogenetic and pharmacogenomic research has attempted the combination of genetic information in relevant genes for the prediction of antipsychotic response with promising results. Pharmacogenetic research has already produced some useful applications, particularly in the detection of side effects related to metabolic alterations. Pharmacogenomic research is relatively new in the field, and it is expected to produce clinically useful results in the next decade. The current applications of pharmacogenetics and pharmacogenomics include individual detection of PMs, selection of population groups for clinical trials, and novel target detection for drug development.

Applications in Individual Prescription

The characterization of an individual's metabolic status is the first and most used clinical application of pharmacogenetics. Most antipsychotic drugs are metabolized by four cytochrome CYP enzymes, namely CYP1A2, CYP2D6, CYP2C9, and CYP3A4 (90,91). Detection of the most common polymorphisms in the genes coding for these enzymes will facilitate the identification of individuals likely to present adverse reactions or treatment failure related to deficient metabolism. Pretreatment genotyping of CYP polymorphisms will allow for the adjustment of therapeutic doses for slow metabolizers and UMs. This practice has already been recommended for a number of antidepressant drugs (92) and will be particularly beneficial in cases where the use of drugs with narrow therapeutic ranges is considered. Several protocols are already standardized for the rapid detection of metabolic polymorphisms, including simple polychain reaction (PCR) techniques (93,94) and DNA arrays for the simultaneous genotyping of the most frequent polymorphisms (95,96).

Preliminary studies incorporating information in drug targets have also proved their value as predictors of therapeutic response. A combination of mutations in a relatively small number of genes resulted in the successful prediction of clozapine response in 76% of the cases (80). Similar strategies are being developed for other antipsychotic drugs, such as olanzapine (47). Tailoring of antipsychotic treatment will incorporate genetic information for the prediction of therapeutic response and drug-induced side effects. Although still under investigation, these strategies will form the basis of future tailoring of antipsychotic treatment according to the individual's requirements.

Applications in Drug Development and Clinical Trials

Pharmacogenomic research will have an obvious impact in drug development. High-throughput technologies involving DNA chips, robotized handling of samples, and computerized analyses permit the investigation of a large number of genes simultaneously and will greatly accelerate the identification of therapeutic targets. These high-throughput technologies can be used to investigate functional alterations (i.e., differential gene expression) in tissue samples from brains of probands, thus identifying putative therapeutic areas. The same high-throughput technologies can be used to investigate drug-induced expression changes of neurotransmitter and receptor proteins in animal and human brains, thus helping to confirm/discard current targets. In addition, taking advantage of the sequence knowledge produced by the human genome mapping project (97), novel targets can be fished out by comparing genomic sequences with proteins of proven therapeutic relevance (98).

Pharmacogenetic applications in clinical trials are already in use. Routine CYP genotyping is carried out to select patients for clinical trials according to their metabolic characteristics. In this way, adverse reactions caused by poor metabolism of the studied drug can be easily detected and prescription could be restricted to population groups with favorable genetic profiles. Although the economic gains may not be substantial as it can result in a reduction of market share, this practice can help to obtain the optimal therapeutic dose for each patient and to avoid adverse reactions caused by deficient metabolism, therefore contributing to the success of the drug and facilitating their approval by regulatory bodies. Further applications of pharmacogenetics, namely identifying patients likely to respond according to their pharmacodynamic profile, may take longer to be introduced in clinical trials. However, this practice can be very beneficial in cases where the use of successful antipsychotics have been found to cause severe side effects in a number of cases (e.g., clozapine). Pretreatment pharmacogenotyping will identify patients likely to show positive response without developing side effects. This practice may help patients to access beneficial treatments, which otherwise would not have been considered.

FUTURE RESEARCH: INVESTIGATIONS ON GENETIC EXPRESSION

The completion of the human genome mapping project showed a lower number of genes (25,000–30,000) than expected. This number can hardly explain the differences between humans and others species (99). To explain this apparent discrepancy, it has been hypothesized that evolution depends not only on the number of genes but other genetic phenomena, such as differential expression, RNA editing, and alternative splicing (100,101). These genetic events play an important role in evolution and can have important implications in the efficacy and safety of drugs (i.e., the most common CYP2D6 functional alteration causes a splicing event). Therefore, future pharmacogenomic research will expand from the study of DNA sequence mutation alone to functional alterations in the hope of better understanding the complexity of drug–target interactions and response variability.

REFERENCES

1. Davis JM, Kane JM, Marder SR, Brauzer B, Gierl B, Schooler N, et al. Dose response of prophylactic antipsychotics. J Clin Psychiatry 1993; 54(suppl):24–30.
2. Kane JM. Factors which can make patients difficult to treat. Br J Psychiatry 1996; 31(suppl):10–14.
3. Prudo R, Blum HM. Five-year outcome and prognosis in schizophrenia: a report from the London Field Research Centre of the International Pilot Study of Schizophrenia. Br J Psychiatry 1987; 150:345–354.
4. Cunningham Owens DG. A guide to the extrapyramidal side-effects of antipsychotic drugs. Cambridge: Cambridge University Press, 1999.
5. Lieberman J, Safferman AZ, Pollack S, Szymanski S, Johns C, Howard A, et al. Clinical effects of clozapine in chronic schizophrenia-response to treatment and predictors of outcome. Am J Psychiat 1994; 151(12):1744–1752.
6. Meltzer HY, Perry E, Jayathilake K. Clozapine-induced weight gain predicts improvement in psychopathology. Schizophr Res 2003; 59(1):19–27.
7. Czobor P, Volavka J, Sheitman B, Lindenmayer JP, Citrome L, McEvoy J, et al. Antipsychotic-induced weight gain and therapeutic response: a differential association. J Clin Psychopharmacol 2002; 22(3):244–251.
8. Chanpattana W, Chakrabhand ML. Combined ECT and neuroleptic therapy in treatment-refractory schizophrenia: prediction of outcome. Psychiatry Res 2001; 105(1–2):107–115.
9. Franchini L, Spagnolo C, Rossini D, Smeraldi E, Bellodi L, Politi E. A neural network approach to the outcome definition on first treatment with sertraline in a psychiatric population. Artif Intell Med 2001; 23(3):239–248.
10. Bertilsson L, Dahl ML. Polymorphic drug oxidation—relevance to the treatment of psychiatric disorders. CNS Drugs 1996; 5(3):220–223.
11. Jerling M, Dahl ML, Aberg-Wistedt A, Liljenberg B, Landell NE, Bertilsson L, et al. The CYP2D6 genotype predicts the oral clearance of the neuroleptic agents perphenazine and zuclopenthixol. Clin Pharmacol Ther 1996; 59(4):423–428.
12. Ring BJ, Catlow J, Lindsay TJ, Gillespie T, Roskos LK, Cerimele BJ, et al. Identification of the human cytochromes P450 responsible for the in vitro formation of the major oxidative metabolites of the antipsychotic agent olanzapine. J Pharmacol Exp Ther 1996; 276(2):658–666.
13. Wooding SP, Watkins WS, Bamshad MJ, Dunn DM, Weiss RB, Jorde LB. DNA sequence variation in a 3.7-kb noncoding sequence 5′ of the CYP1A2 gene: implications for human population history and natural selection. Am J Hum Genet 2002; 71(3):528–542.
14. Sachse C, Brockmoller J, Bauer S, Roots I. Functional signficance of a C/A polymorphism in intron I of the cytochrome P450 CYP1A2 gene tested with caffeine. Brit J Clin Pharmacol 1999; 47(4):445–449.

15. Nakajima M, Yokoi T, Mizutani M, Kinoshita M, Funayama M, Kamataki T. Genetic polymorphism in the 5′-flanking region of human CYP1A2 gene: Effect on the CYP1A2 inducibility in humans. J Biochem 1999; 125(4):803–808.
16. Basile VS, Ozdemir V, Masellis M, Walker ML, Meltzer HY, Lieberman JA, et al. A functional polymorphism of the cytochrome P450 1A2 (CYP1A2) gene: association with tardive dyskinesia in schizophrenia. Mol Psychiatry 2000; 5(4):410–417.
17. Weber WW. Pharmacogenetics. 1st ed. New York: Oxford University Press, 1997.
18. Bertilsson L, Dahl ML, Dalen P, Al-Shurbaji A. Molecular genetics of CYP2D6: Clinical relevance with focus on psychotropic drugs. Brit J Clin Pharmacol 2002; 53(2):111–122.
19. Eichelbaum M, Evert B. Influence of pharmacogenetics on drug disposition and response. Clin Exp Pharmacol Physiol 1996; 23(10–11):983–985.
20. Bradford LD, Kirlin WG. Polymorphism of CYP2D6 in Black populations: implications for psychopharmacology. Int J Neuropsychopharmcol 1998; 1(2):173–185.
21. Kapitany T, Meszaros K, Lenzinger E, Schindler SD, Barnas C, Fuchs K, et al. Genetic polymorphisms for drug metabolism (CYP2D6) and tardive dyskinesia in schizophrenia. Schizophrenia Research 1998; 32:101–106.
22. Lam LCW, Garcia-Barcelo MM, Ungvari GS, Tang WK, Lam VKL, Kwong SL et al. Cytochrome CYP2D6 genotyping and association with tardive dyskinesia in Chinese schizophrenic patients. Pharmacopsychiatry 2001; 34(6):238–241.
23. Scordo MG, Spina E, Romeo P, Dahl ML, Bertilsson L, Johansson I, et al. CYP2D6 genotype and antipsychotic-induced extrapyramidal side effects in schizophrenic patients. Eur J Clin Pharmacol 2000; 56(9–10):679–683.
24. Arranz MJ, Dawson E, Shaikh S, Sham P, Sharma T, Aitchison K, et al. Cytochrome P4502D6 genotype does not determine response to clozapine. Brit J Clin Pharmacol 1995; 39:417–420.
25. Spina E, Gitto C, Avenoso A, Campo GM, Caputi AP, Perucca E. Relationship between plasma desipramine levels, CYP2D6 phenotype and clinical response to desipramine: a prospective study. Eur J Clin Pharmacol 1997; 51(5):395–398.
26. Wrighton SA, Stevens JC. The human hepatic cytochromes P450 involved in drug metabolism. Crit Rev Toxicol 1992; 22(1):1–21.
27. Hsieh KP, Lin YY, Cheng CL, Lai ML, Lin MS, Siest JP, et al. Novel mutations of CYP3A4 in Chinese. Drug Metab Dispos 2001; 29(3):268–273.
28. Dai D, Tang J, Rose R, Hodgson E, Bienstock RJ, Mohrenweiser HW, et al. Identification of Variants of CYP3A4 and Characterization of Their Abilities to Metabolize Testosterone and Chlorpyrifos. J Pharmacol Exp Ther 2001; 299(3):825–831.
29. de Leon JH, Vatsis KP, Weber WW. Characterization of naturally occurring and recombinant human N-acetyltransferase variants encoded by NAT1. Mol Pharmacol 2000; 58(2):288–299.
30. Wikman H, Thiel S, Jager B, Schmezer P, Spiegelhalder B, Edler L, et al. Relevance of N-acetyltransferase 1 and 2 (NAT1, NAT2) genetic polymorphisms in non-small cell lung cancer susceptibility. Pharmacogenetics 2001; 11(2):157–168.
31. Reis M, Santoro A, Suarez-Kurtz G. Thiopurine methyltransferase phenotypes and genotypes in Brazilians. Pharmacogenetics 2003; 13(6):371–373.
32. Larovere LE, de Kremer RD, Lambooy LH, De Abreu RA. Genetic polymorphism of thiopurine S-methyltransferase in Argentina. Ann Clin Biochem 2003; 40(Pt 4):388–393.
33. Ciotti M, Marrone A, Potter C, Owens IS. Genetic polymorphism in the human UGT1A6 (planar phenol) UDP-glucuronosyltransferase: pharmacological implications. Pharmacogenetics 1997; 7(6):485–495.
34. Clarke DJ, Moghrabi N, Monaghan G, Cassidy A, Boxer M, Hume R, et al. Genetic defects of the UDP-glucuronosyltransferase-1 (UGT1) gene that cause familial non-haemolytic unconjugated hyperbilirubinaemias. Clin Chim Acta 1997; 266(1):63–74.
35. Leysen JE. Receptor profile of antipsychotics. In: Ellenbroek BA, Cools AR, eds. Atypical Antipsychotics. Basel/Switzerland: Bikhäuser Verlag, 2000:57–81.
36. Meltzer HY, Gudelsky GA. Dopaminergic and serotonergic effects of clozapine. Implications for a unique clinical profile. Arzneimittelforschung 1992; 42(2A):268–272.

37. Seeman P, Kapur S. Schizophrenia: more dopamine, more D2 receptors. Proc Natl Acad Sci USA 2000; 97(14):7673–7675.
38. Heinz A. Dopaminergic dysfunction in alcoholism and schizophrenia—psychopathological and behavioral correlates. Eur Psychiatry 2002; 17(1):9–16.
39. Kapur S, Zipursky R, Jones C, Remington G, Houle S. Relationship between dopamine D(2) occupancy, clinical response, and side effects: a double-blind PET study of first-episode schizophrenia. Am J Psychiatry 2000; 157(4):514–520.
40. Kerwin RW, Osborne S. Antipsychotic drugs. Medicine 2000; 28(4):23–25.
41. Cohen BM, Ennulat DJ, Centorrino F, Matthysse S, Konieczna H, Chu HM, et al. Polymorphisms of the dopamine D-4 receptor and response to antipsychotic drugs. Psychopharmacology 1999; 141:6–10.
42. Shaikh S, Makoff A, Collier DA, Kerwin RW. Dopamine D4 receptors: potential therapeutic implications in the treatment of schizophrenia. CNS Drugs 1997; 8:1–11.
43. Gurevich EV, Bordelon Y, Shapiro RM, Arnold SE, Gur RE, Joyce JN. Mesolimbic dopamine D3 receptors and use of antipsychotics in patients with schizophrenia. A postmortem study. Arch Gen Psychiatry 1997; 54(3):225–232.
44. Schafer M, Rujescu D, Giegling I, Guntermann A, Erfurth A, Bondy B, et al. Association of short-term response to haloperidol treatment with a polymorphism in the dopamine D(2) receptor gene. Am J Psychiatry 2001; 158(5):802–804.
45. Malhotra AK, Buchanan RW, Kim S, Kestler L, Breier A, Pickar D, et al. Allelic variation in the promoter region of the dopamine D2 receptor gene and clozapine response. Schizophrenia Research 1999; 36(1–3):92–93.
46. Scharfetter J, Chaudhry HR, Hornik K, Fuchs K, Sieghart W, Kasper S, et al. Dopamine D3 receptor gene polymorphism and response to clozapine in schizophrenic Pakistani patients. Eur Neuropsychopharm 1998; 10(1):17–20.
47. Staddon S, Arranz MJ, Mancama D, Mata I, Kerwin RW. Clinical applications of pharmacogenetics in psychiatry. Psychopharmacology (Berl) 2002; 162(1):18–23.
48. Basile VS, Masellis M, Badri F, Paterson AD, Meltzer HY, Lieberman JA, et al. Association of the Msc I polymorphism of the dopamine D3 receptor gene with tardive dyskinesia in schizophrenia. Neuropsychopharmacology 1999; 21:17–27.
49. Segman R, Neeman T, Herseco-Levy U, Finkel B, Karagivech L, Schlafman M et al. Genotypic association between the dopamine D3 receptor and tardive dyskinesia in chronic schizophrenia. Molecular Psychiatry 1999; 4:247–253.
50. Steen VM, Lovlie R, MacEwan T, McCreadie RG. Dopamine D3-receptor gene variant and susceptibility to tardive dyskinesia in schizophrenic patients. Molecular Psychiatry 1997; 2(2):139–145.
51. Lerer B, Segman RH, Fangerau H, Daly AK, Basile VS, Cavallaro R, et al. Pharmacogenetics of Tardive Dyskinesia. Combined Analysis of 780 Patients Supports Association with Dopamine D3 Receptor Gene Ser9Gly Polymorphism. Neuropsychopharmacology 2002; 27(1):105–119.
52. Mihara K, Kondo T, Suzuki A, Yasui-Furukori N, Ono S, Sano A, et al. Relationship between functional dopamine D2 and D3 receptors gene polymorphisms and neuroleptic malignant syndrome. Am J Med Genet 2003; 117B(1):57–60.
53. Kishida I, Kawanishi C, Furuno T, Matsumura T, Hasegawa H, Sugiyama N, et al. Lack of association in Japanese patients between neuroleptic malignant syndrome and the TaqI A polymorphism of the dopamine D2 receptor gene. Psychiatr Genet 2003; 13(1):55–57.
54. Inada T, Arinami T, Yagi G. Association between a polymorphism in the promoter region of the dopamine D2 receptor gene and schizophrenia in Japanese subjects: replication and evaluation for antipsychotic-related features. Int J Neuropsychopharmcol 1999; 2(3):181–186.
55. Liao DL, Yeh YC, Chen HM, Chen H, Hong CJ, Tsai SJ. Association between the Ser9Gly polymorphism of the dopamine D3 receptor gene and tardive dyskinesia in Chinese schizophrenic patients. Neuropsychobiology 2001; 44(2):95–98.
56. Wong AHC, Buckle CE, Van Tol HHM. Polymorphisms in dopamine receptors: what do they tell us? Eur J Pharmacol 2000; 410:183–203.

57. Arranz MJ, Munro J, Osborne S, Collier DA, Kerwin RW. Difficulties in replication of results. Lancet 2000; 356:1359–1360.
58. Hernandez I, Sokolov BP. Abnormal expression of serotonin transporter mRNA in the frontal and temporal cortex of schizophrenics. Mol Psychiatry 1997; 2(1):57–64.
59. Pralong D, Tomaskovic-Crook E, Opeskin K, Copolov D, Dean B. Serotonin(2A) receptors are reduced in the planum temporale from subjects with schizophrenia. Schizophr Res 2000; 44(1):35–45.
60. Meltzer HY. The role of serotonin in antipsychotic drug action. Neuropsychopharmacology 1999; 21(2):s106-s115.
61. Joober R, Benkelfat C, Brisebois K, Toulouse A, Turecki G, Lal S, et al. T102C polymorphism in the 5HT2A gene and schizophrenia: relation to phenotype and drug response variability. J Psychiat Neurosci 1999; 24:141–146.
62. Masellis M, Basile VS, Meltzer HY, Lieberman JA, Sevy S, Macciardi F, et al. Serotonin subtype 2 receptor genes and clinical response to clozapine in schizophrenia patients. Neuropsychopharmacology 1998; 19:123–132.
63. Arranz MJ, Collier DA, Sodhi M, Ball D, Roberts G, Price J, et al. Association between clozapine response and allelic variation in the 5-HT2A receptor gene. Lancet 1995; 346:281–282.
64. Arranz MJ, Collier DA, Munro J, Sham P, Kirov G, Sodhi M, et al. Analysis of a structural polymorphism in the 5-HT2A receptor and clinical response to clozapine. Neurosci Lett 1996; 217:177–178.
65. Arranz MJ, Munro J, Owen MJ, Spurlock J, Sham P, Zhao, J et al. Evidence for association between polymorphisms in the promoter and coding regions of the 5-HT2A receptor gene and response to clozapine. Molecular Psychiatry 1998; 3:61–66.
66. Lane HY, Chang YC, Chiu CC, Chen ML, Hsieh MH, Chang WH. Association of risperidone treatment response with a polymorphism in the 5-HT(2A) receptor gene. Am J Psychiatry 2002; 159(9):1593–1595.
67. Malhotra AK, Goldman D, Ozaki N, Breier A, Buchanan R, Pickar D. Lack of association between polymorphisms in the 5-HT2A receptor gene and the antipsychotic response to clozapine. Am J Psychiatry 1996; 153(8):1092–1094.
68. Masellis M, Paterson AD, Badri F, Lieberman JA, Meltzer HY, Cavazzoni P, et al. Genetic variation of 5-HT2A receptor and response to clozapine. Lancet 1995; 346(8982):1108.
69. Nothen MM, Rietschel M, Erdmann J, Oberlander H, Moller HJ, Nober D, et al. Genetic variation of the 5-HT2A receptor and response to clozapine. Lancet 1995; 346(8979):908–909.
70. Arranz MJ, Munro J, Sham P, Kirov G, Murray RM, Collier DA, et al. Meta-analysis of studies on genetic variation in 5-HT2A receptors and clozapine response. Schizophrenia Research 1998; 32:93–99.
71. Sodhi M, Sham P, Makoff A, Collier DA, Arranz MJ, Munro J, et al. Replication and meta-analysis of alleleic association of a 5-HT2C receptor polymorphism with good response to clozapine. Molecular Psychiatry 1999; 4(1):225–226.
72. Segman RH, Heresco-Levy U, Finkel B, Inbar R, Neeman T, Schlafman M, et al. Association between the serotonin 2C receptor gene and tardive dyskinesia in chronic schizophrenia: additive contribution of 5-HT2Cser and DRD3gly alleles to susceptibility. Psychopharmacology (Berl) 2000; 152(4):408–413.
73. Yu YWY, Tsai S-J, Lin C-H, Hsu C-P, Ynakg K-H, Hong C-J. Serotonin-6 receptor variant (C267T) and clinical response to clozapine. Neuroreport 1999; 10:1231–1233.
74. Reynolds GP, Zhang ZJ, Zhang XB. Association of antipsychotic drug-induced weight gain with a 5-HT2C receptor gene polymorphism. Lancet 2002; 359(9323):2086–2087.
75. Basile VS, Masellis M, McIntyre RS, Meltzer HY, Lieberman JA, Kennedy JL. Genetic dissection of atypical antipsychotic-induced weight gain: novel preliminary data on the pharmacogenetic puzzle. J Clin Psychiatry 2001; 62(suppl 23):45–66.
76. Tsai SJ, Wang YC, Yu Younger WY, Lin CH, Yang KH, Hong CJ. Association analysis of polymorphism in the promoter region of the alpha2a-adrenoceptor gene with schizophrenia and clozapine response. Schizophr Res 2001; 49(1–2):53–58.

77. Bolonna AA, Arranz MJ, Munro J, Osborne S, Petouni M, Martinez M, et al. No influence of adrenergic receptor polymorphisms on schizophrenia and antipsychotic response. Neurosci Lett 2000; 280:65–68.
78. Mancama D, Arranz MJ, Munro J, Makoff A, Kerwin RW. The histamine 1 and histamine 2 receptor genes—candidates for schizophrenia and clozapine response. GeneScreen 2000; 1:29–34.
79. Mancama D, Munro J, Arranz MJ, Makoff A, Kerwin RW. Association analysis of muscarinic acetylcholine receptor polymorphisms in clozapine treated schizophrenics. Am J Med Gen 2000; 96(4):269.
80. Arranz MJ, Munro J, Birkett J, Bolonna AA, Mancama D, Sodhi M, et al. Pharmacogenetic prediction of clozapine response. Lancet 2000; 355:1615–1616.
81. Schumacher J, Schulze TG, Wienker TF, Rietschel M, Nothen MM. Pharmacogenetics of the clozapine response. Lancet 2000; 356(9228):506–507.
82. Winsberg BG, Comings DE. Association of the dopamine transporter gene (DAT1) with poor methylphenidate response. J Am Acad Child Psych 1999; 38(12):1474–1477.
83. Roman T, Szobot C, Martins S, Biederman J, Rohde LA, Hutz MH. Dopamine transporter gene and response to methylphenidate in attention-deficit/hyperactivity disorder. Pharmacogenetics 2002; 12(6):497–499.
84. Arranz MJ, Bolonna AA, Munro J, Curtis CJ, Collier DA, Kerwin RW. The serotonin transporter and clozapine response. Molecular Psychiatry 2000; 5:124–130.
85. Kaiser R, Tremblay PB, Schmider J, Henneken M, Dettling M, Muller-Oerlinghausen B, et al. Serotonin transporter polymorphisms: no association with response to antipsychotic treatment, but associations with the schizoparanoid and residual subtypes of schizophrenia. Mol Psychiatry 2001; 6(2):179–185.
86. Smeraldi E, Zanardi R, Benedetti F, Di Bella D, Perez J, Catalano M. Polymorphism within the promoter of the serotonin transporter gene and antidepressant efficacy of fluvoxamine. Molecular Psychiatry 1998; 3:508–511.
87. Kim DK, Lim S-W, Lee S, Sohn SE, Kim S, Hahn CG, et al. Serotonin transporter gene polymorphism and antidepressant response. Neuroreport 2000; 11(1):215–219.
88. Exton MS, Artz M, Siffert W, Schedlowski M. G protein beta3 subunit 825T allele is associated with depression in young, healthy subjects. Neuroreport 2003; 14(3):531–533.
89. Zill P, Baghai TC, Zwanzger P, Schule C, Minov C, Riedel M, et al. Evidence for an association between a G-protein beta 3-gene variant with depression and response to antidepressant treatment. Neuroreport 2000; 11(9):1893–1897.
90. Coutts RT, Urichuk LJ. Polymorphic Cytochromes P450 and Drugs used in Psychiatry. Cell Mol Neurobiol 1999; 19(3):325–355.
91. Prior TI, Chue PS, Tibbo P, Baker GB. Drug metabolism and atypical antipsychotics. Eur Neuropsychopharmacol 1999; 9(4):301–309.
92. Kirchheiner J, Brosen K, Dahl ML, Gram LF, Kasper S, Roots I, et al. CYP2D6 and CYP2C19 genotype-based dose recommendations for antidepressants: a first step towards subpopulation-specific dosages. Acta Psychiatr Scand 2001; 104(3):173–192.
93. Hersberger M, Marti-Jaun J, Rentsch K, Hanseler E. Rapid detection of the CYP2D6*3, CYP2D6*4 and CYP2D6*6 alleles by tetra-primer PCR and of the CYP3D6*5 allele by multiplex long PCR. Clinical Chemistry 2000; 46(8):1072–1077.
94. Roberts R, Sullivan P, Joyce P, Kennedy MA. Rapid and comprehensive determination of cytochrome P450CYP2D6 poor metabolizer genotypes by multiplex polymerase chain reaction. Human Mutation 2000; 16(1):77–85.
95. Sheffield LJ. The hunt for new genes and polymorphisms that can control the response to drugs. Pharmacogenomics 2002; 3(5):679–686.
96. de Longueville F, Surry D, Meneses-Lorente G, Bertholet V, Talbot V, Evrard S, et al. Gene expression profiling of drug metabolism and toxicology markers using a low-density DNA microarray. Biochem Pharmacol 2002; 64(1):137–149.
97. Lander ES, Linton LM, Birren B, Nusbaum C, Zody MC, Baldwin J, et al. Initial sequencing and analysis of the human genome. Nature 2001; 409(6822):860–921.

98. Whittaker PA. What is the relevance of bioinformatics to pharmacology. Trends Pharmacol Sci 2003; 24(8):434–439.
99. Rubin GM. The draft sequences. Comparing species. Nature 2001; 409(6822):820–821.
100. Bracco L, Kearsey J. The relevance of alternative RNA splicing to pharmacogenomics. TRENDS in Biotechnology 2003; 21(8):346–353.
101. Oleksiak MF, Churchill GA, Crawford DL. Variation in gene expression within and among natural populations. Nature Genctics 2002; 32:261–266.

Index